Fragmented Intimacy

Peter J. Adams

Fragmented Intimacy
Addiction in a Social World

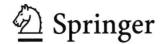 Springer

Peter J. Adams, Ph.D.
School of Population Health
University of Auckland
Private Bag 92019
Auckland
New Zealand
p.adams@auckland.ac.nz

ISBN 978-0-387-72660-1   e-ISBN 978-0-387-72661-8

Library of Congress Control Number: 2007934532

Printed on acid-free paper.

9 8 7 6 5 4 3 2 1

springer.com

Preface

I recall during my early years as a clinical psychologist being asked by hospital staff to speak with a 32-year-old man addicted to alcohol who was being discharged following treatment for pancreatitis. This had been his third admission for the same illness, and hospital practitioners were exasperated by his choice to continue drinking despite being repeatedly told it would cause irreparable damage to his pancreas from which he would be unlikely to survive. I met him in a side-room on the ward. He sat in his pyjamas in the corner of the room, thin and ashen looking, with a worried frown fixed across his face. Our conversation was initially stilted and I was trying hard not to replicate the lectures and sermons he was likely to have already received from hospital staff. As we talked I was able to piece together bits of information about his current circumstances: he lived alone, he was unemployed, and his only family contact was with a brother who visited to check on him occasionally. He started to relax into the conversation and then talked about his long struggles with alcohol: his drinking had begun in his early teens; it had provided him with confidence and friendships; he had had some serious motor vehicle accidents; he had tried to stop drinking but soon continued; he had lost friends, jobs, and family relationships; and in response he had increasingly sought intoxication as a refuge. He admitted this was not the way he wanted to be and declared that this time when he returned home he was going to stop for good. Somehow I felt unconvinced. Although he stared intensely into my eyes as he said this, his words sounded vaguely like something he had stated many times before; somewhat similar to those routine declarations one makes at church services or at New Year's Eve celebrations. I offered to meet with him further, and we negotiated a time later that week. Unsurprisingly, I never saw him again, and several months later I heard he had been readmitted with acute pancreatitis and had subsequently died.

This was one of my first solid encounters with the power that addictions can exert in a person's life. I had been brought up in a home free from the effects of addictions, so this early professional exposure left me with many troubling questions. What could we have done differently? Could we have locked him up for his own protection? Could we have developed a secure monitoring regime to prevent his drinking? Was there a psychological strategy that we could use to switch his commitment to drinking? Maybe there is a drug that we could use that might help him change? Somehow none of these possibilities seemed viable, and when I searched my psychology texts I found they offered little in terms of satisfactory directions. I was left wondering what inner force could be so powerful that a person would knowingly risk everything including his life. On the surface it appeared to violate all we know about the human struggle for survival, and it was hard to think of any organism that would work so consistently on its nonsurvival. As my career led me into further—and similarly humbling—exposures to people struggling with addictions, I found my initial let's-get-in-and-fix-it attitude tempered progressively through recognition of the scale of the problem. I encountered with increasing regularity the many dramatic ways addictions impact on others living close by: partners feel trapped in loveless marriages, children suffer abuse and neglect, parents face ongoing loss and despair, and friends encounter deceit and betrayal. The question troubling me then widened to, How is it possible that over the course of many years such a large number of people in our communities willfully and knowingly pursue relationships with something addictive to an extent that it causes significant harm to them and the people they love? What is the psychological and social infrastructure that makes this possible?

Writing and reading are two contributory parts of the social event of written communication. While the act of writing and the act of reading seldom occur simultaneously, writers and readers still form a social connection via a variable time delay, and it is worth at this point to consider some of the factors that might influence both parties in their willingness to engage with this book. On the writing side, my primary motive for undertaking this project was to provide a clear description of what it might mean to view addictions as social events; in other words, to bring the diverse world of social theory closer in order for it to shed light on the perplexing question of why addictions persist. To this end, the book provides a step-by-step guide to looking at addictions in terms of relationships and family systems and extends this understanding onto interactions within wider social networks. On the reading side, the book is worth exploring because it opens up what readers will discover is a radically different way of looking at addictions. Rather than a solitary experience, addictions are seen as forming, intensifying, and dissolving in a social world. Accordingly, the book has something to offer both the professional and the lay reader. For professional readers, including specialist addiction practitioners, general health workers, and community professionals, it provides a uniquely systematic account of how addictions could be approached in social terms. The final chapters also outline how these might translate into self-help strategies, community responses, and improvements in clinical practice. For lay readers, including those struggling with addiction, family members, or people simply curious about this major social issue, the book provides an accessible account of what is happening in addictive contexts and how each person involved might respond.

Peter J. Adams, March 2007

Acknowledgement

I want to acknowledge the contributions and generosity of several people. First, I want to thank my partner, Jude, and our four children for putting up with my preoccupations. Next, I am very grateful to my parents, Bob and Nelly, for their support and for providing me with a physical location to write. I am grateful to my close work colleagues John Raeburn, Barbara Docherty, Samson Tse, Robert Brown, Helen Warren, Janie Sheridan, and Janet Fanslow, for their ongoing support and encouragement. I want to particularly acknowledge the contributions of Helen Keane, Glenn Laverack, Alison Towns, and Pam Armstrong, who generously gave of their time in reading and providing feedback on the initial drafts. I am also indebted to overseas colleagues who generously provided me with locations to visit during the writing, particularly Francesco Piani and Paola Gosparini in Italy, David Korn and Phil Lange in Toronto, and John Strang and Robert Patton in London. Finally, I am grateful to the University of Auckland and the School of Population Health for providing me with the study leave without which I would never have found the time.

Contents

Contents

PART II: PROCESSES

PART III: FAMILIES AND COMMUNITIES

PART IV: APPLICATIONS

Part I
Theory

Chapter 1

Addiction in Perspective

Filled with mingled cream and amber; I will drain that glass again; Such hilarious visions clamber; Through the chamber of my brain; Quaintest thoughts, queerest fancies; Come to life and fade away. What care I how time advances? I am drinking ale today

(Edgar Allan Poe[1])

In these early years of the twenty-first century we find ourselves constantly immersed in talk about addictions. Newspapers and television regularly present disturbing items on the rising negative effects of addiction. When the country is not waging a "war on drugs," it is struggling with drunken driving, youth drug crime, increases in pathological gambling, alcohol destroying families, spates of Internet addiction, and so forth. Increasing numbers of popular books on addiction appear in book stores with titles such as, *Codependent No More; Woman, Sex, and Addiction: A Search for Love and Power;* and *Workaholics: The Respectable Addicts.*[2] Many people with high media profiles regularly succumb to addictions; the tabloids and magazines revel in details on fallen movie stars, television celebrities, sports heroes, community leaders, and politicians. Self-professed alcoholics and drug addicts often bare their souls on syndicated television talk shows, detailing stories on the horrors of being addicted and its impact on loved ones.

In each if these contexts the understanding of what is meant by "addiction" conveys slightly different meanings. At times addiction is mentioned casually in phrases such as, "I'm addicted to chocolate" or "Golf is my addiction"; at other times it is taken more seriously: "Addictions are leading more and more people into crime"; "Addiction drives most of our corruption"; and at still other times, it is referred to in a manner that is nuanced with menace and judgment: "We must stamp out all addictions"; "Addicts are weak and worthless people." Addictions are simply an increasing part of public consciousness.

Another driver for the constant reference to addictions is the mounting evidence that they are commonplace, and that they directly affect large numbers of people and their loved ones. For example, national surveys in the United States indicate that 2 percent of the adult population is struggling with addictions to alcohol and 1.5 percent with addictions to other drugs.[3] Furthermore, the increased availability of opportunities to gamble adds a further 1.5 percent with addictive problems associated with gambling.[4] These figures assume that people disclose their consumptions accurately to interviewers (usually on the telephone), which for particularly sensitive subjects

3

P.J. Adams, Fragmented Intimacy: Addiction in a Social World
© Springer 2008

like illicit drugs and gambling is likely to lead to an underestimation in the reported prevalence. Adding to this underestimation are the unknown numbers of people with problems associated with potentially addictive and compulsive behaviors related to eating, sex, and work. With this in mind and allowing for some crossover between addictions, a reasonably conservative estimate of addictions to alcohol, other drugs, and gambling would be about 3 to 5 percent of the adult population. While this may still seem a small proportion, its significance multiplies when the focus is widened to include friends and family whose lives are seriously affected by the addiction of a loved one. Various claims have been made about the typical number of other people affected; common claims are that at least four other people are seriously affected by one person addicted to alcohol and/or drugs, and maybe five for those addicted to gambling.[5] Given that some of those addicted may belong to the same family and that such estimates have yet to be firmly established, a reasonable but conservative assumption would be that the lives of at least two people are severely affected. Taken together—persons with an addiction and those closest to them—this means that at any one time something in the region of 9 to 12 percent of the population, or roughly person in ten, can be expected to be experiencing serious disruptions in their lives because of addictions.

In contrast to the widespread concern and talk about addiction today, it is easy to forget that the notion of people acquiring an ongoing condition called "addiction" has had a relatively short history.[6] As a concept, it emerged just over a century ago as a way of referring to people who despite numerous attempts at change appeared to return habitually and helplessly into inebriation. This central idea of an ongoing condition involving loss of control over alcohol use was interpreted over subsequent years as a compulsion, a habit, a behavioral disorder, a disease, or a medical condition. Since each of these terms draws on different theoretical understandings, what one person might mean when referring to as an addiction differs from what others might mean, and this varies according to educational background, context, and belief. It can even vary in meaning within the same sentence, as in, "I have no control over this

Under-standings of addiction vary according to background and context

habit," which mixes ideas of choice and compulsion. This flexibility and variability poses problems in definition, and depending on how the term is used, may reveal more about the speaker's background than about a common meaning. Indeed, definitions of the concept have fluctuated between medical interpretations of disease or dependence and psychological interpretations of compulsion or behavioral disorder, and sometimes more commonplace understandings of it as a bad habit or compulsive drive.

Currently the two loudest voices on what is an addiction are speaking from two very different vantage points. From one vantage point, looking from the outside, are the addiction scientists and clinicians who draw on definitions based on their professional backgrounds in medicine and psychology. From another vantage point, looking from the inside, are those with direct experience of addictions who attempt to depict an inner world of torment, confusion, and despair based on their own personal encounters.

Turning first to the scientist/clinician, Marc Schuckit broadly describes the term *substance dependence* as referring to the "central role that the substance has come to play in the individual's life, evidence of problems relating to controlling intake, and the development of difficulties (especially physical and psychological problems) despite which the individual continues to return to the substance."[7] Note how this medically oriented definition tries as much as possible to locate addiction within an individual person or patient. Another imperative for the scientist/clinician is to use descriptors that are clear and observable and lend themselves to measurement. For example, in the *Journal of the American Medical Association* Morse and Flavin defined alcoholism as "a primary, chronic disease with genetic, psychosocial and environmental factors influencing its development and manifestations. The disease is often progressive and fatal. It is characterized by impaired control over drinking, preoccupation with the drug alcohol, use of alcohol despite adverse consequences, and distortions in thinking."[8]

Both these descriptions owe much to the original World Health Organization[9] definition that in 1952 sought a consensus between experts on what was meant by an addiction to alcohol (see inset box). More recently, Arthur Blume[10] has organized the key parts of these definitions into three critical elements: (1) compulsive use, (2) loss of control, and (3) continued use despite adverse consequences. These three elements are used as a guide for clinicians to categorize whether or not a client is addicted.

For those experiencing addiction the goals of clarity and measurement matter less than communicating the experience of addiction. For example, the handbook of Narcotics Anonymous describes drug addictions in the following way:

> **1952 WHO Definition of Alcoholism**
> "Alcoholics are those excessive drinkers whose dependence on alcohol has attained such a degree that it shows a noticeable mental disturbance or interference with their bodily or mental health, their interpersonal relations and their smooth social and economic functions, or who show the prodromal signs of such development. They, therefore, require treatment."

> Our disease isolated us from people except when we were getting, using and finding ways and means to get more. Hostile, resentful, self-centered and self-seeking, we cut ourselves off from the outside world. Anything not completely familiar became alien and dangerous. Our world shrank and isolation became our life. We used in order to survive. It was the only way of life that we knew.[11]

Here addictions are characterized with reference to mental states, to emotions, and to an altered inner stance on the outside world. They typically describe this reorientation as involving a range of deteriorations and losses. As described in brochures by the renowned Betty Ford Center:

> Chemically dependent persons develop an intense relationship with their drug of choice. It grows subtly until it becomes so consuming no other meaningful relationship can exist. Persons with no other relationship—no other important elements in their lives—are said to be spiritually bankrupt. They have lost communication with the larger world around them and have become locked into the lonely world of self-centeredness.[12]

Addiction here is described as not only involving loss of relationships and connections with the world, it also involves the ultimate loss of the inner core of the self: a person's spirituality.

The interpretations of the scientist/clinician and those experiencing addictions mark two extremes on a continuum of perspectives on addictions. The approaches that people take to addiction typically fit somewhere along this continuum and tend to incorporate some aspects of the scientist/clinician outside-in perspective and some aspects of the experiencer's inside-out perspective. For instance, common psychological approaches to addiction try to combine observations of how people behave with understandings of what they are thinking.[13]

In a similar vein, this book draws on understandings from both vantage points but it does so with a new twist: it explores the nature of addiction as essentially a social event. Accordingly, the term *social* occupies a central position throughout the book. As with addiction, there are many senses to the term *social*, but here it primarily is used to refer to the way people connect with other people and with other things in their lives. The refocusing of attention onto connections and relationships has important implications. It draws attention away from thinking of addicted persons as separate individuals standing alone by themselves and promotes the view that such people occupy an intersecting points in the net of relationships. At this stage in the book, this shift in orientation may seem somewhat curious, but as the content unfolds, the power of what this means will slowly emerge. In a social world, addictions involve the progressive intensification of one relationship—the relationship to an addictive substance or process—at the cost of other relationships. When a person's social world is reorganized around this singular and dominant relationship, the new structure entails progressive deterioration in connections with the world around. Furthermore, the relationships that are most affected by these deteriorating connections are those with people who are closest and most loved, and consequently it is in the realm of intimacy that addictions are most actively destructive.

A social perspective focuses primarily on the relationships between people

Dangerous Consumptions

Addictions comprise one dimension of a population's relationship to drugs, gambling, and other dangerous consumptions. Other dimensions include the nature of heavy nonaddictive consumptions, the cultural meanings associated with these consumptions, the way they are manufactured and marketed, and the manner in which a community or a nation chooses to enjoy or limit such consumptions. Each dimension involves issues and studies in their own right. For example, the heavy but nonaddictive consumption of alcohol, while not leading to the same intensity of problems as addictions, does arguably cause more widespread harm through drunkenness, injuries, sexual coercion, crime, relationship conflict, and so on.[14]

As a consequence of the flexibility of different ways of thinking about addictions, they are increasingly identified across a broad variety of dimensions of living. Besides alcohol and other drugs, the term *addictions* is now regularly extended to other excessive consumptions in activities as diverse as gambling, eating, body enhancement, shopping, sex, pornography, intimate relationships, work, Internet use, computer games, and exercise, and the list keeps growing. As a result, writers on addiction are gradually widening their focus to include more than alcohol and other drugs.[15] Jim Orford contends that the traditional focus on physically enhanced addictions has

> "narrowed our sights upon excessive drug use, and particularly upon a few categories of drugs thought to have major 'addiction' potential, and have prevented us from developing a satisfactory science of addiction in the more generally understood lay sense of that word. In particular they have hindered a useful cross-fertilization of ideas between alcohol, drug, gambling, eating, and sexual behavior studies."[16]

According to this inclusive approach, differences between each form of addiction are outweighed by their commonalities. Their processes, particularly their psychological processes, share much in terms of motives, thinking, and consequences. For example, an addiction to alcohol results in similar losses of friends and relationships as does an addiction to sex. More can be gained by combining forces in studying the intricacies of all these forms of addiction than by remaining attached to their differences.

This broadening of the use of the term *addictions* has attracted criticism on a number of grounds. In the first place, treating any consumption as potentially addictive could convey the impression of trivializing the tragic effects of hard-core addictions. Excessive consumptions of food and sex and excessive shopping cannot really be compared to the devastation experienced with addictions to substances such as alcohol, amphetamines, or opiates. In the second place, bundling addictions together tends to obscure the diverse character of specific consumptions. For example, each drug group has its own biological and psychological idiosyncrasies: heroin develops quicker tolerance, alcohol promotes depression, cannabis has a longer withdrawal, and so forth. Each small difference can have significant effects in how the product is consumed and its consequences for a person's lifestyle. A final major criticism concerns the way broader understandings potentially relabel normal behavior as pathology, thereby broadening and elevating the role of addiction experts to consultants on general living.[17] As Helen Keane puts it:

A broad approach to addictions risks overlooking their differences and complexities

> "The development of new and wide-ranging addictive pathologies cannot help but strengthen the hold of medical expertise and therapeutic authority over people's conduct and desires. Addiction attribution encourages the routine application of standards of the normal and the healthy to almost all aspects of our lives."[18]

She cautions against this unnecessary and unqualified widening of the gaze of experts. Indeed, her suspicions appear well founded when writers such as Patrick Carnes and associates argue that

"the biggest challenge will come to us as addiction professionals. If each patient is
to receive the depth of treatment in each addiction and the breadth of treatment
necessary across issues, the 28-day program loses its legitimacy. We envision a
three- to five-year process involving many specialties and formats."[19]

Mindful of these cautions, this book adopts a conditionally inclusive
approach to addictions in which the nature of the object of an addiction has
been left intentionally open but with some provisos. In later chapters the
reasons for this will become more apparent, but to explain it briefly, from a
social perspective the main identifiers of addictions are not derived from
aspects of the product being consumed. Addictions are identified by a particular pattern of connectedness with the world. This pattern involves the
progressive intensification of one relationship to the detriment of all other
relationships and in a way that leads to multiple levels of harm. This pattern

Addictions
involve a
particular
pattern of
connected-
ness with the
world

is as clearly observed with addictions to alcohol and illicit drugs as it is with
addictions to gambling and to some extent to sex and compulsive eating.
This pattern is less obvious when it comes to tobacco. In terms of health,
addiction to tobacco is arguably the most important of all addictive processes. For example, as high as 21 percent of the annual death toll in the
United States can be attributed to smoking-related disease.[20] Despite its
importance, tobacco addiction is not extensively discussed in this book.
While there are social dimensions to tobacco use, the overriding physical
nature of this addiction eclipses the social processes. An addictive relationship to tobacco tends to involve some rearrangement of a person's social
world, such as socializing more with other smokers, but the main binding
force is the physical addiction, and a smoker's social world does not undergo
the same level of rearrangement that is common in addictions to consumptions such as alcohol, cocaine, or gambling.

A further caution regarding discourses on addiction relates to the overex-
tended use of theory for its own sake. Addictions as a complex domain provide an excellent playground for academic theorizing. Here I am mindful of
a cautionary note provided by George DuWors:

All schools, theories, disciplines, and therapies tend to value their specialty at the
expense of links stressed and studied by other schools. Virtually all of the schools
fight over the corpus delicti of the near-dead alcoholic. The alcoholic, his family, and
society are consumers of theories about his destructive behavior (and theirs) that
compete for recognition, utilization, and cash.[21]

The application of theory needs to account for itself in terms of its potential
to make a tangible difference to those affected. Accordingly, this book is
written with the strong conviction that the social dimensions of addiction are
genuinely important in looking at ways to reduce suffering associated with
addictions—suffering experienced both by persons with addictions and by
their immediate loved ones. The strength of the theoretical dimensions of
the book emerges most clearly in the last part of the book when discussion
moves on to explore applications to families, communities, and services.

Overview of This Book

Several features of this book have been included to help the reader access its central message. Although the book leads the reader into new territory, it still draws heavily on a wide range of familiar sources to support each step. These sources include the outcomes of research studies into addictions, scholarly studies of related ideas, works on history and culture, as well as new applications of other fields of study such as health promotion and philosophy. To avoid the clutter created by including this reference material in the body of the text, all references have been placed in the endnotes at the end of the book. The main content is written in a style that seeks to engage and communicate with academics, clinicians, students, and general readers interested in addictions. But this intention is complicated by the challenges that *A social* occur as a natural consequence of venturing into new territory. Familiar ways *vocabulary* of speaking about addictions do not lend themselves easily to talking about *helps avoid* addictions in a social context, and their use can lead to ambiguity and confu- *confusion* sion. For example, adopting a word like *recovery* is liable to trigger nonsocial *with particle* understandings that cut across intended social descriptions of change; it *terminology* implies disease processes at the level of the individual or single organism. For this reason, this exploration of a social approach to addictions moves consciously away from words associated with previous understandings and replaces them with a limited number of new words. While the reader may find this initially challenging, in the longer run, persisting with the new words will improve overall clarity and consistency. To increase familiarity and comfort with these new words, each one is introduced and explained clearly, and for more detail the reader is encouraged to make use of the glossary at the end of the book.

The book is divided into four parts, each of which examines addiction from a different angle. Part I, Theory, outlines the conceptual frame for understanding addictions in a social world and examines how, in social terms, addictions emerge in families. Part II, Processes, focuses on the social processes associated with intimacy and addictions and examines common ways these manifest in families and other social networks. Part III, Families and Communities, discusses opportunities for initiating change in a world fragmented by addictions. Part IV, Applications, explores how individuals, families, and communities might combine forces to prevent and challenge the addictions in their midst.

Here is a brief summary of the chapters of each part. The four chapters in Part I provide an overview of a social interpretation of addictions. Chapter 2 outlines what is meant by the term *social world* and introduces its relevance to health and well-being. It explores how basic assumptions about addictions determine how addictions are thought to work, and it illustrates this by contrasting biological and psychological approaches, which focus on the person as an isolated individual, with social approaches, which emphasize the importance of relationships. Chapter 3 develops a simple framework for understanding the many ways relationships provide the basis for how people define and identify themselves. It examines how the strengthening of an addiction happens in parallel with the weakening of other relationships in such a way that people end up feeling isolated and socially fragmented from those around them. Chapter 4 looks in detail at the phases a person moves through in becoming addicted, in suffering from its effects, and then in attempting to change. It explores how deteriorating relationships prompt a series of crises that lead eventually to an interest in change. It then illustrates the difficulties posed by having to continue to function within social networks while at the same time trying to reform them.

In the chapters in Part II, the reader is invited to shift from a position above looking down to a position looking in through relationships to see how addictions interact with intimacy. Chapter 5 examines the central role intimacies play in a social world. It identifies four strands of intimacy that in varying combinations enable a person to form diverse and flexible forms of intimacy with other people as well as with pets, inanimate objects, places, ideals, and mood-altering drugs. Chapter 6 explores how developing an intimacy with an addictive object interplays with intimacies within a family. Chapter 7 focuses in detail on the use of violence and other controlling tactics to manage potential threats to an addiction.

The chapters in Part III combine the overview perspectives on addiction outlined in Part I with the internal analysis of intimacy developed in Part II. Chapter 8 examines the manner in which addictions fragment relationships between individuals in a family as well as disrupt links to other social layers in the neighborhood, workplace, and community. Chapter 9 looks more closely at the experience of loved ones living close to a person with an addiction. Family members often feel trapped in an ongoing cycle of attempts at change and disappointing returns to the status quo. The cycle only appears to reinforce the

Content of the book works progressively from theory to application

power of the addiction. Nonetheless, opportunities are identified in the potential for combined effort to reduce fragmentation and provide a stronger impetus for change. Chapter 10 details the various pathways that people associated with an addiction might take in the long process of reconnecting into to a social world.

The four chapters in Part IV examine applications of social understandings to how individuals, families, communities, and other combinations of people can respond to addictions in their midst. Chapter 11 provides an overview of social approaches that families might make use of in challenging an addiction. Since the change process involves a long difficult journey, and professional assistance is only available in short bursts, the chapter outlines strategies that families can use to address their own struggles. Chapter 12 looks at the ways volunteer networks, local communities, and other networks can make use of empowerment and community capacity-building strategies to support change. It focuses on three examples: a Canadian volunteer network of support groups, the Croatian/Italian community movement that provide a network of clubs to support families in change, and an indigenous Māori approach that utilizes the strengths of cultural processes to enable the rebuilding of social interconnections. Chapter 13 focuses on the role of addiction practitioners (and other health practitioners) in facilitating the change process. It questions the current overreliance on one-to-one counseling and recommends broadening the skill base to include abilities aimed at engaging families and communities. It also explores how social perspectives could be incorporated into assessment and intervention planning. Chapter 14 concludes with an overview of the social approach and an outline of directions for development.

Companion Relationships

Since this book's account of addiction in a social world calls on a range of concepts and ideas, a series of inset boxes are provided to help locate these concepts and ideas within the lived experience of those affected. Most of these boxes provide dialogues that capture some of the real-life tensions and dilemmas that people encounter. To help give these descriptions a narrative focus, all depictions in these boxes are derived from addictive contexts involving four separate companion relationships; two couple and two parent–child relationships.[22] The following descriptions of these relationships introduce the narratives that are woven into the inset boxes over the course of the book.

Four companion relationships provide a parallel account of lived experiences

Bert and Joan

Bert and Joan have been married for 21 years. It has been a troubled relationship, particularly with each increase in Bert's involvement with heavy drinking. Bert manages a large store selling building supplies and houseware products. After work he likes to join his friends at a local bar where he drinks and engages in raucous banter until the bar closes. Some evenings he prefers to remain at home, drinking whiskey and watching sports on television, then falling asleep in his armchair. Whether he goes out or stays at home, Joan is woken up in the early hours of the morning when he stumbles noisily into bed and starts interrogating her about her day. She dreads that time, and has hoped for years that their two children, Donald and Fiona, are too deeply asleep to hear the noise and arguments that inevitably follow. She has seen it as her role to shelter the children from Bert's excesses and to try to provide them with the stable and loving environment that she grew up in. Her elderly parents are unaware of the extent of problems they are experiencing, but she has confided with her closest sibling, Mary.

Joan feels frightened and trapped in the marriage. Bert is regularly drunk and openly abusive toward her at home, and because of this she has gradually lost contact with her friends and family. She fantasizes daily about leaving and setting up her own home, but she stays, trying desperately to maintain stability for her children, particularly as they are both at vulnerable times in their lives.

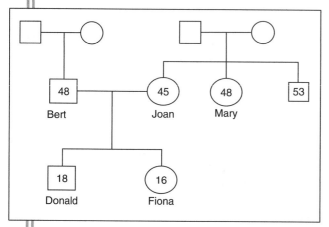

Donald at 18 is looking seriously at options for employment next year. He is shy and withdrawn, with few friends and low confidence in stating his needs or in making decisions. Fiona, on the contrary, is full of confidence, and at 16 is already involved in a serious relationship with a boyfriend. Lately she has been going to parties and coming home early in the morning drunk and disheveled. Joan realizes that it will not be long before both children go their separate ways, leaving her alone with Bert. Her one consolation is her full-time job as an elementary school teacher. Shortly after her children started school, she had begun helping her children's teachers in class and found she enjoyed the involvement. She then contributed more regularly as a teacher's aide. When the children moved on to middle school, she decided she wanted to become a teacher. She then enrolled part-time in teacher training and while it was a constant struggle for her to balance the demands of learning with those of her home life, she finally graduated and was offered a position at the same school she had been working in. She is proud of this achievement, and knows from feedback that she is good at her job.

Figure 1.1 Bert/Joan genogram

Bert, too, feels he is facing a challenging time in his life. He recently missed out on an anticipated promotion to regional manager for the building supply company; the company said his relationships with staff were too authoritarian. At 48, he now feels his career has stalled and he is trapped in a dead-end job. What business would invest in retraining an overweight man approaching 50 with poor staff relationship skills? He resents his wife's success in her new career. Why did she need to work anyway? He brought in enough money for the family, and besides it worked much better when she remained at home to look after the house and care for the children. Outside the home he endeavors to convey an open friendly stance with his work colleagues and his drinking friends, but inside he feels his efforts are increasingly empty and meaningless, and his friendliness is becoming more difficult to maintain. Added to this, he feels progressively disconnected from his home life; he does not understand his children, there is little tenderness left between him and Joan, and he feels increasingly as though he is staring into his home from the outside.

Cathy and Dion

Cathy and her son Dion live together in a cramped inner-city public-housing apartment. Cathy has a well-formed addiction to opiates, which she developed in her late twenties after meeting Robert, Dion's father. At first Robert introduced her slowly to the pleasures of injecting heroin, confining her use largely to special occasions. As she developed a taste for the drug, she pressured him for more regular use and soon joined him in his activities associated with the drug's importation and distribution, the proceeds from which enabled both of them regular daily access to high-quality heroin. She was 2 months pregnant with Dion before she recognized the signs, too late to change anything. It was painful to watch Dion's drug withdrawal in the hospital, but despite these temporary misgivings she was soon back with

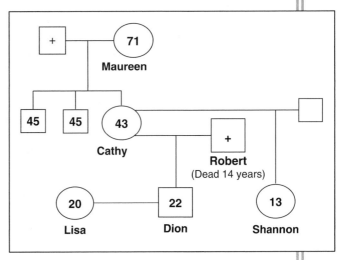

Figure 1.2 Cathy/Dion genogram

Robert pursuing their daily rounds, with baby Dion tagging along.

When Dion was about 8 years old his father suddenly disappeared. Cathy is unsure why, but suspects he may have died of an overdose during one of his many travels abroad. As her own links to Robert's associates were dwindling, she entered into a series of relationships with other heroin users in the supply network; this ensured her continued access to the drug distribution system. In one short-lived relationship she became pregnant again giving birth to her daughter, Shannon. The new baby lived with them episodically but was usually in foster care because of her Cathy's use. At times Cathy grew worried about the effects of her lifestyle on her children, and accordingly made some attempts to change, at one stage restricting her use to morphine and at another joining the local methadone program. Nonetheless, she always remained firmly enmeshed in the network of other heroin users and knew in her heart that she was not ready to leave.

Dion grew up in this disorganized world with remarkably few negative effects. He became an outgoing and confident young man, mixing well with most people and adjusting without complaining as his mother moved between cramped living situations and different partners. The last three years in their current flat had been the most stable period he can remember, and he is reluctant to upset the situation by leaving. He also worries about how his mother would cope without him. When she gets into bad moods she often talks about how pointless her life is, that he is the only good thing left in it and that she would kill herself if he were not around. He only half believes her, but he is genuinely concerned about the threat of overdoses and about her becoming sick from poor hygiene and nutrition. In the meantime, his life is moderately comfortable. He receives unemployment benefits and is studying art and design part-time at a local community college. Influenced by what he has observed with Cathy, he maintains a high level of fitness and avoids all drug use, including alcohol and tobacco. He is in the early stages of a relationship with Lisa, who now shares his small bedroom, where together they plan out their dreams of traveling abroad.

While Cathy remembers the many periods of pleasure associated with her heroin use, she is now growing weary of constantly striving to maintain her supply. She is tired of the ongoing fear of police raids, of violence from suppliers, and the ever-present menace of drug withdrawal. She has seen many of her friends die from overdoses, infections, and AIDS, and she herself had contracted hepatitis C from an infected needle and is now beginning to suffer from its effects. It frightens her to think of living a life without heroin, and she has no idea what she would become if she were to enter a straight world. But she now feels there must be a calmer alternative to her current chaos. If only she could pull herself out of this hole, make new friends, find a well-paid job, find a partner who cared about her, and silence all her thoughts of worthlessness and hopelessness.

Danny and Jack

At 56, Jack has no intention of giving up his work as a dairy farmer. His father worked the same land well into his seventies, as had his grandfather before him. He always hoped his son Danny would do the same, but Danny has chosen to break with this tradition and follow a lifestyle that he and his forefathers would have difficulty understanding. Danny works as an assistant to a local builder and travels with him to building projects around the community. Of most concern to Jack is Danny's apparent lack of solid commitment to anything in his life. He drives fast cars, stays up late, drinks heavily, smokes cannabis regularly, and shows little interest in spending time either on the farm or with his wife and children. Jack helped him build a house on one corner of the property, vaguely hoping it would help him settle down, but Danny's erratic lifestyle continued. Jack's disappointment grew even more intense following the death of his own wife to liver cancer, leaving Danny as his only close relative.

Danny resents his father's old-fashioned devotion to the farm and what he sees as an oppressive expectation of his taking it over eventually. He married Julie when he was 20 after she fell pregnant with their eldest daughter, Adrienne. They subsequently had two more children, but throughout he maintained little involvement with their upbringing, leaving Julie to provide the care while he sought work. The move into the house on his father's property seemed only to reduce his involvement; he identified even less with home life, and spent much of his free time fixing cars and socializing with friends. Heavy alcohol and cannabis use had been commonplace in his teens, but as many of his friends straightened out, got married, and took on mortgages, he and a small hard-core group stuck resolutely to a routine of drunken Friday and Saturday evenings. These were typically long evenings that usually ended with him col-

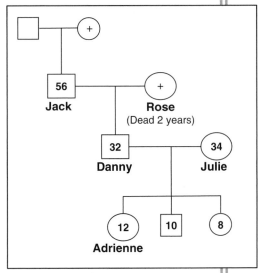

Figure 1.3 Danny/Jack genogram

lapsing and sleeping on other people's couches. He is also finding that the more difficult things become at home, the more attractive these drinking sessions become. He looks forward to them each week, anticipating an interlude in which, once he has had three or four drinks and perhaps some cannabis, he enters another world where the worries of home life drift away into the background.

Jack can see Danny's life slowly deteriorating into a pattern of partial commitments and heavy drinking. He had seen it all before. His own mother had been alcoholic and he can painfully recall her slow deterioration into intoxication and hopelessness. Unlike Danny, her drinking occurred more discreetly at home, but like him her drunkenness resulted in increasingly embarrassing incidents, ones that led friends and families to withdraw all contact. He could now see that Julie is increasingly pursuing a family life separate from Danny. Jack can also recognize that she considers Danny more a hindrance to bringing up the children, and he fears that she might leave and he could lose all contact with his grandchildren. He desperately wants to help his son realize what is going on before it is too late, but whenever he gently asks about either his lifestyle or his relationship, Danny invariably shouts at him, slams doors, and refuses to meet or speak with him for days and sometimes weeks. As occurred with Danny's mother, Jack feels compelled to watch helplessly as his son's social world disintegrates.

Jacinta and Wendy

Jacinta and Wendy have lived as a couple for just on 18 years. Their home environment is in turmoil because of Jacinta's strong attachment to gambling on slot machines. Jacinta had previously been married but after two disappointing years of quarrel and conflict she left her husband, determined never to commit to a long-term relationship again. Her resolve was short-lived. She met Wendy on an overseas vacation trip, discovered that they shared much in common, and found herself falling progressively in love with her. They were initially very happy together, but as the years rolled by they both began talking more openly of their regrets at not having had children. With the support of a gay friend, Jacinta became pregnant and they soon welcomed the birth of their son, Elliott. His early years were the happiest in their relationship; they were both totally focused on savoring each step in their son's development.

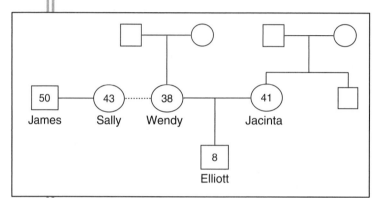

Figure 1.4 Jacinta/Wendy genogram

Since Wendy, who had trained in health administration, had the higher earning capacity, she continued to work full-time in her job as a hospital manager. Jacinta gave up her full-time job and found part-time work as a supermarket checkout supervisor, which allowed one of them to be at home when Elliott came home from school. Despite this shift, Jacinta felt unfulfilled in her work and was silently envious of the close bond Wendy was forming with Elliott.

Jacinta recalls her first encounter with slot machines when a group of friends took her to a casino while they were on an overseas vacation. She remembers putting some coins into the machine and while she initially enjoyed anticipating the outcome, she could not understand why people found them so attractive. But then, later in the evening, as her friends were talking of moving onto a nightclub, her last dollar coin returned a jackpot; the money kept pouring out and out—*kerchunk, kerchunk*—until just over eight hundred dollars in coins had spilled into the tray and onto the floor. Her friends were amazed; everyone was looking at her; she was in rapture and to celebrate she bought them all expensive cocktails. Later she tried to return to the machines, but her friends dragged her away to a nightclub. Nonetheless, the memory of elation at her first big win pursued her and she kept returning several times a week to play the slot machines in her own neighborhood. She was trying constantly to reconnect with her first high, but, unfortunately, it was never quite the same. Sure, she had some wins and these helped bolster her enthusiasm, but mostly she returned home with losses ranging between two to three hundred dollars per evening.

A year later, her gambling had claimed all her savings and a large proportion of Wendy's. She then resorted to spending their money for rent and food, which led inevitably to arguments with Wendy. She tried hard not to go gambling anymore, but in the evenings found the call of the machines too irresistible. She started borrowing from friends and family, promising to return the loans as soon as possible. When this never happened, her friends gradually dropped all contact, leading her to begin skimming small amounts at work from the supermarket's income.

Tracking back from her childhood, Wendy can recall many periods of pain and upset in her close relationships. During her adolescent years she struggled with her emerging sexual identity, trying out different arrangements in a series of ill-fated relationships. At 18, by this time clear about her sexual preference, she was deeply hurt when her parents, a conservative and churchgoing couple, discontinued any contact when she told them she was a lesbian. Following this rejection, she drifted in and out of other relationships until she finally met and settled down with Jacinta. While she maintained some good friendships, particularly with Sally and James, her closest bonds were with Jacinta and Elliott, and their little family was crucial to countering her previous encounters with dislocation and rejection. Consequently, as Jacinta chose to spend more and more time out in the evenings, Wendy could feel the foundations of her life beginning to crumble. Added to this, when she discovered that Jacinta had been intentionally deceiving her and secretly spending household finances on gambling, she felt doubly abandoned. The discovery was reinforced further when she heard from friends about other unpaid loans. Mistrust and suspicion had entered her safe haven and she was again feeling adrift in a world of uncertainty and fear.

Discussion

These four relationships—Bert/Joan, Cathy/Dion, Danny/Jack, Jacinta/Wendy—are discussed throughout the book in the inset boxes. Their stories are developed through snippets of relevant conversations that help illustrate the content in the main text. The conversational snippets for each relationship interconnect and form four parallel stories of addiction that resolve in various ways later in the book. While the content of the book and these parallel addiction narratives do not purport to have all the answers to the challenges of addiction, they do open up a new and, I believe, helpful way of looking at the social world in which addictions occurs.

Conversational snippets will illustrate the social world of addictive contexts

Chapter 2

A Social World

> *Historically, culture is a particular way of being in fundamental situations: birth, death, love, work, giving birth, being embodied, growing old, speaking. People have to be born, to die, and so forth, and a people arises in response to these tasks, to these calls, as it understands them. This understanding, this listening, and the resonance that is granted it, is at the same time what a people is, its understanding of itself, its being-together. Culture is not a system of meanings attributed to fundamental situation on the basis of conventions, a project or a contract; it is the being-there that is people.*
>
> *(Jean-Francois Lyotard[1])*

When Captain James Cook and his crew landed in Tahiti on April 13, 1769, after sailing through the bitter weather of the South Pacific, a whole new world opened up not only to them but also to the many people in different parts of Europe who subsequently read accounts of their voyages. Cook himself represented the best of the British Royal Navy; he was a brilliant cartographer, a strong leader, and someone who was deeply respectful of other people and their cultures. Others on board included artists, botanists and one key ambassador of European culture, Joseph Banks. He was a man of aristocratic upbringing and with broad interests in both the arts and the sciences and it was his writings that provided Europe with a window on a new way of interpreting this and their own world.

At first, the voyagers encountered the new world as both enthralling and perplexing. They were immediately struck by the natural beauty of the place and its people. The crew enjoyed the absence of European restrictions on lifestyle and sex, and several sought to establish their homes on the islands. But much of what they encountered was hard to understand. For example, Polynesian interpretations of ownership seemed to differ from their own, and the crew was increasingly angered by the constant accessing of their possessions. This they interpreted as "stealing" and they had difficulty appreciating the very different approach Tahitians had to property. Such different interpretations led to bitter disputes and at times bloody confrontations.

William Robertson Sights Tahiti

"We saw the whole coast full of Canoes, and the country had the most Beautiful appearance it's possible to Imagine. From the shore side, one two and three miles Back, there is a fine Level country that appears to be laid out in plantations, and the regular-built Houses seem to be without number; all along the Coast, they appeared like long Farmer's Barns, and seemed to be all very neatly thatched, with Great Numbers of Cocoa-Nut Trees.... This appears to be the most populous country I ever saw, the whole shore-line was lined with men, women and children all the way that we sailed along."

(Master of the ship *Dolphin*)

Nonetheless, besides these first contact misunderstandings, what Banks recognized was that the natural beauty and order of this apparent Garden of

P.J. Adams, Fragmented Intimacy: Addiction in a Social World
© Springer 2008

Eden made somewhat of a mockery of European attempts to construct a utopian world (see inset box above).[2] For some time, Enlightenment Europe had championed the role of reason and advanced civilization in building the ideal society. Already the challenge of Romanticism was claiming that the ideal world cannot be constructed, instead it emerges from the beauty and order of the natural world.[3] Europeans with all their advanced culture and technology were misguided to think their way was superior, and the Banks accounts of encounters in the South Pacific appeared to confirm this position. The encounter between the two worlds was important both for opening up new possibilities and for appreciating one's own interpretive frameworks.

Worlds, Paradigms, and Assumptions

Before exploring approaches to addiction, we need some conceptual tools that enable comparisons between the different approaches. Three terms will be employed for this purpose: *worlds, paradigms,* and *assumptions.* A *world* is understood here as a total environment that involves a complex of relationships within which people live, think, and interact (see the inset box below for common examples). As with the first contact between two separate cultures, worlds can often emerge as a result of two physically separate environments. Long-term separations enable very different ways to emerge of looking at the world. However, in an age of high physical mobility and mass communication these physically separate worlds are less common, and the separation is more likely to emerge from adherence to different cultural and belief systems. For example, in large cities people of different cultures occupy the same physical environment but at the same time live separately in parallel worlds; they share the same space and time but experience events quite differently. While these differences are often driven by culture and ideology, they are also affected by more subtle variations in background that have impacts on outlook. For example, people brought up in a home riddled with tension and conflict would be expected to experience their world with higher levels of anxiety than would people up in a happy and stable home environment.

The term *paradigm* refers to the conceptual system out of which a particular world is constructed. Paradigms[4] involve clustered ways of approaching experience that incorporate systems of interlocking forms of seeing, thinking, and talking. They are on the whole larger overarching systems that enable the smaller conceptual units—such as theories, models, arguments, approaches, and discourses[5]—to operate. Their relative size and scope is important. Their expansive overarching character often

> **Everyday Worlds**
> • "Caught between two worlds"
> • "The wonderful world of science"
> • "A ghastly world of death and destruction"
> • "Your world is different than mine"
> • "A world within a world"
> • "We belong to the new world"
> • "Welcome to my world"
> • "She's in her own little world"

means they fade into the background, while in the foreground attention is dominated by specific theories and models. For example, Captain Cook and his crew immersed in a Eurocentric view of the world had little awareness that their way of seeing things was determined by their own perspectives, and this prevented them from appreciating the different cultural practices of Polynesians. The elements of a paradigm also tend to entail a range of diverse linkages with these smaller conceptual units that make them difficult to pin down and describe. For example, well-formed theories tend to make specific predictions about aspects of a world, and these predictions are often testable; someone could go out into the world and check their accuracy. However, paradigms with their diffuse and interlocking ways of approaching experience are often difficult to define, nonspecific in what they refer to, and certainly do not lend themselves to testing and validation.

Paradigms themselves are resourced by sets of underlying basic *assumptions*. To use the crude metaphor of a glass fish container, if each major assumption provides the substance for a glass wall, the paradigm is then composed of the interlocked structures of several walls that are required to create a container, and the "world" becomes the fluid environment in which the goldfish swims. Accordingly, assumptions are unavoidable elements within a paradigm that simultaneously limit and enable how a paradigm functions. For example, the

Assumptions simultaneously limit & enable how paradigms function

most celebrated—and most disputed—contrast in assumptions between two paradigms occurred in the sixteenth-century Copernican Revolution during which thinking switched from the assumption that the earth was at the center of the universe to the assumption that the sun was at the center. In hindsight, this switch seems relatively simple and self-evident, but at the time, for those wedded to the assumption of the earth at the center, the switch was inconceivably huge. Over previous centuries astronomers had established an elaborate array of theories and models that explained the regularity of movements by the heavenly bodies. The new assumption of the sun at the center would entail having to abandon these theories and reshape from scratch a whole new paradigm from which to interpret what is observed. Furthermore, the assumption of the world at the center was linked with other domains of knowledge such as theology, physics, and medicine. To relinquish this assumption would require them to entirely rethink what it might mean for humans and their world to no longer be at the center.[6]

Four Features of Paradigms

There are four critical features of paradigms that are worth examining before moving on to applying paradigms to addictions. The first important feature is that they are "incommensurable"[7]; aspects belonging to two separate paradigms are incommensurable when they cannot be legitimately compared with each other because their use and meaning function differently in one contextual system than they do in the other. Since the assumptions within a paradigm contribute strongly to specific meanings, attempts at one-to-one translations lead inevitably to misunderstandings. For example, Tahitian and Maori use of the term *aroha* (*alofa* in Samoa, *aloha* in Hawaii) roughly translates into English as "love," but the one-to-one translation of an important word like this is riddled with problems. In Polynesian eyes, *aroha* links up with other aspects of how Polynesians see the world and how they understand the connection between the individual and the broader collective. Its use signals the many ways in which specific instances of love partake in a grander collective process of universal love. This means that equating it to the narrower European notion of love misses out on the range of other important nuances appreciated by the speaker of each Polynesian language and thereby loses many of its vital associations and meanings. One world is carved up differently than the other world in such a way that any one-to-one translation of this and many other key words misses out on meanings and interrelationships between concepts. While in a peripheral manner they could function as roughly equivalent, their full meanings are incommensurable because they are derivative of different systems of assumptions.

A second critical feature of paradigms is that their basic assumptions are untestable. In essence, fundamental assumptions are leaps of faith; they involve ways of looking and thinking that are necessary for research and theory, but are themselves unfalsifiable. For instance, in the European scientific paradigm of "objectivism,"[8] one basic assumption is that knowledge, to be knowledge, needs to be reproducible and objective; if it is not solidly established, it remains merely a matter of opinion. However, this assumption itself is not testable; besides, it would be impossible to conceive of a way of testing it. It is not only a strongly held belief but also a fundamental commitment to a way of looking at things, a commitment that lays out the ground rules for acquiring knowledge and sharing it[9]; it will be defended by adherents of the paradigm regardless of what happens. Proponents have invested much of their time and talents into it being the case, and to shift away from this assumption would involve cutting frighteningly loose from the enterprise of science as they know it.

Basic assumptions in a paradigm involve fundamental leaps of faith

A third critical feature is that different paradigms offer different opportunities for seeing and understanding how things fit together. This provides the counterweight to the paradigm inertia that result from dependence on one system of assumptions. Different paradigms involve cutting up what we observe in different ways, and exposure to them will generate alternative ways of seeing and thereby stimulate alternative ways of responding.[10] For example, when James Cook and his crew returned to England, his exposures in the South Pacific contributed significantly to supporting a paradigm switch to the Romanticism that was sweeping Europe at that time. Up until then, the European Enlightenment had propelled an overriding interest in the human capacity to use rationality to create a civilized world. Those who accompanied Cook were able to point to a natural and primitive world could manifest high degrees of order and beauty, and this challenged assumptions of the superiority of their rationally constructed social order. Rather than viewing the natural world as something to be tamed or conquered, Cook's voyages supported an interest in nature as something that civilized society seeks to negotiate an ongoing and reciprocal relationship.

The fourth and final feature is that paradigms are slow to change. Their essential untestability and incommensurability mean both that it is difficult to convince people of the need to shift and that the prospect of a new world opens up as daunting and unfamiliar. Furthermore, particularly for core supporters of a paradigm, why should they shift? It is what they know and it has successfully helped explain things in the past. Besides, they have conducted all their research and theorizing within that paradigm and to move on from it could negate all that effort. Thomas Kuhn, in his analysis of how paradigms behave, argued that for major paradigm changes, the reluctance of adherents to convert leads the majority to stick doggedly to what they know and to repel challenges by adapting the old paradigm in ways that ensure its survival.[11] Consequently, the time it takes to complete a paradigm shift is the time it takes for determined adherents either to be removed or die out. This in most contexts would take decades.

Dominant and Alternative Paradigms

Paradigms vary in strength and scope. In some situations paradigms compete vigorously as equal combatants that contest with each other for adherents. When these contests occur, societies benefit because the multiple ways of looking at things enable all parties to become aware of their assumptions, and they are constantly challenged to reflect and justify their various positions. Unfortunately, pluralistic environments require considerable effort and commitment to maintain, and historically these periods tend not to last long before one paradigm begins to edge into a more dominant position than the others. For this reason, pluralistic environments can be seen to function in most cases as periods of transition from one dominant paradigm to another. Strong examples of pluralistic periods occurred in classical Athens, Song-dynasty China, Moorish Spain, and Vienna of the 1900s.[12] Each of these periods was followed by changes into new orthodoxies. As one paradigm gains dominance it also increases its access to political and institutional systems and processes. The environment is no longer a level playing field, and the adherents of alternative paradigms are relegated to subsidiary and marginalized roles such as those of playing the critic, the curiosity, the clown, or even the outcast roles of radical or crackpot. For example, when Russia embraced Marxist-Leninism, it enabled the socioeconomic assumptions incorporated into this paradigm to be constantly reinforced through the media, political structures, and ways of speaking. Only

Dominant paradigms are reinforced by ways of speaking and behaving

one voice could be officially heard, and with this advantage, alternative paradigms soon faded away.[13]

Such dominance also typifies academic contexts, where dominant paradigms attained levels of dominance that eclipsed other alternatives. Examples of this occurred with behaviorism in psychology, structuralism in anthropology, and analytic approaches in philosophy. Perhaps the most practical outlook is to accept that at any particular time one paradigm is likely to dominate others, and that the main task is to ensure there is a healthy stock of alternative paradigms ready at hand when the dominant paradigm flounders or capsizes.

The dominance of a paradigm can reach a point where it is so completely ingrained into ways of thinking and seeing that its adherents are unaware of the extent of their allegiance. Once a paradigm takes strong hold, institutional systems, ways of speaking, professional practice, and even the design of buildings and clothes work together to reinforce its central assumptions. For example, the dominance of medical interpretations of mental health has been strengthened by basing services in places called "hospitals," provided by "doctors" and "nurses" who administer "treatments" to "patients" affected by mental "illness".[14] Attached to each of these words are embedded assumptions pointing to the similarities between mental well-being and physical well-being. The similarity is reinforced repeatedly at several levels—in concepts, language, buildings, images, clothes—to a point that the similarity becomes so familiar it appears to be self-evident and factual. At this point a paradigm has achieved such dominance that adherents are no longer aware of it as a paradigm and unreflectively assume it to be a solid part of the fabric of reality. It also means that alternative conceptions can no longer be seriously entertained[15]; they are mere opinions or viewpoints, while the familiar paradigm is solid and factual. In some ways the process can be likened to goldfish swimming in water without appreciating that the water is there and that they are wet. The paradigm has become so familiar, so omnipresent, that awareness of its existence fades and the possibility of alternatives dissolves into obscurity.

A paradigm can attain such dominance that adherents no longer realize they inhabit it

The Particle Paradigm

This book contrasts two paradigms that are used to understand addictions: the "particle" paradigm and the "social" paradigm. One paradigm is dominant, the other is emergent. One has enabled a vast array of research programs, the other has yet to attract research attention. One is more suited to health service environments, the other is suited more to community environments. Both paradigms provide a basis for understanding and explaining addictions and both provide useful platforms for designing and implementing interventions.

The term *particle paradigm* refers here to a cluster of assumptions that revolve around the idea that the self is primarily an individual object and that this object—or particle—is the appropriate focal point for understanding addictive processes. Other selves, too, are viewed as individual objects and together they move about within an environment connecting, disconnecting, and influencing each other, but always moving as discrete objects—objects with their own boundaries, attributes, and potentialities. The image this conjures up is that of a billiard ball traveling through absolute space, bumping into other billiard balls, and moving forward as a result of net forces generated by each ball's weight and momentum. As with the balls, the reasons for people to behave as they do can be explained in terms of principles and processes happening at the focal point of the individual object. Attributes of the ball, such as mass, inertia, and angle of movement, account for where it will move next, just as attributes of people, such as intelligence, character, and attitude, account for how they will behave next. Similarly with addictions, according to a particle perspective, addictive behavior emerges as a response to the internal and external forces that impact on the addicted person. Environments, relationships, and social influences are seen as important, but only inasmuch as they are understood as attributes or factors attached to the primary particle. The key focus is on how the various internal and external forces are integrated at the point of the individual.

Particle approaches to addiction focus on the attributes of people as primary particles

Two key dimensions of human existence lend themselves most strongly to this individualistic focus: the person as an organism and the person as a psychological being. With respect to the former, most organisms function as discrete autonomous units. They are bounded by membranes behind which they have evolved physiological systems and organ systems that enable them to maintain life, to reproduce, and to adapt to environmental changes. Humans, as organisms, share these qualities, and the discipline of medicine has led the way in developing increasingly elaborate ways of supporting and managing the survival of each separate human organism. Humans also operate as individual psychological beings. They think, remember, sense, and feel—each of these contributing in a complex way to how they actually behave. The discipline of psychology has grown rapidly over the last century and now offers a broad range of ways of relating psychological processes to human behavior. As with medicine, the discipline's primary focus is on the person as an individual, as a behaving particle. Both disciplines explore different dimensions of the person, but share a common preoccupation with the person as a primary particle. In approaching addictive behavior through the bifocal lens of medicine and psychology, the orientation naturally conforms to a focus on the person as an individual particle.

Origins

The story of the emergence of the particle paradigm over the last two centuries parallels the story of the ascent of the disciplines of medicine and psychology. It was during the nineteenth century's development of medicine as self-consciously scientific that particle orientations began to gain a firm foothold. As medicine cut away its links with theology, astrology, and natural philosophy, explanations of addictive behavior in terms of religious and relational concepts such as evil, diabolical forces, and destiny became isolated from their mythico-religious roots and soon lost their currency. Instead, toward the end of the nineteenth century, the two emerging disciplines of psychology and medical science vied to provide alternative understandings. Their debates were fluid and the terminology shifted and changed.

Psychology & medicine have propelled the adoption of particle assumptions

Mariana Valverde's (1998) detailed account of this period discusses how at first the psychological constructs of *will* and *habit* were applied by clinicians to those of their patients who regularly appeared with recurring alcohol inebriation.[16] Their patients were seen to suffer either from a weakness of will or an excess of habit. Later, clinicians working in different countries struggled to describe what they observed using a mixture of psychological and medical terms; examples include *monomania of the will, dypsomania, habitual inebriation,* and *the habitual drunkard*.[17] Despite this rapprochement, in the first half of the twentieth century leading figures in medicine in both Britain and the United States launched an ongoing campaign for recognition of addictions as primarily a medical issue. The following new terms emerged with progressively heavier reference to medical concepts: *disease of inebriety, alcoholism, addiction,* and ultimately *alcohol and drug dependence*. This culminated in the World Health Organization's[18] consensual recognition in 1957 of alcohol and drug dependence as a syndrome with the following definition:

> Drug addiction is a state of periodic or chronic intoxication produced by the repeated consumption of a drug (natural or synthetic). Its characteristics include: (i) an overpowering desire or need (compulsion) to continue taking the drug and to obtain it by any means; (ii) a tendency to increase the dose; (iii) a psychic (psychological) and generally a physical dependence on the effects of the drug; and (iv) detrimental effects on the individual and on society.[19]

The medical use of the term *dependence* emphasized the biological dimensions of addiction, such as tolerance and withdrawal, and firmly anchored understandings to the perspective that addiction or drug dependence emerges primarily from the individual as a discrete organism.

In the last three decades of the twentieth century, the strengthening discipline of psychology, supported by its improved scientific research methodologies, reasserted its contribution. Its leading proponents—Nick Heather, Alan Marlatt, Jim Orford, Carlos DiClemente, and Bill Miller, to name only a few—examined the various ways in which addictive behavior can be understood in terms of learning and adaptation to challenging environments. Earlier psychodynamic and other internal psychologies had contributed episodically to the study of addiction, but their role was minimal compared to the advances in medical approaches. But with the rise of behaviorism during the 1960s, people struggling with addictions were beginning to be studied in terms of behaving particles, and this then led on to psychological explanatory concepts such as *conditioned responses, reinforcement contingencies, and cue exposure.* Later, shadowing the rise of cognitive psychology, internal psychological processes regained a foothold and behaving particles became behaving-thinking particles. A new range of concepts were closely defined and studied, and led to terms such as *causal attributions, self-efficacy,* and *motivational set.*

Despite the ongoing sparring and occasional skirmish between medical and psychological studies of addiction, the rivalry is best seen as a sideshow. The main performance is reserved for the consolidating dominance of the particle paradigm. Both medical and psychological traditions emphasize the nature of addiction in terms of people as particles. For medicine, the idea of a person reduces naturally to the notion of an organism, a complex organism for sure, with psychological, emotional, and social attributes, but at a fundamental level primarily an organism. For psychological orientations, while expressing some discomfort with the language of disease,[20] their emphasis on the person as an individual does not pose any essential threat to the particle orientation. On the contrary, their focus on the person as a behaving or thinking individual reinforces a particle orientation. Together the alliance between these two traditions has enabled the particle paradigm to attain almost complete dominance in the study of addictions.

The "Biopsychosocial" Model

The biopsychosocial model is a relatively recent variant of the particle paradigm that has evolved primarily to accommodate the rise of psychological study of addiction, and, to a lesser extent, recognize the relevance of social and cultural influences. Advocates for the particle paradigm of both the medical and psychological persuasion ran into a problem.[21] While remaining firmly wedded to explanations grounded at the level of the individual, it was becoming clearer from a number of quarters that social factors played a significant role in both the origins and course of most addictions. Addiction research and theory identified with increasing importance the roles of culture, social position, community influences, and family dynamics.[22] Explanations could not be contained adequately within the bounds of the person, and vague reference to environmental influences no longer sufficed. Since both addiction research and theory were heavily invested in the paradigm, their challenge was to find a way to accommodate social processes without transforming the paradigm itself. Their response led to formulation of what they referred to as the biopsychosocial model of addiction.[23]

The central advantage of a *biopsychosocial* model is that it recognizes the complex and multileveled nature of addictions.[24] It encourages medical and psychological approaches to work side by side, and it recognizes the legitimacy of social orientations. Its key challenge is to find a way of communicating between the three orientations. As Carlos DiClemente puts it:

The biopsychosocial model rescues the particle paradigm from needing to change

> The biopsychosocial model clearly supports the complexity and interactive nature of the process of addiction and recovery. However, additional integrating elements are needed in order to make this tripartite collection of factors truly functional for explaining how individuals become addicted and how the process of recovery from addiction occurs.[25]

Note how in this quotation DiClemente relates the model back to how "individuals become addicted." Forging links between biomedical and psychological approaches is relatively easy because both share a common base of particle assumptions. However, the social dimensions of being human cannot be reduced to variables, factors, or influences attached to individual particles. Social processes sit less easily on a bed of particle assumptions. Instead of looking at addiction as a social event in itself, social influences themselves become condensed, abstracted, and particularized so that they can fit in with the biopsychosocial frame. The frame fails to acknowledge that adopting a truly social orientation on addiction requires a move away from the particle assumptions inherent to biological and psychological theories.

The Social Paradigm

In contrast to the particle paradigm, the social paradigm shifts the focus of attention away from people as discrete individuals and toward viewing people in terms of their relationships. This simple move catapults understanding into a different conceptual environment involving a significant shift in how personal identity is understood. The whole emphasis moves from seeing people in terms of qualities, attributes, and potentialities, to seeing people in terms of the nature of their relationships with other people and with other objects. As the switch from seeing the earth as the center of the universe to seeing the sun as the center radically changed ways of thinking, so the switch from people-as-particles to people-in-relationships has implications for how we understand ourselves. When looking through a social lens, social involvements are no longer seen as *A social* mere factors or influences; they are seen as actively constituting personal *orientation* identity and as such they take on a primary rather than derivative role in *focuses on* making sense of human realities. *people*

When it comes to reorienting addictions into a social world, the move *in their* also involves a fundamental shift in focus and interpretation. Instead of *everyday* viewing addiction as an attribute attached to a particular addicted person, *relationships* the central idea involves understanding addiction as a social event. The next two chapters will develop what this means in more detail, but the following provides a brief summary. When people become addicted, they enter into a very intense relationship with the object of their addiction. Since, as social beings, most people maintain a broad range of relationships with other objects (including people, processes, and things), the intensification of one particular relationship has consequences for other relationships within that social system. For example, preoccupation with one object consumes time and resources at the expense of other surrounding relationships. As this preoccupation intensifies, other relationships deteriorate and slowly an addictive social system emerges, with the addicted person strongly and rigidly attached to one object and only peripherally attached to other objects. In social terms, what is important here are not the qualities and attributes of the objects involved, but rather the nature of the relationships and the qualities of the interplay between the various objects.

Origins

A social interpretation is new to the field of addictions, but it has a strong history in other contexts. Its genealogy can be traced back into different traditions that share this common interest in the relationships between particles rather than the particles themselves. It is beyond the scope of this discussion to explore all the influences that contribute to a social orientation, but, in brief, the major influences can be organized into four major genealogical lines: philosophy, social theory, health theory, and social practice. Each is summarized briefly in the following subsections.

From Philosophy: Knowledge Is Situational

In his major work on rhetoric, the mid-nineteenth century philosopher Friedrich Nietzsche (1844–1900) acknowledged that although certain "truths" appear over time to have a universal significance, they cannot be abstracted away from their origins in human experience and human relationships.

What is truth? A mobile army of metaphor, metonymies, and anthropomorphisms, in short, a sum of human relations that were poetically and rhetorically heightened, transferred, and adorned, and after long use seem solid, canonical, and binding to a nation.[26]

Here Nietzsche is questioning an underlying assumption of a specific theory of knowledge called objectivism (also variously called empiricism, realism, and positivism): the belief that knowledge to be knowledge needs to be universally true and true across all time (see inset box for common assumptions).

Knowledge Assumptions

Objectivism assumes knowledge to be:

- *Universal*
  Stable across time, culture, ideology gender, and other circumstances
- *Reducible*
  Portions of knowledge can be reliably combined to give an adequate picture of the whole
- *Univocal*
  Capable of unambiguous expression, free from the complications of multiple views of reality
- *Containable*
  Able to be captured in propositional form and stored for others to access
- *Transportable*
  Units of knowledge can be transferred between contexts and still retain their essential meaning

These assumptions have dominated the pursuit of knowledge over the last two hundred years—the same period in which the particle paradigm has flourished. The relationship is not accidental. Objectivist assumptions are essential in developing approaches within a particle paradigm because they justify the emphasis on separated particles without reference to context. Objectivism was consistently opposed by a diverse range of philosophers that included important figures such as Georg Hegel, Edmund Husserl, Soren Kierkegaard, and Martin Heidegger. Their opposition provided an initial platform for the birth of the postmodernist movement and its various manifestations. Postmodernism[27] (also called postmodernity or later modernity) is a loosely connected cluster of academic traditions that share a common interest in questioning the primary assumptions of objectivism. Knowledge is seen as context specific rather than universal and is linked irreducibly with *Social context is critical* language and social context. Within a world where human relationships, *to the meaning* social context, and language are paramount, confining one's focus to a *ing of human* particle orientation will result in overlooking much of the detail that *interaction* makes human interaction meaningful.

From Social Theory: Social Involvements Constitute Situations

The energy and diversity of modern social theory can be at times overwhelming. Much of it is indirectly or directly related to the challenges posed by postmodernism. The streams of activity include various schools of French philosophy, large parts of North American sociology and anthropology, a lively network in British social psychology, as well as a range of activities in social geography, culture and gender studies, and literary criticism.[28] To touch briefly on one of the early figures, the Viennese born American sociologist Alfred Schutz (1889–1959) managed through his teaching and writing[29] to coax other sociologists to begin looking more closely at how people's situations in everyday life affect their experience as a whole. In his book *The Phenomenology of the Social World*,[30] he connected the domain of personal meaning with the domain of action and explored how these are constituted through the interaction of experience and the social world. Sociologists influence by his work (students such as Peter Berger and contemporaries such as Harold Garfinkel) adopted his shift from an emphasis on overarching structural processes (such as "class" and "market") to an emphasis on the experience of social involvements, and went on to develop theories and methods that examined how value and identity is often derived from the particularities of specific situations. Those who followed, and many from other social theory traditions, have helped sketch the fine detail of how people experience their situatedness in everyday life, and the complex dynamics of social interrelationships.

From Health Science: Strength Emerges from Social Involvement

A third genealogical line, and one that will be cited again when discussing communities in Chapters 9 and 12, is the strengthening view that personal health and well-being are strongly associated with social processes. Three main disciplines have contributed to such an orientation: public health has contributed through its recognition of the importance of wider determinants of health,[31] psychology has contributed through its development of the concept of *resilience*,[32] and health promotion has contributed through its study of the processes of community empowerment.[33] Public health research is encountering with increasing regularity the extent to which a person's relative position on a social gradient—varying from wealthy and integrated to poor and marginalized—can have a marked impact on major indices of health. For example mortality rates for most major diseases are higher for those lower on the gradient. These observations connect with research in psychology and education, which has found that a broader focus on factors affecting strength and resilience may provide better direction for intervention than the narrower focus on risk factors and on what is going wrong. For example, adolescents are less likely to suffer mental health issues when they maintain stronger social connectedness, spiritual connectedness, and cultural involvement.[34] These two themes, social determinants and resiliency, come together in the concept of empowerment. When people have a sense of control over the way they approach issues that confront them, they are more likely to come up with solutions that suit their circumstances, more likely to own and maintain their chosen responses, and as a consequence more likely to be successful. For example, broad-based capacity-building strategies with impoverished inner city communities are demonstrating surprising effectiveness and durability.[35]

The nature of social involvement is a major contributor to health

From Social Practice: Personal Identity Is Derived from Social Connection

A fourth genealogical line can be identified in the quiet creep of social approaches into the realms of psychological counseling and psychotherapy. Examples include systems theory, family therapy, ecological theory, narrative therapy, and a range of other language-oriented or rhetorical approaches.[36] These approaches share a common interest in exploring how relationships rather than the qualities of individuals contribute to psychological well-being. A key early figure in this movement was the American anthropologist Gregory Bateson (1904–1980). He examined closely how reciprocal communication processes between people provide a powerful impetus into how they experience the world. He labeled his approach as "cybernetic" because he saw language and communication as the medium in which relationships form, and that a study of the way information passed between people could explain many aspects of how people respond to each other. Bateson's work contributed to a broad range of clinical interventions, from his influence on the social processes associated with schizophrenia, to language-oriented hypnotherapy, to couples and family therapy. His influence on service interventions with addictions is most apparent in various applications of systems theory, language approaches and family therapy.

Switching to a Social World

The various genealogical lines listed above weave together into the fabric of a social paradigm, but the leap into this world is no easy matter, especially for those of us who have lived and breathed particle assumptions for long periods. The switch to viewing addictions as a social event entails a letting go of particle assumptions and leaping out into a different way of seeing human affairs. By way of illustration, the above figure presents the bare outline of a cube that the reader can look at from two perspectives. First, look at it with the square to the left as the front of the cube. Now, shift to looking at the square to the right as the front. Try switching again, and again. Each switch involves a radical transformation of how the cube is perceived. Neither perspective has precedence over the other; both are equally valid, and adopting one does not negate the possibility of the other. Note also that during the course of switching it is difficult to think of the cube in one way

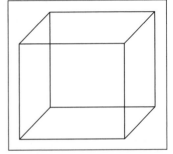

Figure 2.1 Multiperspective cube

while seeing it in terms of the other. The two perspectives are not open to being mixed or blended; the cube is seen one way or the other, not somewhere in between. These features illustrate aspects of what happens when switching from a particle to a social paradigm. The perspectives they offer are valid in their own way, but they are not open to being merged or blended. Switching requires letting go of assumptions from one and taking on assumptions that belong to the other. Attempts at transporting assumptions from one frame into the other blocks the transition.

It is surprising that given the vibrancy of social approaches across many disciplines, more has not been made of them in the study of addictions. Their absence raises concerns that the particle paradigm may have attained sufficient strength for it to be considered completely dominant—a situation where adherents are so embedded in it they may be unaware of the strength of their allegiance. Indeed, in certain contexts, such as hospital addiction services or addiction research units, it is often difficult to encounter discussions that step outside of particle assumptions. Talk tends to focus almost exclusively on counting and treating affected particles. Nonetheless, in other contexts, such as in twelve-step groups, residential programs, and community contexts, the focus on individuals is never entirely secure. The addiction field has managed to retain a strongly diverse range of influences with perspectives derived from culture, religion, and popular psychology. While these influences are insufficient to challenge the dominance of the particle paradigm, they have by contrast brought into relief the opportunity for alternative perspectives.

A Guide to Paradigm Switching

This book is written with the paradigm switcher in mind. It assumes—perhaps falsely for some—that the predominant influences on the reader's thinking about addictions are derived from particle assumptions. While the initial experiences of entering new zones will seem stimulating and exciting, there is a strong risk of this turning into annoyance and disappointment once disorientation occurs in the new terrain. To reduce the effects of disorientation the following provides a five-point guide to working with the ideas in this book:

1. Questioning old assumptions, beliefs, and explanations: The book invites readers to let go of old assumptions, ride with the flow of ideas presented here, and see where the voyage leads. There will perhaps be parts of the book that are difficult to swallow, but their place in the broader schema will become more obvious as the book proceeds. Particle assumptions are so deeply embedded into both public and academic discourses on addiction that clashes and misunderstandings are inevitable. As in the example in the inset box, Captain Cook's early contacts with New Zealand Maori[37] challenged both parties to engage in new experiences but from an old conceptual base. The primary orientation in this book invites readers to move from seeing addiction as an attribute of a person to seeing it as a relationship among other relationships. All other content in the book flows from this central idea. While progressing through each chapter, readers are urged to keep linking back to this central idea of addiction as a social event. Whenever the content clashes with the reader's own beliefs, it may be helpful to pause and to reflect on whether the disagreement relates to an attachment to particle assumptions. Such attachments might be put aside, at least temporarily, to allow enough space for a social interpretation of addiction to establish its potential.

> **A Maori First View of Captain Cook**
> "A vessel came there [a bay in New Zealand], and when our old men saw the ship they said it was an *atua*, a god, and the people on board were *tupua*, strange beings or 'goblins.' The ship came to anchor, and the boats pulled on shore. As our old men looked at the manner in which they came on shore, the rowers pulling with their backs to the bows of the boat, the old people said, 'Yes, it is so: these people are goblins; their eyes are at the backs of their heads; they pull on shore with their backs to the land to which they are going.' When these goblins came on shore we (the children and women) took notice of them, but we ran away from them into the forest, and the warriors alone stayed in the presence of those goblins; but, as the goblins stayed some time, and did not do any evil to our braves, we came back one by one, and gazed at them, and we stroked their garments with our hands, and we were pleased with the whiteness of their skins and the blue of the eyes of some of them."

2. Changing the vocabulary: Vocabulary is a potent device for reinforcing the primary assumptions of a particular paradigm. As described in the inset box, considerable confusion ensued when William Hodges, the artist on Cook's ship, engaged a young Maori woman to pose for a painting.[38] To assist the process of switching paradigms and to avoid confusing crossovers with particle assumptions, this book makes use of a limited set of new words and phrases that reinforce the relational nature of addiction. Words such as *relapse* and *recovery* are embedded in particle thinking and tend to focus attention onto qualities attached to the person and thereby convey little of a relational view of addiction. They will be replaced with relational words such as *reversion* and *reintegration*. This also applies to the term *addiction*. From now on, instead of using *addiction* as a noun (object word), which implies some form of disease process within the individual, this book will refer to the term *addictive relationships*, in which *addictive* as an adjective qualifies a certain type of relationship without conjecturing on internal processes. For the same reason, other terms qualified by *addictive* include *addictive substance/process* to refer to the object of an addictive relationship, and *addictive system* to refer to the immediate set of relationships surrounding an addictive relationship. Other terms used will be explained as they arise, and a glossary for reference is provided at the end of the book.

> **Early Misunderstandings**
>
> "Language difficulties at first gave rise to a misunderstanding between the girl and the painter, for she, having been paid well to go down into the saloon, imagined that she ought to give satisfaction, in the way she understood it, as soon as possible in return for her gift.... She was astonished when signs were made for her to sit on a chair; such a novel way of doing things struck her as absurd, but she promptly volunteered a prone position on the chair for the painter and his companion. To her further surprise she was eventually put in a correct position, just sitting on the chair with nothing to do; whereupon, to the wonderment and entertainment of herself and the two savages with her, she quickly saw her likeness appearing in a red crayon drawing."

3. Openness to new territory: An important drawback to consider when switching from an established paradigm to an emerging one is the latter's lack of opportunity to establish its central ideas. A well-established and dominant paradigm, such as the particle paradigm, has had ample time to embed its assumptions, to refine its language and ideas, and to develop its main explanations. An emergent paradigm is caught between partially relying on language and concepts from the previous paradigm, and partially grappling with developing its own terminology and way of thinking. Furthermore, it lacks the support of established research programs to credential its main assertions. Nonetheless, this very drawback is also its key advantage. As commentators on science have observed, well-worn paradigms tend in the end to fill up their territories for discovery.[39] In a crowded research space, studies become increasingly elaborate, making them either too expensive or too repetitive to pursue; they become tired and overly elaborate, and they eventually run out of steam. A new paradigm (such as viewing addictions in a social world), while it lacks the supports and refinements of older paradigms, has the advantage of opening whole new territories for exploration and

discovery. As suggested by Joseph Banks on board Captain Cook's Endeavour (see below inset box), the opportunity for new territories presupposes a willingness to venture out into unknown seas.[40]

4. Connect ways of thinking to ways of experiencing: Paradigm switching is not a process that can be achieved by thinking alone; shifts in values, meanings, and perceptions also play a role. True voyages of discovery cannot rely solely on the mind because old ways of thinking are strongly immersed in old assumptions. New ways of thinking often rely on prior exposure to new ways of perceiving the world as occurred with Galileo's use of the telescope and behaviorism's use of the Skinner box. For example, in his experience of sailing across the vast expanses of the Pacific, Captain Cook began to appreciate the immensity of the achievement of ancient Polynesian explorers who had spanned out in frail vessels across thousands of miles of ocean (see inset box[41]); he had to see this to really appreciate it. Similarly, to activate the senses and the imagination, throughout this the series of boxes containing diagrams, vignettes, internal monologues, dialogues, and testimonials placed alongside the main text provide a more concrete means to illustrate key points. These boxes are intended to assist paradigm switching by introducing perceptual and experiential elements that trigger associations between the texts and experiences in everyday life.

> **Venturing Out**
>
> "When I look on the charts of these Seas and see our course, which has been Near a streight at NW since we left Cape Horne, I cannot help wondering that we have not yet seen land. It is however some pleasure to be able to disprove that which does not exist but in the opinions of Theoretical writers, of which sort most are who have wrote any thing about these seas without having themselves been in them."

> **Cook Marvels at Polynesian Voyaging**
>
> "How shall we account for this Nation spreading it self so far over this Vast ocean? We find them from New Zealand to the South, to these islands to the North [Hawaii] and from Easter Island to the Hebrides; an extent of 60 degrees of latitude or twelve hundred leagues north and south and 83 degrees of longitude or sixteen hundred and sixty leagues east and west, how much further is not known, but we may safely conclude that they extend to the west beyond the Hebrides."

5. Managing expectations and sticking with them: In contrast to the example of a switch in perspective as depicted in the cube diagram (see previous inset box), the switch into a social world is unlikely to make sense immediately. This particularly applies to those who have been immersed in particle orientations for a long time. The process of letting go particle assumptions will take time, and it is this period of time between two worlds that can cause problems. When attempting to step between different sets of assumptions there is typically a long period of standing with one foot in one world and one foot in the other. This period of transition can often result in experiences of confusion and discomfort caused by a muddling of the values and meanings from both worlds. While this is unlikely to reach the level of discomfort experienced by Captain Cook and his crew (see inset box, above[42]),

> **The Discomforts of Voyaging**
>
> "The Sea is now tempestuous, the Decks are never dry, all the Ship moist & damp; my Cabin cold & open to the piercing winds, full of unwholesome effluvia and vapours, every thing I touch is moist & mouldy & looks more like a subterranean mansion for the dead than a habitation for the living. In the Captain's Cabin there are broken panes, the apartment full of currents & smoke… if to this we add that there the pitching of the Ship is more felt, than any where else it will clearly appear, that these Expeditions are the most difficult task that could be imposed on poor mortals."

some level of confusion should be anticipated. The challenge for the reader is to remain immersed long enough in the reorientation outlined in this book for its merits to emerge.

The next two chapters provide an overview of how a focus on relationships can improve our understanding of the power of addictive processes.

Chapter 3

Addiction and Connecting

It is not his body but his brain that is drunken. He may bubble
with wit, or expand with good fellowship. Or he may see intellectual
specters and phantoms that are cosmic and logical and that take
the forms of syllogisms. It is when in this condition that he strips
away the husks of life's healthiest illusions and gravely considers
the iron collar of necessity welded about the neck of his soul.
This is the hour of John Barleycorn's subtlest power.

(Jack London, "John Barleycorn"[1])

The previous two chapters have outlined the importance of addictions and introduced the basic assumptions underlying the social paradigm that comprises the orientation for this book. This chapter explains the vital role of social connections in forming identity, the process of entering into an addictive relationship, and how this is likely to impact on other people.

Connecting to the World

A key tool for understanding the function of relationships in a social world is the concept of social connection.[2] As explored in the previous chapter, relationships rather than particles form the substance of a social world, and one way of depicting relationships is to think of them in terms of connections. A person connects with other people, with other things, with imaginary objects, with things in the past, and with things in the future. Connections can happen in very many ways: they can be stronger or weaker; they can be static or dynamic; they can merge, divide, branch, and braid; they can disconnect, reconnect, partially connect, and connect intermittently. Above all, as an outcome of linking up, both parties to a connection—the connector and that to which one connects—derive something from the link in terms of who or what they are. The connection adds to the raw material upon which identities are derived. Each connection plugs into a wider system of connections and it is this web of interconnections from which the social world is composed.

Identity and Social Connection

Consider for a moment how one might respond to the question, "Who are you?" It is an important question and attempts at answering it can often

P.J. Adams, *Fragmented Intimacy: Addiction in a Social World*
© Springer 2008

lead a person down perplexing and bewildering pathways. As depicted in Figure 3.1, it is a question that, without reference to anything else, is difficult to answer. In this diagram the particle "me" hangs in absolute space with very little else to refer to. It is simply a location for existence, an empty vessel with which all aspects of the world might engage. In addition, this "me" remaining there alone, without further description or context, provides little guidance regarding what it is to be me.

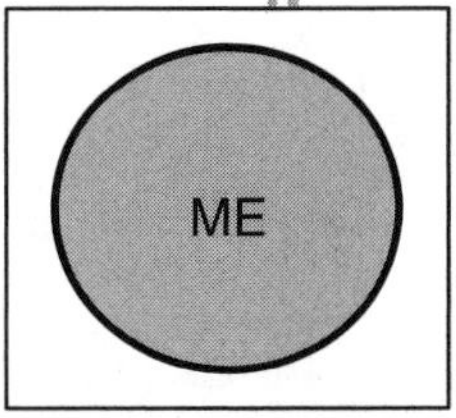

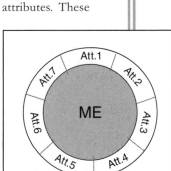

Figure 3.1 Me Alone

When it comes to saying more about me, there are several ways in which it could be tackled. One way would be to describe me in terms of aspects attached to me—personal attributes such as "I am impulsive," "I am wise," and "I lack confidence." In Figure 3.2 the object "me" is depicted as surrounded by a range of attributes. These attributes are wrapped up within me as a set of potentialities similar to the way in which the properties of a solid object, such as a piece of iron, carry attributes such as weight, density, and conductivity. However, most attributes, other than aspects such as appearance, are not immediately observable; they usually function as shorthand for something else. They identify a potential way of behaving based on a long series of observations. The heavier weight of lead cannot be seen, but when it is held it presses more strongly onto a hand than steel, and when heated it transfers this heat less quickly than with copper. Similarly an outgoing person is more likely to engage in conversation and a loner will typically prefer solitary to social activities.

Figure 3.2 My attributes

The presence of these attributes is usually identified by watching how a person responds and behaves over time. Their use relies on a common historical understanding of what the attribute category means and how that person's or thing's behavior conforms.[3] Inferences made from these observations are communicated to others and fed back to the person concerned. They are useful because they help us organize what we look at things and assist us in making predictions about how things may happen in the future. However, in the context of the current discussion, there is a more important aspect to how attributes are identified. The majority of observations from which attributes are drawn are derived from observations of how people and things behave within relationships. They are derived from how people and objects are seen to interconnect, and it is this system of relationships that provides meaning and context for discerning their value and importance.

For example, consider the situation when a day-care staff member refers to a child as "aggressive." Her judgment is based on a series of observations of how that child interacts with other children. Her conclusion is not derived from observations of the child alone; her judgment is based on how she sees the child interacting and responding to situations and other children. Interestingly, her use of the term *aggressive* is highly salient because it will have significant consequences regarding how that child's interactions would be viewed by others and how others will respond in the future.

> ### Jacinta/Wendy: Who Are You?
>
> Jacinta is thinking back to when, shortly after the collapse of her marriage, she took off by herself on her first trip overseas. She recalls how early in the trip she landed in the Burmese (Myanmar) capital Rangoon and was surprised by the unfamiliarity of local ways of living and relating. As she sat looking at a grand pagoda, she wondered how she might relate to the people around her. She began talking to an old Burmese man who had learnt English during British rule. At one point he says, "I know little about your country and I'd really like to know who you are." This seemed a straightforward question, but when she tried to answer it, she had to think hard.
>
> "People say I'm sociable, curious, and caring," she responded, but it seemed clear that despite his genuine interest he was not making much sense of this. She said, "No, that's no good." She thought for a moment and said, "I have two aging parents."
>
> "How many brothers and sisters have you?"
>
> "One sister, and she has two small children."
>
> "That's important, children. They are our future. I have fourteen grandchildren."
>
> "Wow," she was thinking hard of other things they may have in common. "I work in a bank, counting money."
>
> "Money, that's important, particularly when like me a person has very little."
>
> As they continued, she found that she could relax and that there was plenty to talk about when she talked of herself in terms of her connections.

The way we construct the nature of our personal identities is primarily constructed not from descriptions of attributes and properties but from observations of the way we connect and relate to each other. We derive our understanding of attributes from what we observe in the relationships. By way of illustration, imagine you have been catapulted onto an alien planet where everything is unfamiliar and you know no one. On this planet are aliens who can communicate through a language converter, and both you and they are keen to understand each other. How would you begin to explain your identity to these alien beings? It would be difficult to talk only in terms of yourself as a particle or a solo entity, because most of the references to properties and attributes rely on a common history. What is more likely to be the case is that you would end up speaking about the things and people that you connect with. It is easier with strangers to talk about connections than properties: "I am a father" becomes "I have an enduring connection to my children"; "I'm an architect—I have a long-term connection to helping people design buildings"; "I'm asthmatic—I have an enduring relationship to breathing difficulties"; and so forth (see above inset box). In this situation it is easier to talk in terms of relationships than in terms of qualities or attributes because the attributes are derivative constructions, short-hand references to a series of observations of how people and things behave within relationships.

Processes of Connecting

As outlined above, the main alternative way of understanding personal identity involves seeing the self through its range of social connections to the world. In the simple connection depicted in Figure 3.3, "me" is connected to a "job," and the relationship between me and my job involves some form of meaningful bond and emotional investment. The person "me" invests time and energy into work and through this activity a sense of being linked emerges. Over time this sense of linkage strengthens and consolidates, and the person becomes confi-dently aware of the connection and incorporates it into what is understood as "me," that is, my identity. In looking more closely at how social connections operate, four important features are apparent:

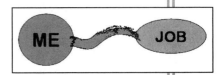

Figure 3.3 Simple connection

1. Varying forms: A person can be connected to a wide variety of different objects. The most familiar form of connection involves relationships with people: "I am married to Geoff," "I am the son of Jane," "I am employed by Kate." Connections can also be made with things: "I built this house," "I holiday in this yacht," "I love this diamond ring." In addi-tion, connections can take many other forms than simple relations with people or things. A person can be solidly connected to a wide range of other objects such as connected to activities (work, hobbies, interests), connected to aspects of the body (important body parts, outward appearances, health issues), connected to animals (pets, horses, farm animals), connected to places (homes, cities, the land), and connected to wealth (earnings, savings, investments). A person can also be effectively and often strongly connected to more abstract and esoteric objects such as being connected to ideals (socialism, post-structuralism, moral virtue), connected to collective identities (nationhood, ethnicity, Catholicism), connected to the past (ancestors, deceased friends, child-hood memories), connected to the future (retirement, future achieve-ments, an idealized future spouse), and connected to spiritual entities (God, a guiding presence, an inner power). Connections to the future are an interesting example of how abstract connections can operate in that the object of the connection need not exist yet and may remain for long periods in the imagination of the connecting person. One of the strongest connections for students is connection to the professionals that they will become. Law students, for example, are constantly relating to and building their lives around the future prospect of themselves liv-ing and working as lawyers.

2. Varying intensities: While connections can be "on" or "off", major shifts in how people connect tend to occur slowly, the strength of each connection varying along a continuum between points of strength and points of weakness. In other words, changes in connec-tivity tend to behave less like a light switch (on or off) and more like a volume control, varying slowly along a continuum from quiet to loud. This slow undulating pattern to social connectivity is important. It means that even when circumstances suddenly change to the object of a connection, the connection itself is likely to remain active for

Connections vary in form and intensity, and transfer positive and negative meanings in both directions

some time and only gradually reduce its intensity. For example, when Bert retires, while this will entail him immediately to stop going to his workplace, he may still find himself waking at the same time, preparing the same breakfast, and vaguely thinking as if he should be setting out for work. It may take him some time before his daily routine adapts to the new reality.

3. Bidirectional transfer: The majority of social relationships operate as two-way interactional connections. Not only is there investment of time, energy, and emotion, but also, in return, people derive a sense of who and what they are. For example, Joan works as a teacher at the local school. She devotes the majority of her waking hours during the week to her teaching. This sizable time input pays off in that her students and her school benefit from her efforts, but she, too, derives a considerable amount of satisfaction from her achievements, a sense of belonging to a collective of similar professionals and a meaningful involvement with her pupils. All these feelings add to her ongoing sense of identity as a teacher. It is this and other active and bidirectional involvements with such connections as work, home, friends, and family that make it possible to construct a personal identity.

4. Negative and positive transfer: The flow of value between a person and other objects in a social system can be both positive and negative, and both add to the meaningfulness of the connection. For example, at work Danny finds that during most weeks he feels either that the job is going well or that it is reasonably tolerable, which means on the whole he feels comfortable in his role. But there are some weeks that are not so easy. At these times the work might appear boring and repetitive and work relationships might fray. Both the positive and negative aspects of Danny's connection to his job give this connection its value, and the flow of negative and positive experiences help generate the substance and meaning of the relationship. To look at another example, the flow of communication in most marriages is both positive and negative. There are times when the relationship is going well and communication is easy, but there are also inevitably periods of miscommunication and tension. Both the good times and bad times in a marriage—while it survives—are accepted as part of what it means to be married. Both add to the sense and the value of being connected.

Bidirectional involvements contribute to a person's sense of identity

A System of Normal Connecting

Each of us lives in an environment of multiple and multilevel connections. Over the course of a lifetime we build up complex networks of connections that provide the substantial base for our social identity. In a social world, connections can even be seen as providing the raw material for personal identity.[4] Figure 3.4 provides an example of some of the main connections a person is likely to experience as important in his or her life. The connections selected are connections at a high level and under each one lays a network of other levels of smaller connections. For example, the connection to family brings with it connections to the various friends of family members, connections to shared interests and activities and connections to common venues such as holiday locations and meeting places. Furthermore, this set of high-level connections is undergoing constant fluctuation and change. The combination varies from person to person and across the course of a life. For example, linkages to the past tend to be more important at an older age than during adolescence, and

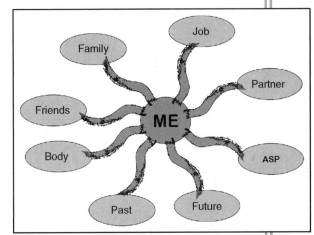

Figure 3.4 Normal system of connecting

correspondingly the younger person may have a stronger affiliation to the future than the older person. Similarly, for those people who avoid connections to people, their connections might be more oriented to animals, the natural environment, or activities such as reading or browsing the Internet.

The other key feature in Figure 3.4 concerns how the person, "me," is part of a system of linkages. Being part of a system carries a number of consequences. First, it means that wherever an object is connected, it is linked, whether directly or indirectly, with everything else within that system. Second, as a consequence of this interconnectedness, any changes to connections in one part of the system will have consequences for another part. For example, in Figure 3.4 separation from a partner will change how family members interact both with the person and the estranged partner. Third, when changes occur within a system, a ripple of relationship adjustments occurs to accommodate that change in a way that enables the system to continue to function. In other words, systems are adaptive; they adjust to change by reconfiguring relationships. Finally, the interconnected adaptations of systems provide a base for personal strength and resilience. This capacity of system is central to health and well-being and will be explored in more detail later in Chapters 8 and 9.

Initiating Connections with Addictive Potential

Also represented in Figure 3.4 is a connecting point labeled "ASP", and which stands for *addictive substance/process*. The term has been chosen to represent connecting objects that have the potential to form addictive relationships.

‖
*Drugs are part
of the world of
everyday
connections*
‖

Common objects with addictive potential include alcohol, tobacco, prescribed minor tranquilizers (benzodiazepines), and arguably food. It is also possible to engage addictively with objects other than substances, and certain activities or processes are gaining greater recognition for their addictive potential. These particularly include activities such as gambling, sex, and work.[5]

For a large proportion of people in modern societies, relationships with substances and processes with addictive potential are a normal part of everyday life. They are accepted either because they are necessary to life (such as sex and work) or because on balance societies, or subsocieties, have deemed them acceptable for their ability to facilitate pleasure (such as alcohol and cannabis). Indeed, for most people these connections function much like any other connection. They are one of an array of linkages in which a person might invest time and energy and from which is derived meaning and identity. For example, a regular drinker of beer enjoys spending many hours drinking with his friends and he knows that his choice of beer brand conveys something about him as a person and the types of people with whom he wishes to associate. Furthermore, since drinking is so commonplace, even when he decides to abstain, he is still surrounded by many people who continue to drink, and through connection to them he maintains indirect connections to drinking. For example, Joan has for health reasons decided not to drink, but her partner Bert continues to drink regularly. For Joan, Bert's absences when drinking, his increased liveliness when drinking, and his spending of their money on drinking all serve to connect her in various ways to alcohol.

Patterns of Fragmentation

The main threat to the integrity of a system of connections is the process of fragmentation. This process involves the progressive intensification of one relationship, which leads to corresponding reductions in the significance of other relationships. In a social system the intensification of one or a set of relationships at the expense of others has major consequences for other people within that system, and is likely to result in a loss of overall social connectedness and to lead ultimately over time to the prospect of progressive disconnection and fragmentation.

Connection Intensification

A person's system of social connections is constantly changing as connections strengthen and weaken and as needs and contexts vary. Involvements are dynamic and continually responding to changes both inside and outside the system of connectedness. For example, people who intensify their involvement with work by devoting 60 hours rather than 40 hours per week are likely as a consequence to weaken other connections such as spending less time with friends or family. While in normal living connectedness to addictive substances/processes[6] is one among many other varieties of connectedness, these connections have a notable capacity for sustained rapid intensification. For most types, this capacity has both psychological and biological dimensions. The psychological dimensions will be explored in more detail in Part II of this book, but in brief, psychological intensification can be viewed as a consequence of the capacity of addictive relationships to control

> **Cathy/Dion: Keeping Going**
> Cathy is speaking with her friend next door.
> "You know what keeps me going through the day?"
> "Wanting to see you're children happy?"
> "Well, maybe in the long term. No, what matters at each moment is knowing that this evening I can use drugs to escape."
> "Not very noble or ambitious."
> "Who needs noble when all you want is a place to feel good about yourself."

feelings. Over a long period, a person can begin to rely on the capacity of addictive substances/processes to manipulate how they feel. This is particularly important in managing negative emotions. As illustrated in the inset box, below, Cathy finds that by injecting heroin in the evenings she achieves some reprieve from ongoing emotions like sadness, guilt, fear, and resentment. This reprieve does little to address any of the underlying issues driving these feelings, and on waking up each morning they greet her with the same intensity. Nonetheless, during the day, despite being clear-headed, she is reassured by knowing she can still return to that island of numbness that evening. Slowly the contrast between the sober and intoxicated world intensifies her commitment to heroin as a means of controlling her feelings.

As discussed in the introduction, substances with physically addictive potential (such as tobacco, alcohol, and opiates) have a particular capacity to promote intensification because emerging connections are enhanced by biochemical processes. A key ingredient to the intensification of biologically enhanced addictive relationships is the buildup of tolerance. Tolerance involves adaptations of the body's nervous system to the presence of a drug, which over time means increasing amounts of the drug are required to have the same level of effect it had previously. With mood altering drugs the key effect involves the control of emotions: "I drink because it makes me feel relaxed, merry, confident, and sociable." However, as use of and reliance on the drug increases, more and more quantities are required to elicit the same emotions: "I need to drink more than before to feel relaxed or sociable." As increased amounts are required, progressively more time and energy has to be devoted to the obtaining drugs and in using them: "I now need to find $1000 per week for heroin compared with $500 four months ago." It serves little purpose maintaining this type of relationship if it no longer has any effect, and for it to have any value one simply must keep adjusting to the requirements for greater consumption. This increased investment of time and energy comes at the cost of other connections. Out of necessity, the system of social connectedness is progressively pared down to allow the tolerance-affected relationship to persist. This biological process, coupled with the psychological processes, makes these connections particularly prone to rapid intensification.

Addictive relationships can be biologically & culturally enhanced

Cultural Intensification

Perhaps as a corollary to their ability to affect how people feel, addictive substances/processes are deeply culturally embedded with layers of meaning and signification. For example, the historical roots of alcohol use in European cultures, and its modern interaction with manufacturing practices through advertising and other promotion, imbues alcohol with charged symbolic meaning. Alcohol is firmly embedded in major ceremonies (such as weddings, funerals, Christmas and other commemorative banquets),[7] it plays an important role in how people socialize (such as at office parties and gatherings of friends), it is firmly linked to gendered activities (such as football or track betting for men), and it is celebrated in literature, humor, and even in national identity (such Irish Guinness and German lager). Similar cultural meanings are built up around gambling,[8] and, within illicit drug-using subcultures,[9] drugs can take on highly valorized meanings with links to rituals of distribution and consumption and they frequently evolve a hybrid vocabulary of their own. These historical strands of meaning instill extra significance to entering into strong relationships with addictive substances/processes. In certain contexts it becomes normal for a particular group to engage intensely with them. The link with them becomes a source of pride, self-esteem, and even of social status. It is a relationship that signals hospitality, generosity, and sociability. It is a relationship that should be displayed, paraded, and celebrated. All these increase the likelihood of engaging with the addictive substance/process with intensity and meaning.

Drug use is valued by most cultures as a part of how people engage & connect

Responses to Disconnection

Just as intensification can result in deterioration in connections elsewhere, so deterioration in connections can lead to intensification. One type of event that illustrates the process well is abrupt disconnection. When attachments that were strong and vibrant suddenly cease, powerful emotional responses are likely to be experienced.

This is easily observed with small children when they lose something they are strongly attached to, such as their favorite cuddly toy. Something that had always been available when going to sleep is no longer there and its absence prompts prolonged wailing and howling. Similarly, in the adult world the sudden disappearance of objects of strong attachment will prompt complex emotional responses (see inset box). A car is stolen, a limb is lost in an accident, a pet dies, fertility ceases, friends emigrate; these losses create a big hole, an absence that elicits a volatile mix of emotions: sadness, anger, remorse, frustration, anxiety. At least part of the response stems from the confusion associated with being attached to something that is no longer there. Other parts are driven by the need to replace or compensate for its missing value. Since most connections serve a

Connections can deteriorate & separate

variety of functions, their absence triggers a search for replacement. For example, having a car stolen requires its replacement or finding some other means of transportation, and the death of a pet calls for other objects of affection. Staying connected to an absence and expecting one's needs to be met is ultimately unsustainable.

> **Danny/Jack: Julie Leaves**
>
> Danny arrives at his father Jack's house in a disturbed state.
>
> "Dad, I arrived home from work yesterday afternoon sensing something was wrong. All the curtains were drawn and shoes were missing from their usual huddle beside the front door. On walking inside I found all the furniture and appliances—even the pictures on the walls—had been removed."
>
> "This is terrible."
>
> "At first I wondered what sort of monstrous burglar would strip a house so thoroughly, but on the empty kitchen bench I find a letter from Julie stating she had left with the children and gone somewhere unknown to me and don't bother trying to find them."
>
> "Look, you can stay here with me, as long as you like."
>
> "All today I've been looking for her, but without success. My life now was in such turmoil. I feel her and the children leaving is more than just an absence. It is like a present absence. If she had gone and that was it, it would have been far easier. But at every moment, I'm walking around next to this big empty hole."
>
> "It's bad now, but it'll get better, son."
>
> "I used to wake up with her lying next to me, I came home from work with her sitting at the table, I went out for a walk with her beside me and I sat next to her on the couch watching TV. Now her absence is there in the bed, at the table, on the street and on the couch. Her absence is there all the time. It's more than I can bear."

The deterioration in a relationship does not only occur in the form of sudden disappearance. Disconnection also takes the form of slow deterioration in its quality and integrity. For example, a more typical pattern with close friends is a gradual loss of involvement. Often without any major incidents or negative intent, friendships simply fall away because of changes such as shifts in interests or locations, or becoming too busy. With these gradual disconnections feelings may be more subdued, but emotions are still active, sadness and regret may occur from time to time, and the need to find ways of compensating for the deterioration remains an issue.

The Role of Addictive Substances/Processes

As described in an earlier inset box (see above), the sudden loss of a partner is, in the early stages, likely to lead to high levels of emotional distress. This is represented in Figure 3.5 where the disconnection with a partner is seen not to simply disappear but hangs out unattached, or more accurately, attached to a place where there was something but now there is nothing. The lack of connection, or this connecting to an absence,

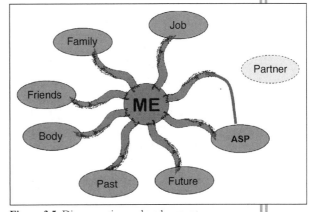

Figure 3.5 Disconnection and replacement

leads to a very troubled psychological state. The person is responding regularly to something that is not there. For example, when Danny's wife and children left him he could choose to compensate for the loss by devoting more time to other connections, such as spending increased hours with family or friends, or working longer hours. He might actively seek to replace the connection as soon as possible with another partner, but this takes time and is fraught with the dangers of transposing the qualities and expectations of the previous relationship. He might also actively maintain his orientation to the absence by pretending or continuing to act as if it still exists. This strategy typically leads to acute distress and he is unlikely to maintain this beyond a few days or a couple of weeks because the tension between what he ideally wants and what is patently the case becomes increasingly unsustainable.

In seeking to compensate for what was provided by the weakened or lost connection, the ideal connecting object is one that is immediately available and works effectively. Alcohol, drugs, and other activities involving mood controlling processes have a range of powerful qualities that make them the ideal replacement for lost or deteriorating connections. As illustrated in the inset box, above, whenever Danny feels down about the loss, he knows from past experience that it will only take two or three cans of beer to be transported emotionally to another place. Alcohol has the capacity to numb painful feelings, it helps in forgetting distressing memories, it fills in time, it can fit conveniently in with most busy or chaotic lifestyles, and above all it works fast and reliably. Other replacement alternatives are more cumbersome. The sympathetic ear of close friends can provide some relief, but they are frequently unavailable at critical times, particularly those hard hours in the middle of the night. Family members can provide support, but their involvement can be complicated by their own agendas and complexities. Spending hours at work or on hobbies helps to distract attention away from the haunting absence, but in a partially depressed and distressed state this requires considerable effort, and can lead to exhaustion and fatigue, which introduces another level of vulnerability.

It is the reliability and convenience of alcohol and other mood-altering substances/processes that forms the basis of their suitability as the other pole in an addictive relationship. This is important not only during episodes of consumption, but also for the times in between. Awareness that the opportunity for involvement is there at hand can make a sizable difference to the sense of strength and confidence with which the remainder of life is

---

Danny/Jack: Reliable Refuge

When arriving home one Friday evening, Jack asks his son, "How are you coping, Dan?"

"I find my week hard going. I'm particularly missing Julie and the kids. My boss expects so much: do this, do that, run here, run there. 'Yes sir, no sir, anything else sir?'"

"Yeah, they never let up."

"I'm also finding it hard living here with you. You're always on my case about getting another job and helping around the farm. You also keep hassling me about my drinking."

"But you're hitting it more than I've ever seen you before."

"I have to. All these hassles. I feel the pressure building up during the week but I stay in charge, 'cause I know on Friday, from 5 o'clock on, I will begin drinking with my mates. It's always there and it always works. After four or five cans I feel calm, around at a friend's house we start raving and having fun. All that other stuff doesn't matter anymore. Tonight and Saturday night I'll be happy and that will be enough to get me to stay in charge through the next week."

taken on. Similar to the way wearing a parachute makes a difference to the attitude and confidence of a test pilot, the knowledge in itself that an alternative place of retreat exists, a refuge from emotional ordeals, increases the sense of self-assurance and resilience in which all aspects of life are encountered. This effect is dependent on the reliability of the mechanism. The same ongoing levels of confidence would not be achieved if the pilot believed the parachute would only open sometimes. The reliability is critical to its becoming the favored relationship within the circle of connections. For example, if taking Valium affected one's mood on only two out of three occasions, then its reliability is questionable and its competitive edge over other relationships is compromised.

Patterns of Deterioration and Intensification

While the initial drivers for forming a strong relationship to an addictive substance/process may vary, once the course is set, the configuration of relationships that emerge follow a similar pattern. Biological, psychological, and cultural intensifiers combine to attract the replacement of deteriorating connections to the addictive relationship. As the connection to the relevant addictive substance/process intensifies, its importance in the system increases and more time and energy are expended in maintaining and protecting that increasingly vital relationship.[10] This of course comes at the expense of other previously important relationships. Just as one section of a garden deteriorates when available time is concentrated on other parts,[11] so intensification of the addictive relationship leads to further deterioration in the quality and integrity of other relationships, which in turn promotes intensification of the *A push-pull* addictive relationship.[12] The process repeats itself in a cycle of deteriorating *process* connections, disconnections, intensifications, and replacements. The push of *propels* deterioration and pull of intensification combine to propel a push–pull proc- *deterioration* ess that is hard to resist. For those affected it often creeps up unexpectedly because they are unaware of the interplay with other areas of their lives. The process is often well advanced before they realize they are locked onto a track they never intended and from which they have no idea how to exit. The central effect is a gradual reconfiguration from a system of diverse connections to a system of connections focused around the intensifying axis of one relationship, the addictive relationship.

Looked at in this way, what is surprising is that, in the formation of most addictive relationships, the process can take such a long time. With alcohol, for example, it may take many years of drinking, even decades, for an addictive social system to fully emerge.[13] Reasons for its typically slow formation lie in the way the rest of the social world responds to signs of reconfiguration. Relationships are two-way processes, and the person or other objects at the other end of a relationship are also plugged into social systems that involve other people. These people have an investment in preserving the integrity of their connecting relationships. They rely on these connections as a source of their own identities. For this reason, people in the world around will often resist and contest a deterioration in connectedness. For example, when faced by the withdrawal of a close friendship, most people are unlikely to passively accept the loss and will seek to restore the friendship through increased contact, offers of help, and emotional appeals, particularly when they see other parts of their friend's life progressively deteriorating.

On top of resistance from other people, while biology, psychology, and culture play a role in intensification, they also play a part in moderating the process. Most cultures emphasize the importance of social engagement, and staying connected is encouraged through regular gatherings, rituals, and social practices. Social disengagement is on the whole not condoned, and efforts will be made to restore deteriorating involvements. Furthermore, people at the center of an addictive system will themselves experience psychological discomfort with major disengagements, particularly in the early stages. In the past they have devoted much of their time and emotions to important connections such as spouses, children, and careers, and it runs contrary to the whole thrust of their lives to allow them to slip away. Added to this, the deterioration of social connections also has implications for physical and mental health and well-being. For example, any loss of engagement with activities involving physical exercise will affect health and fitness, intoxication will increase the probability of motor vehicle accidents, excessive use of drugs will have implications for the health of major organs, and the loss of contact with people will increase a person's vulnerability to anxiety and depression. In time, warning signs of deterioration in a person's physical and mental well-being will signal the need to protect and restore these fraying connections.

Biological and social factors can also help moderate intensification

The Advanced Addictive System

Figure 3.6 depicts the later stages of an addictive system where most of a person's connections have deteriorated as a result of the ongoing intensification of an addictive relationship. Previous relationships have been gradually replaced by strengthened connections to the addictive substance/process. The addictive relationship has now become the central axis within the system. Admittedly, the diagram presents a bleak picture. People's quality of life would be severely compromised were most of their connections to be co-opted into the ever-strengthening relationship to addictive substances/processes. The majority of people in addictive relationships have not, as yet, progressed to this late stage, and most manage to retain a scattering of weakened connections. However, there are usually plenty of signs that their systems are moving in this direction: close friendships are weakening, health is deteriorating, conflict is occurring regularly at home and work, extended family members have dropped contact, and the person tends to think very little about the past or the future. Nonetheless, even for those people who have succumbed to persistent intoxication, they usually retain some ways of connecting meaningfully with the world. For example, the person in Figure 3.6, has retained some connection with family, even if it is a volatile and mostly negative relationship to one parent.

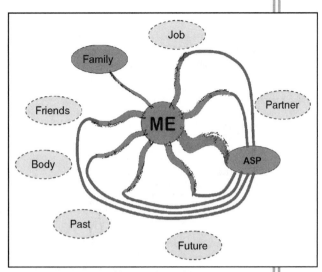

Figure 3.6 Late-stage addictive relationship

As a consequence of the increasing and dominant strength of the relationship between the person and the addictive substance/process, it begins functioning more and more as a central axis around which other relationships operate. Notice how in Figure 3.6 the relationship between "me" and drugs ("ASP") has intensified in two ways. First, as a consequence of disconnection elsewhere, the direct relationship has consolidated (represented by a thicker line). Second, what were previous connections to other objects have now been transferred to connections with drugs (represented by diverted connections). This second way of reconnecting has some interesting facets. Some of the replacement connections (to drugs) may still carry some of the outward features of their previous connections, when in reality their primary function is to support the drug connection. For example, a man in the development of an addictive relationship to alcohol can appear to be connecting strongly with a group of friends. He meets and drinks with them regularly and clearly enjoys their company. But the appearance of friendship and intimacy is deceiving. His previous long-term friends, those who genuinely cared about him, have gradually dropped away in favor of an assortment of casual acquaintances who are heavy drinkers, booze mates, people with whom he can drink heavily without feeling abnormal. These connections have a residual or secondary function and lack meaning because they occur mostly when intoxicated, and whenever trouble occurs members in the group are the first to back away from each other. A similar process of mimicking normal connectedness can be observed with spouses and other close family members, and the use of them to camouflage an addictive relationship will be explored in greater detail in Chapters 5 and 6.

If the social system has been reconfigured around one critical relationship, it starts to operate more as a primary axis about which other less salient relationships hang. This complicates issues of personal identity. The person and his or her addictive world have become intertwined to such an extent that it is difficult to consider personal identity without strong reference to addictive matters. The person, "me," and the addictive substance/process (ASP) now share the center of the system with an almost equal level of importance, and what applies to the person applies in many ways in a similar way to his or her connection to the addictive substance/process. As argued in Chapter 2, if a person's identity is derived substantially from social connections, then his or her identity in this system is derived from the addictive relationship. The identity of "me" must by necessity be tangled up within the relationship between "me" and ASP. For example, for an intravenous heroin user the activities associated with both acquiring and using drugs can become so dominant in that person's life that the prospect of not using is difficult to imagine. Using has been such an integral part of daily activity that it is frightening to consider a nonusing lifestyle[14]: "I am a drug user; this is what I know and my whole life revolves around using." "I cannot begin to imagine myself as a nine-to-five, dinner-on-the-table, home-loving straight person." In this way the interaction between the social world and personal identity work together as further impediments to change.

The initial push–pull pressures that lead into what later becomes an addictive relationship can be various. It might relate to experiences of trauma such as war or sexual abuse.[15] It might be driven by physical dependency or social processes such as peer pressure or group conformity rituals. It could be a response to bereavement, social isolation, parental conflict, or cultural oppression.[16] Alternatively, a person may have simply slipped into the relationship without any major pressure; perhaps it was more a matter of a pattern of behavior that over time took on a life of its own. Whatever the initial reasons, from a social perspective, once intensification of the addictive relationship is underway, the interplay between the strengthening addictive relationship and deteriorating connections feeds itself, and the initial reasons for the relationship are absorbed by the strength of this circular and self-perpetuating process. Based on this social understanding of addictions, the next chapter explores what it might mean to undertake reversing this process.

Cathy/Dion: Octopuses

Occasionally in winter Dion makes a point of visiting the ocean shoreline. He is particularly fond of walking around the rocks at the end of a beach where he can stare down into the turbulent waters buffeting the rocks below. Looking down into the depths he sometimes imagines octopuses moving around in the seaweed, spreading their tentacles and picking up bits to eat.

He thinks to himself, "Really, I know little about their habits, but I wonder what it must be like for them during a major storm. Waves would crash onto the shoreline, picking up any unattached objects and crushing them mercilessly."

He pauses to consider this a bit more and thinks, "To avoid getting hurt, an octopus would need something to cling to as much as possible to avoid being dashed against the rocks. Each tentacle would need to wrap around something stable and hold firm. This contrasts with calm times, when it is possible to move around without much need for attachments."

Walking on further he thinks about how this in some ways resembles how he normally handles stress. "When things are going fine I move about with little regard for all the connecting points that surround me. When things get rough—when I'm down, feeling rejected, suffering a major disappointment—I suddenly find myself valuing my connections to family, friends, and work. I call on them in a variety of ways to help me through the hard times. Each connecting person can provide me in different ways with the strength to endure."

Dion then starts to think about his mother Cathy. "I wonder what it would be like if my only connecting point had been one rock. What would happen if that one rock became detached? Wouldn't I be terrified that without that one big attachment I would end up crushed?" With an overwhelming sense of sadness he faces the question, "How could Mom possibly change?"

Chapter 4

Responding to Addiction

Lying awake on a bench in the town belt,
Alone, eighteen, more or less alive,
Lying awake to the sound of clocks,
The railway station clock, the Town Hall clock,
And the Varsity clock, genteel, exact
As a Presbyterian conscience,
I heard the hedgehogs chugging round my bench,
Colder than an ice-axe, colder than a bone,
Sweating the booze out, a spiritual Houdini
Inside the padlocked box of winter, time and craving.

(James K. Baxter, "The Cold Hub")

James K. Baxter struggled throughout his life with his addictive relationship to alcohol. His concept of a "cold hub" or inner nothingness captures something of the social emptiness that lies at the core of addictive systems. The previous chapter outlined how within a social system the rising dominance of an addictive relationship feeds off deteriorations in relationships elsewhere. This leads to experiences of fragmentation for other people in the system. This chapter explores the prospect of change. It outlines change as a slow and difficult journey involving periods of crisis, moving forward and reverting back and rethinking before the pathway for reintegration is established.

The Prospect of Change

The normal multiconnected social system described in the previous chapter is by necessity constantly interacting with connections to other systems. The dynamic waxing and waning in the strength of these connections enables the system to maintain its flexibility and to adapt to changing circumstances. By contrast, the addictive system is less responsive to its surroundings. Its configuration pivots around one central axis: the relationship to the addictive substance/process. This one connection takes on primary importance that ends up dominating all other points of connection. Its centralized solidity provides the system with strength, but it comes at the cost of a weakened capacity at adaptation. This results in three interlocking characteristics that provide obstacles to change: rigidity, isolation, and self sufficiency.

51

P.J. Adams, *Fragmented Intimacy: Addiction in a Social World*
© Springer 2008

Rigidity is an important characteristic of the addictive social system. A rigid system's strength relies on tight and static bonds within that enable it to withstand stress from outside. So, too, relationships in the addictive world tend to be managed in ways that reduce the likelihood of bending to pressure from outside. This applies particularly to the relationship with the addictive substance/process; if that bond was to weaken, the system as a whole would be put at risk and consequently the relationship must be protected at all costs. This demand for protection leads to an all-or-nothing, you're-either-for-us-or-against-us response to the outside world. Changes introduced from outside are viewed more as threats than opportunities, and the connections within are typically enlisted to shore up and resist any pressure to change. For example, following a person's arrest for driving while intoxicated, his or her family members might be enlisted to support the legal defense by contributing money, character endorsements, and perhaps even lying on the witness stand. The contributions are not voluntary acts given in the spirit of family love and loyalty. Those in the system know that noncompliance will result in punitive consequences such as being chastised, abused, and potentially cast out from the system altogether—banished to join the ranks of "hostile others." Since rigidity contributes significantly to the negative experiences of family members, later chapters explore its effects in more detail.

A direct consequence of a system's rigidity is a tendency toward isolation. Interconnections in the world around continue to change, form, re-form, and vary in intensity, but a rigid system is unresponsive to this fluidity. To hold its strength it needs to protect itself from the vagaries of the outside world, and it does this by preserving the bonds within its grasp and by maintaining the strength of its boundaries. Consequently those connected into the addictive system find themselves increasingly recruited into routines of protection and isolation. For example, children growing up in addictive family systems often avoid speaking to friends about their home life, or exaggerate or lie about the normality of relationships at home, and they are unlikely to invite friends over to visit or play. Similarly for adults (as described in the inset box), Joan has opted to manage her home environment in ways that conceal what is really happening. Such behavior adds to the isolation of the whole system and further strengthens the rigid bonds within the family.

> **Bert/Joan: Maintaining Appearances**
>
> Joan is speaking with her sister Mary about Bert's drunken behavior.
>
> "It would be very embarrassing if others saw how Bert blunders around at home when he's had a few too many."
>
> "I've seen him like that occasionally."
>
> "I work hard to keep the house tidy, inside and out. I warn the children not to talk about our home life with their friends and teachers. I invite people to come to visit only during the day, when he has had less to drink. At night I make sure all the curtains are drawn and I try to keep him in a positive mood so he will not start shouting or throwing things. If he does, I clean the mess up quickly."
>
> "That's good, Joan, but people will eventually find out what's really going on."

Since isolated social systems cannot rely on other systems for assistance, the addictive system is forced to rely primarily on its own resources. As the addictive relationship strengthens, the system of connections grows increasingly self-sufficient and self-perpetuating, and despite the lack of balance and flexibility, the arrangement has its own internal logic. The progression of deteriorating connections conveys to the person in the addictive relationship the impression that the world outside is becoming increasingly hostile and that people are becoming envious and perhaps resentful of the ever-strengthening relationship to the addictive substance/process. The person feels increasingly besieged and disempowered by the social world around. With little else to turn to, this pressure results in an even stronger reliance on the addictive relationship, leading in turn to further deteriorations in other connections and further reliance on the addictive relationship. In this way the addictive social system feeds its own slow pattern of social detachment.

> **Cathy/Dion: Problem or Solution?**
> Cathy is trying to explain to Dion how she views her drug use.
>
> "To me my drug use was never a problem. I saw it more as a solution to a problem than a problem in itself."
>
> "That's not how I see it. When you get into heavy use, you don't look after yourself: you look sickly, you have no money, you hurt yourself, sometimes you're beaten up… there's all sorts of things that go wrong."
>
> "Of course; but the idea of stopping always seemed rather moronic. I did stop once and everyone patted me on the back and congratulated me for being so strong. To them I'd seen the light and everything was going to sort itself out."
>
> "I remember. Things did get better."
>
> "But I found life without drugs anything but a solution. I felt very unhappy. No, I've never had a problem with taking drugs. It was the rest of the world who had the problem."

Why Change?

If an addictive system is so self-sustaining and resistant to change, what could possibly shift it from its fixed position? The system itself has no need for change and it certainly is not open to gentle suggestion or persuasion. As illustrated in the inset box, the problem is often identified with the outside world rather than the addictive substance/process. Despite multiple insults and coordinated attacks from the outside world, the relationship carries on regardless; it seems the harder people try to pull at what binds it, the tighter and tighter the knot becomes. Consequently, most people in addictive relationships sustain them over long periods and many are locked into them until they die.[2] So, given the self-supporting strength of addictive relationships, what could possibly challenge this tight and self-sufficient configuration? What forces might create some movement within this rigidity?

With a rigid structure, the opportunity for change emerges when, despite its strength, small stress fractures begin to appear and spread across its surface. Pressure increases and small cracks become larger cracks. The system itself lacks the flexibility to respond adequately to these emerging gaps, other than to quickly cement over the cracks and try to disguise them. Yet some cracks are too wide to cover over. As feared, these wide persistent cracks challenge the integrity of the structure as a whole and put the entire system into crisis. The following discussion outlines three common varieties of threats that have the capacity to put an addictive system into crisis.

The first variety relates to threats to the dependability of the addictive relationship. As discussed in the previous chapter, the reliability and availability of the addictive substance/process is a critical ingredient of its attractiveness. Other connections are simply less convenient and harder to gain benefits from. But should this reliability fail, given its central role, the entire system is likely to go into crisis. Over time the reliability of the addictive relationship can encounter fundamental challenges. For example, physical tolerance can threaten an addictive relationship to drugs. The person may reach a point where consuming larger and larger amounts no longer has the same emotional effect. This might lead to a point at which the body's capacity to absorb a drug is outstripping what is required psychologically (see inset box). Another example relates to threats in the supply of the addictive substance/process. This can occur when incarcerated, or when an illicit drug supply dries up, or when a person's access to primary resources such as money or mobility is restricted. One further example of a threat to reliability occurs when the level of stress and distress is beyond the capacity of the addictive substance/process to moderate. This might occur during periods of severe bereavement. For instance, the situation in which heavy drinking sessions no longer numb and console; instead they end up as sessions involving intense sadness and deep depression.

A second common variety of threat to the addictive system is a direct conflict of interest between the addictive relationship and another significant relationship within that system. As mentioned earlier, most addictive relationships remain connected to other relationships, particularly family relationships, and it is only after many years that total domination within the system is achieved. In the meantime the addictive relationship can coexist with other strong relationships as long as they refrain from challenging it. For example, a mother in an addictive relationship to cocaine seeks simultaneously to provide the best upbringing for her two children. In her mind she is managing this well and pretends to herself that the time and effort she is putting into acquiring and using cocaine is having minimal impact on the children. This view is not shared by her ex-husband. While visiting he notices her increasingly inappropriate behavior, the children talk of her long absences and their worry about her getting hurt, and they seem increasingly anxious and vigilant. One Sunday he finds the children unattended while she is locked in her room, clearly drug affected and hiding from the world in a disturbed emotional state. He would like her to continue providing the care, but he is too perturbed by the effects of her intoxication to stand by and let it continue. Somewhat reluctantly, he engages a lawyer to sue for custody on

---

Danny/Jack: When It Stops Working

Danny is finally talking to Jack his father about his drinking.

"You know, the worst moment in my life occurred about a year ago, February the fourth to be exact. It happened a few months after Julie left and I was drinking really bad."

"Yeah, I remember you were all over the place."

"As usual I was in a bar, knocking back bottles of beer followed by whiskey chasers. I just kept drinking and drinking, wanting desperately to get to that place of numbed nothingness. I was feeling the effects on my body but my mind wasn't getting to where I wanted to be."

"That must have been scary."

"I kept trying but time was running out. I knew it wouldn't be long before my body would give out and I would collapse, and still my head wasn't getting there. I remember very clearly that feeling of terror spreading through me as I realized I was not going to get there in time."

the basis of her addiction. In her mind, her bond with her children means everything and she cannot imagine life without caring for them, but she realizes that should the case proceed she is unlikely to retain custody. The dilemma she now faces is the choice between either the addictive relationship or her ongoing relationship with her children—a terrible choice, because both directions would lead to unbearable loss and hardship.

Another variety of threat occurs when the social networks immediately surrounding the addictive relationship start asserting their own strength. This is tricky, particularly in a system with rigid internal and fragmented external connections. A person acting on his or her own is unlikely to possess sufficient strength and influence to mount a genuine challenge. However, action by a collective, a coordinated event, could pose more of a contest. Such action could happen in several different ways. For example, an adult daughter may decide she wants to challenge her father's regular drunkenness, but instead of directly challenging him, she opts to work on setting the scene. She begins by talking it over with her other sister. Once she is on board, they both work on their mother. Slowly, after considerable discussion, they develop a common strategy, and vow to back each other up. In another example, a gambling counselor provides the catalyst for coordinated action. The counselor has met on several occasions with family members and has gradually engaged them in a common understanding of the mother's gambling. As a team they plan a coordinated strategy, checking out with one another its effects as they go along and backing one another up as required.

For well-developed addictive social systems, one or two challenging episodes will not in all likelihood be sufficient to unsettle the strength of the addictive relationship. One blow from a sledgehammer is unlikely to crack a large concrete block, but with multiple blows the rigidity of the block betrays its own strength, small hairline fractures form, and with more blows these enlarge into discernible cracks. Many challenges, including the examples above, will be of insufficient strength, but with multiple challenges over time the cracks begin to appear and the incentives and opportunities for change begin to emerge.

A single challenge to an addictive relationship is unlikely to threaten its rigidity

Personal Crisis as Systemic Crisis

It makes little sense to others that the addictive relationship's exaggerated connectedness should continue. It has already clearly compromised many aspects of living—work, health, and home—and without it there would at least be some chance of rectifying the damage. From the outside it is very simple: remove the addictive relationship and the strife would cease. The addictive substance/process is the problem and it simply must be eliminated. From inside it is a different matter. So much of life is now invested and

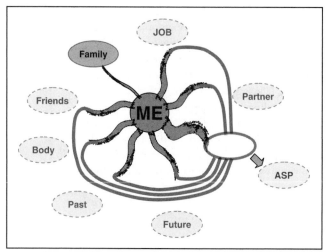

Figure 4.1 Abstaining

entangled with the addictive relationship that elimination is not really that simple anymore; it has major consequences for the system as a whole. As can be seen in Figure 4.1, the orientation of connections has shifted from a spread of separate involvements, to a focus on the one big connection. The prospect of forfeiting this one relationship would understandably threaten the person's identity as a whole. How would it be possible to survive any major difficulties with the one source of strength removed? Furthermore, removal of the addictive substance/process would lead to the simultaneous disconnection of a string of replacement connections. This would leave a number of connecting links dangling without attachments. Considering the distressed experienced with the loss of one major connection, it would pose enormous difficulties for a number of connecting points to be simultaneously cut adrift.

The person at the centre of the addictive system finds him or herself caught in an intensifying dilemma. For example, in the inset box Danny is finding himself under increasing pressure to change. On the one hand, he is hearing from everyone around him the same chorus about the benefits of stopping. On the other hand, inside himself he senses an intensifying reliance on the drug for daily survival. As the pressure mounts it seems like the whole world is conspiring to make the addictive relationship more difficult. But the worse it gets for him outside, the more he relies and values the addictive relationship on the inside. The outside and inside worlds are on a collision course, which will ultimately need to be resolved by a decision in favor of one or the other.

Deep within, perhaps at a pre-awareness level, the person senses the seriousness of attempting to remove the addictive substance/process from the system. He or she senses that it is not a simple matter of surgical removal. Everything would have to change, and the whole network of connections would be disrupted. The person would

---

Danny/Jack: Ganging Up

A few weeks after alcohol began failing him, Danny is talking more to his father about how he is feeling.

"Everyone's on my case. The doctor keeps lecturing me, the boss hassles me, Julie threatens to stop letting me visit the children… even my friends are dropping big hints."

"Yeah, maybe they have a point."

"I know you're on their side too. It's like the whole world is ganging up on me. Things keep going wrong. Dope is more expensive; I keep getting chest infections; I feel drained of energy a lot of the time."

"It's only going to get worse."

"Thanks, Dad. I'm trying to hold things together and you come up with that pessimistic shit."

be driven to embark on a journey into an alien and frightening world, with no guarantees of safety, and totally exposed to the fierceness of everyday life. It therefore makes ultimate sense to resist, avoid, deviate, and oppose any events that might lead to such a disconnection. What from the outside is often identified as *denial*, from the inside is seen as a life-and-death struggle to preserve a structure that is seen as necessary for survival. When pushed many other possibilities will be embraced—attending psychotherapy, taking medication, changing jobs, or moving to a new home—but the central relationship to the addictive substance/process is beyond negotiation. Discussion and problem solving skirt endlessly around the key dilemma, but the decision is too frightening to confront because, from within, it is patently obvious that changing this would entail unstitching the system as a whole.

Setting Out and Setting Back

Setting out to reconstruct multiple connections with the world is much like setting out on a long and challenging journey. It is not just a weekend trip. It resembles more an epic voyage where the route is uncertain and many challenges are faced along the way. It is the voyage of Odysseus in quest of the Golden Fleece, the biblical Exodus in which Moses led the Israelites across the Sinai desert, Captain James Cook's quest for the great southern continent, and Frodo Baggins' long journey to destroy the Ring in *Lord of the Rings*. It is a journey involving slow progress, sometimes moving in circles and sometimes moving backward. It inevitably involves deviations and detours, and at many points it tests the traveler's fortitude and commitment.

Change involves a journey with many deviations & detours

First Attempts at Change

Over time, and perhaps through a series of crises, a person in this situation will be persuaded by the force of circumstances to make some sort of attempt at disconnecting with the addictive substance/process. For example, a woman in a strongly addictive relationship to alcohol might feel cornered enough by the loss of work, risks to health, and threats to her marriage to consider making an attempt at abstinence. She successfully stops her drinking; that was reasonably straightforward. Her health improves, she has fewer arguments with others, and for the first month everything appears to be sorting itself out. However, as soon as she experiences any sort of stress, she finds she has few resources to help moderate its effects. She might enter periods of feeling intensely bored or lonely;

perhaps accumulated relationship tensions are beginning to filter out at home; perhaps she finds normal everyday stresses, without the prospect of reprieve, impossibly difficult to endure. Whatever the trigger—and it does not need to be major—lacking other easily accessible connections, she is likely to experience an almost irresistible pressure to fill in the empty space with drinking again. Where else in her fragmented connections is she going to find strength? The prospect of restoring the familiar system built around drinking hangs enticingly above her, calling her constantly back to a way of life she knows will get her through and keep her operating adequately.

From another angle, it is hard to imagine how a world without the addictive relationship might compete realistically with the emotional potency and convenience of an addictive substance/process. Minor tranquilizers, for example, are ever ready to provide comfort in a world that appears perpetually rough and hostile. Alternative connections would take some time to establish and tend to come with other baggage. For instance, it would take a considerable amount of time and effort to renew friendships sufficiently before they would be able to provide the same level of support and comfort as tranquilizers, and with a poor previous history these friends are likely to be hesitant and reluctant to reenter trusting friendships in which they have been previously hurt. The addictive substance/process responds without reservations. The person knows that after a few pills, after a few drinks, after some time gambling he or she will be transported to a place of peace, where the chaos around seems less important and where the world seems to accept the person as normal and not as evil or weak.

The potency of the addictive relationship competitively blocks forming new relationships

Another possible response to crisis is attempting to change while still retaining significant connections to the addictive substance/process. For example, while still continuing to use or drink heavily, attempts are made to restore relationships with friends and family members. This is a possibility, particularly with strong physically addictive substances such as heroin or minor tranquilizers, but on first attempts at change this course is unlikely to meet with success. The problem is that the task of rebuilding relationships is fraught with its own difficulties and challenges. For example, reconnecting with friends may involve facing past grievances and grappling with personality tensions. When processes like this become difficult, people naturally call on the strength of connections elsewhere in their systems. Since the addictive relationship still remains the strongest connection, people inevitably are drawn into using it as a means of managing the emotional volatility involved in rebuilding. This entails increased consumption of the addictive substance/process, which in turn upsets the rebuilding process because the effect of intoxication is most likely a major cause of the relationship's deteriorating in the first place. Consequently, for genuine first attempts at change, most people require at least a temporary separation from the addictive substance/process in order to avoid undermining any progress they make.[3]

Replacement

In an ideal world, the task of rebuilding would involve stopping the current activities, clearing the site as much as possible, and building the new structure from scratch. But people do not inhabit ideal worlds. Their need for housing continues, their need for a place to connect with others continues, and they may have strong reasons for retaining much of the old structure. This complicates matters and increases the time and effort required for progress. Those involved are caught in a delicate balancing act between keeping things going and trying to introduce changes. Neurath provided a commonly used nautical metaphor for such change.[4] Most of the planks on a wooden ship have rotted and need to be replaced; unfortunately, there is nowhere to come ashore, so they must be repaired while remaining afloat. The task requires the careful removal and replacement of each plank one by one, with additional plugging and bailing to ensure the boat does not sink. It is a complicated procedure, and by the end most of the ship's planks have been replaced.

The person modifying an addictive social system faces a similar task, but an even more complicated challenge because it is not only substance (planks) that requires replacement but also the system's structure. The addictive relationship provides the central spine running through all connections and holding them together. It cannot be reshaped all at once or the integrity of the system as a whole would fall apart. To keep everyday life going, something is required in the interim to hold the structure in place while the connecting planks are reformed.

In recognition that the process of reconnecting will take a long time, probably years, the most practical way to survive the early stages is to replace the absence of the addictive substance/process with something else, ideally something equally potent in terms of managing stressors. The availability of replacement options also matters in terms of attempting change in the first place. For example, in the situation where a man clinging to the side of a cliff is being asked to move, the command for him to let go one hand and shift it further along to another handhold just out of sight would require a high degree of trust. He needs to believe that there is actually another stable object to cling to and that this new position will lead him closer to safety. Similarly, the person shifting away from an addictive relationship requires some reassurance that a replacement is at hand and that it will be reliable and stable enough to support things when reliance on the addictive relationship is loosened.

An obvious danger in replacing the addictive substance/process is that the replacement ends up filling the empty slot on a long-term basis and as a consequence the configuration of connections remains the same. This type of replacement—static substitution—can occur in two major ways: substitution with a similarly addictive object or substitution with an entirely different

The process rebuilding of social connections will take considerable time

---

Danny/Jack: Seesawing

Danny is chatting to Jack as they wash the dishes.

"Dad, I worry about the amount of alcohol I go through."

"Yep, I've been…"

"Okay, okay. But look I've managed to cut down; I'm drinking every second evening and I'm not getting completely wasted."

"That's great, Danny. Well done."

"It is great, I'm feeling better, but now I'm smoking more dope during the day, and it's really expensive."

"Oh. Well, maybe on dope it'll be easier to change altogether."

"I don't think so. If I cut down smoking dope I'd end up back drinking heavily again."

---

object. Replacement with a similarly addictive object is a tempting prospect because chances are it will temporarily reduce hostility from the outside world. In the inset box, Danny's attempt to reduce his drinking results in a greater reliance on his cannabis use, and as a result at least some of the problems associated his drunkenness subside and for a short period his friends and family seem less concerned. Nonetheless, as his emotional reliance is transferred from alcohol to cannabis, and as his level of biological tolerance to cannabis rises, many of the same problems reemerge. Without any changes to his system of connections, the replacement has little value and he has few reasons to justify not returning to the more familiar drug.

Replacement with objects other than addictive relationships can take many forms. The main requirement is that the object be highly meaningful to the person and have immediate potency. Without these qualities, the substitute is unlikely to compete sufficiently with what it replaces. Replacement objects can take the form of people such as the love for a key family member (a spouse, a child), loyalty to a deceased mentor, commitment to a group or a team, a therapeutic engagement, a sense of a guiding spiritual presence and a major activity (such as work hobbies etc). For example as depicted in the inset box below, a person might initially choose to replace the addictive relationship by spending as much time as possible at work. Work then becomes the central source of meaning and identity, and it helps keep the person preoccupied and diverted away from linkages with the addictive substance/process. As with substituting with an addictive substance/process, these replacement objects can perpetuate the configurations within an addictive social system without engineering significant change.[5] Work becomes an obsession, and there is little time or energy for activities outside work. For Jacinta her work and other projects have replaced her gambling, but it is not going anywhere because there is no space for rebuilding other connections. The replacement hangs within the same configuration, waiting with little to prevent the return of the previous addictive relationship. In another example, a person might attempt to short-circuit the slow process of reconnection by jumping into a closely intimate and possible

---

Jacinta/Wendy: Replacing Gambling

Over dinner Jacinta and Wendy are discussing Jacinta's recent attempt to stop gambling.

"Jacinta, don't get me wrong, but since you stopped playing the machines, I really haven't seen much of you."

"That's great encouragement."

"Why do you have to spend so much time working and stuff?"

"It keeps me thinking of other things."

"But you spend every evening working on projects. I don't even know what you're doing. At least when you gambled you had some nights off, and I knew what you were up to. Now I have no idea, and nothing seems to have changed here."

"Look, you wanted me to change, and I have! These projects keep me from thinking about other things."

"Yes, but how long will this go on for? I don't really see anything else changing."

sexual relationship early in the process. This is a dangerous path.[6] The person chosen for intimacy could end up filling the space vacated by the addictive substance/process, and thereby perpetuating the one-axis relationship configuration. Furthermore, in order to fill the space adequately the replacement relationship is likely to require considerable reshaping and managing that may lead to unsustainable idealization or to the other person feeling controlled.

Transitional Replacement

For someone in a well-formed addictive system, the odds are very low of surviving for any length of time with an unattached addictive relationship.[7] Unfortunately, it is an extended length of time that is the main ingredient required for rebuilding alternative connections. For example, reconnecting to family members is likely to involve considerable time and heartache. During that time the pressure to resort to an addictive substance/process will be close to irresistible. The unattached sober world is unfamiliar, scary, and feels very unsteady—not the kind of feelings that encourage confidence in approaching things differently. Some form of transitional replacement is a necessary part of holding things together long enough for the slow process of building opportunities for reconnection to get underway.[8] What distinguishes transitional replacement from static substitution is that its primary purpose is for the reliance to move beyond itself. It is there as a temporary phase, a bridge to a world where it either becomes one among many strong attachments or is discarded as no longer necessary. Most people attempting it will typically find the first two years very difficult.[9] The slow process of rebuilding normal connections, coupled with the overriding temptation to revert back to the previous addictive configuration, opens out as an arduous and at times frightening journey. There is often little room for other things, as the all-consuming task of staying on-track unfolds. The following discussion briefly introduces three examples of transitional replacement, and the process is discussed more fully in Chapter 9.

Transitional replacement provides a bridge to reintegration

One common form of transitional replacement is with a counselor, psychotherapist, or other addiction practitioner. Following the brave decision to embark on a voyage of change, those attempting the change entrust themselves to the therapeutic relationship for guidance and support. Their regular meetings involve story telling, emotional disclosure, checking out of alternative realities, close examination of thinking processes, and careful planning of a course of reconnection. While therapeutic approaches vary widely,[10] at their center is the practitioner–client relationship, and this involvement aims to serve two critical functions. First, it provides a temporary space for the client to experience acceptance, validation, and care.

This serves to replace some of the features provided by the addictive relationship. Second, it enables the therapeutic relationship itself to provide a launching pad for a process of resocialization. The practitioner fosters a safe level of managed intimacy within which the client explores honest, direct communication, and grapples with the issues of moving from controlling people to trusting them. Ideally, in time, this managed intimacy spreads to forming genuinely close relationships within the client's own social networks as the opportunities arise.

Another commonly employed form of transitional replacement is drug substitution for addictive relationships to opioids (heroin, morphine). Instead of obtaining heroin illegally, another longer-acting opioid is provided legitimately, usually through local health services.[11] Ever since the early 1960s, when Dole and Nyswander[12] provided people in addictive relationships to heroin in New York with methadone as an alternative, research has demonstrated repeatedly that health gains could be made by substituting prescribed opioids for illicit opioids. The benefits extend to the person's health (less infection and reduced overdoses), the well-being of communities (improved family and community participation), and society in general (less crime and fewer health costs). A key dimension to the effectiveness of opioid substitution is the way it enables users to begin disentangling their social world from the illicit underworld that supplies the drug.[13] They are no longer tied up in the daily processes of obtaining large amounts of cash, finding suppliers, scoring drugs and then injecting them. Furthermore, the dose they take is regulated and appropriately administered, thereby reducing the chances of overdose, poisoning, and diseases, particularly HIV and hepatitis C. They now have the space—physically, mentally, and emotionally—to gradually build up a normal world of connectedness. This space enables them to take on regular jobs, to put adequate time into the care of their children, to make new friends, and to gradually partake in normal social relations.

Replacement with opiates is complicated by the biologically enhanced nature of the relationship. As with tobacco, overcoming the physical addiction is a challenge in itself. It remains a controversial topic,[14] but for some, the space it provides does enable the building of sufficient connectedness for the relationship to opiates to shift to one among many in a person's system of connectedness.

A third common route is via the fellowship offered by Alcoholics Anonymous (AA) and what it has parented in similar fellowships such as Narcotics Anonymous, AlAnon, and Gamblers Anonymous. Alcoholics Anonymous for many provides a powerful transitional replacement, with AA meetings serving several functions at once. Attendees are encouraged to go to meetings regularly ("ten meetings in ten days"); this fills in time and increases the vigilance required to avoid reverting back to addictive patterns. While some people attending might recoil at the high reliance on attendance (see Danny's response in the inset box), the meetings provide an accessible place to receive messages of acceptance, being cared about and supported,

Transitional replacement provides a launching pad for social reconnection

and where one's troubling emotions are listened to and validated.

The regular availability of meetings is critical because the competitive edge for addictive substances/processes is their availability and reliability. The fellowship provides a ready-made social world that often extends beyond AA meetings. It is not uncommon for AA members to socialize outside meetings, join in common events, and even share accommodation together. Perhaps the most important dimension to the approach is its emphasis on spiritual connectedness. At its core lies a 12-step program that advocates a process of change involving a handing over of oneself to a powerful spiritual force, a "higher power," that not only replaces the connection vacated by alcohol but also provides the platform for launching back into a world of genuine connectedness. The "higher power" could be construed in many forms: a loving God, an important relationship, the natural world, and others. It is believed that without this strong inner connection, it will be extremely difficult for a person in an addictive relationship to relinquish control. This strong inner connectedness can be carried everywhere and used as the base strength for the long task of rebuilding other connections.

> ### Danny/Jack: White Knuckling
>
> Following urging by Jack, Danny had started attending a local Alcoholics Anonymous meeting.
>
> "How're the meetings going, Danny?"
>
> "Oh, I've stopped going. I know, I know, I was getting something out of them. But what I heard was starting to get me down."
>
> "Get you down?"
>
> "Well, I know it's important to keep going. But the same guys there kept on ranting about being sober for twenty years, how they go to meeting four times a week and how AA means everything to them."
>
> "Well, at least they are not drinking!"
>
> "Well, yeah? Hello?" Danny replies with a hint of sarcasm. "And where are their lives? They spend more time at meetings than with their family. As far as I can see they're just as obsessive about AA as they were about drinking. I don't want to be like that."
>
> "No, no, I understand. There are people like that, 'white knucklers,' they call them. People who just stop drinking, who substitute AA for their drinking but don't change anything else."
>
> "Hmm, well, I don't need to be around them while I'm changing."

For each of these three examples, it is still possible for the process of transitional replacement to flounder in static substitution. Considerable effort is required to keep one's life functioning while at the same attempting to restore multiple connections. It may take more than one attempt before the importance of the process of reconnecting is recognized and to realize that replacement is merely a staging post on the path to social reintegration.

Reversion

Reversion[15] occurs when people who had previously set out to reduce the strength of an addictive relationship change their minds and opt to revert back into the addictive social system. Reversions come in many forms. Some involve dramatic collapse with huge loss of face and considerable distress both to the person reverting and to friends and family. Other reversions sneak up stealthily and involve a slow but steady deterioration in commitment to change. Others occur silently and privately—perhaps in the lonely

> **Danny/Jack: Smooth Reversion**
>
> Danny is discussing with Jack his first attempt at change.
>
> "Dad, when I got back to drinking again last month, it didn't happen the way I expected. It wasn't dramatic, not a big deal."
>
> "Yeah, funny that's how my mom described it, too."
>
> "I stopped drinking and smoking dope and everything seemed fine. I wasn't under any sort of pressure; I was talking more with Julie and the kids, work was going well. I really had no excuse, but one day it just happened. I slipped, just a matter of course, as if nothing had happened."
>
> "And you have no clue why?"
>
> "Yeah, and looking back now, I guess I really had no idea what I was getting into. It seems that when I change I need to do a lot more than just stopping my drinking and drug use."

hours of the night—and other people may have little idea of what is happening. It might take family members months and sometimes years before they fully appreciate its extent. Many reversions appear to happen almost as a matter of course, like a homecoming, a natural return, a gentle turning back to a system of connections that are normal, familiar, and even comforting (see inset box). What also surprises people during a reversion is how despite their prior efforts they revert quickly to a similar intensity of connection to the addictive substance/process as they had before they attempted to change. The previous patterns of behavior reestablish themselves swiftly as if nothing had happened in between.

This is not so surprising from a social perspective. As discussed earlier, change requires the slow rebuilding of a normal system of connectedness during which the imprint or template for the addictive social system remains in place. As soon people renew their commitment to the addictive substance/process, this background framework reasserts its presence, for there is usually little in the way of strong alternative connections to prevent its return.

Reversions are highly probable events, particularly during the first attempts at change. Research into interventions for addictions indicates that the majority of those who complete programs are likely to revert to their addictive social systems within a year after discharge. In the largest study of interventions for addictive relationships to alcohol—Project Match[16]—952 outpatients and 744 residential program aftercare patients were randomly assigned to one of three of the leading forms of intervention for addiction.[17] When the project interviewed participants 1 year later, it found that despite their exposure to treatment, for all three types of program approximately 70 percent of participants had reverted in varying degrees to their addictive social systems. Other well-conducted studies come up with similar findings.[18] Despite the enormous strides people make during intervention programs, once they are left alone to continue their own lives, most struggle to make the change stick, and many will revert to the addictive system fairly quickly.

A constructive way to view reversion is to think of it less as a failure and more as a part of the process of preparing for change.[19] The first major attempts at change take people on a voyage into new and unfamiliar territory. As explorers venturing into a new land, the likely obstacles and pitfalls are unknown and the explorers may find themselves lulled into a false sense of security. They may not yet appreciate the ruggedness of the mountain range they have to climb, or how many provisions they should take, or how physically fit they would need to be, or what noxious insects and plants are waiting to infect them. The scope of the undertaking and the dangers involved have yet to be encountered. Furthermore, since most addictive social systems take considerable time to form because of the long passage of time, a person entrenched within such a system may have difficulty recalling the nature of a world of normal multiple connectedness. Since it is only partially remembered it may take some initially unsuccessful attempts for the person to gain a full appreciation of the nature of the task and what it is going to take to rebuild a normal system. In this way a reversion can be seen as a necessary phase in orienting the person to the time, energy, and commitment that will be required for changes to persist.

Making It Stick

Reintegration

Reintegration[20] is the journey of progressive reconnection that moves the person in the addictive configuration back to the normal world of multiple connections. By its very nature reintegration takes a long time. It is composed of a series of small steps of accumulating connectedness to the world around. Figure 4.2 puts this into perspective by summarizing the sequence of events described so far. The addictive relationship is initiated through a combination of enhancers associated both with the target substance/process (such as physical tolerance) along with psychological and cultural enhancers (such as the high value of drugs in youth culture). Intensification of this connection grows interactively with increasing deterioration in other connections. This leads to a gradual fragmentation and loss of quality and integrity in relationships with people around. These people begin to resist and challenge progressive fragmentation, which in turn leads to some form of crisis. This crisis or a series of crises prompt an attempt at change. However, the change process is more difficult than expected because

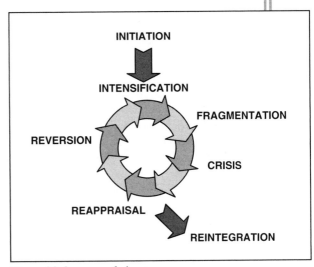

Figure 4.2 Summary of phases

the demands for rebuilding relationships were not fully appreciated and such rebuilding will typically take a long time. Attempts at replacement without reintegration lead to preservation of the addictive configuration that in time facilitates a full reversion to the addictive system. The sequence is repeated with further intensification, fragmentation, crisis, and reappraisal. Following another reversion the cycle may repeat itself a few further times before the person finds an adequate transitional replacement that enables enough time to begin the long process of progressive reconnection or reintegration.

The concept of reintegration describes the restoration process. In contrast to terms such as *recovery* and *rehabilitation, reintegration* is not derived from particle paradigm or medical conceptions of the person as an isolated individual. Reintegration emphasizes structural linkages and thereby better depicts the importance of relationships and the social nature of the process. Unlike recovery, reintegration also implies obligation both of the person in the addictive relationship and those within the social network to participate in the change

Recovery belongs to individuals, reintegration belongs to a social world

process. If the world outside refuses to provide opportunities for connection, the process of change would be unlikely to occur. For example, when a man in an addictive relationship to gambling decides to stop gambling, he is responsible for making that decision and in initiating the change, but he is unlikely to progress far if the world around him refuses to engage in reconnections. Others will naturally be cautious because of past disappointments and deceptions, but if he remains totally shunned and treated as a pariah, he will have nothing to rebuild his world with. Hence, during reintegration the onus is not only on the person in the addictive relationship to initiate and pursue change, but is also on others to enable and participate in this reconnection process. The nature and issues associated for both parties with this process of reconnecting is explored in considerable detail in Chapter 10.

Cascading Reconnections

As eluded to earlier, in the fragmented world that surrounds the person in an advanced addictive social system, the journey into a socially connected world is a slow journey and typically one involving multiple ordeals and challenges. Consider, for example, the length of time it might take recent immigrants to build a circle of trusted friends, particularly when they know no one in their new land. Such immigrants would arrive knowing that it would be a matter of years before their social connections would mature into close and trusting relationships. With little else to go on, they would begin their reintegration by mixing with people through work and common interests. Conversations at coffee breaks turn into sharing outside interests, which in turn leads to meeting up after work, leading to meeting with other friends, then to forming social groupings, then to active friendships, leading eventually to the prospect of forming enduring and intimate friendships.

This slow but cascading pattern of forming connections—often plagued by doubts and loneliness and riddled with disappointments—is a well-trodden path and one that most immigrants accept as a consequence of leaving their previous social networks.

For people seeking to leave or emigrate from addictive social systems, the nature of this process is obscured by the impression that strong connections with the world still exist. In time it becomes apparent that the quality of these connections is weak—all except for the addictive relationship from which they are attempting to escape. It may take several attempts before they begin to recognize that as with immigrants they face a lengthy process of creating social opportunities before quality relationships can emerge.

Reintegration creates a pathway to intimacy

The path to restoring intimacy can be pursued in two directions: restoring previous connections and creating new ones. The majority of addictive relationships have not reached the stage where all relationships have lost their integrity. Even in advanced addictive configurations (as illustrated in the previous chapter) close family members are still likely to be maintaining some level of communication.[21] Nonetheless, while it makes sense to begin the reconnecting process with these relationships, progress with them can be very slow. Immediate family members who witnessed previous false starts and broken promises, and felt deceived and hurt, will be understandably reluctant to reciprocate signals of affection. For example, a son who had as a child been on the receiving end of the parent's drunken verbal abuse may take a long time before he is willing again to open up in a trusting fashion to the parent. Furthermore, relationships outside the immediate family may not be worth pursuing. For example a drinker may have progressively replaced important friendships with a circle of less significant drinking companions. Besides their ongoing commitment to drinking, these relationships may lack the potential for a genuine commitment to intimacy. Older friends may have drifted away; they have new circles of friends and new interests and may lack interest in reconnecting. Accordingly, for many of those in addictive systems, reintegration on the basis of previous connections may be too complex and slow, and the process will require a parallel strategy that will deliver connectedness more quickly.

A second direction for restoring connections resembles more the path pursued by immigrants and involves building connections from the ground up. Here the logical place to start is by engaging in new activities, hobbies, or interests that enable increased social involvement. These activities may lead in time to strengthening social connections that stretch out beyond the activities themselves. As the circle of multiple connections evolves, some points of connection mature and attain higher levels of intensity and meaningfulness. This is likely to be new territory—or long forgotten territory—for those leaving an addictive system. Emotionally they may experience some reluctance, some trepidation about the looming closeness, particularly as it is unshielded by the opportunity to retreat to the addictive relationship. For this reason, care is required to avoid any crisis of confidence that might lead to reversion. It is important to tread carefully, one step at a time, and take on only as much as seems manageable. Bit by bit the emergence of more intense and meaningful social connections sets up the opportunity for higher quality close relationships. These new connections open up the prospect of intimacy, and it is the nature of intimacy and addictive relationships that will be the focus of Part II.

Part II
Processes

Chapter 5

Becoming Intimate

Again she struggled with it, fighting him with her small, fine eyes, with the plush arrogance of a top dog, with her nascent transference to another man, with the accumulated resentment of years; she fought him with her money and her faith that her sister disliked him and was behind her now; with the thought of the new enemies he was making with his bitterness, with her quick guile against his wine-ing and dine-ing slowness, her health and beauty against his physical deterioration, her unscrupulousness against his moralities—for this inner battle she used even her weaknesses—fighting bravely and courageously with the old cans and crockery and bottles, empty receptacles of her expiated sins, outrages, mistakes.

(F. Scott Fitzgerald, "Tender Is the Night")[1]

In the above extract F. Scott Fitzgerald illustrates the subtle interpersonal dynamics that are often intertwined in lifestyles associated with addictive processes. Part I of this book introduced the switch from viewing addiction in terms of human particles to viewing addiction as a social event. Part II moves in closer to the core of addictive relationships and examines the processes associated with forming, maintaining, and ending social connections in addictive systems. In particular, Part II explores the nature of intimacy as a special form of social connectedness. Addictions understood within a social world operate most strongly in the zone of intense sociality, namely at those points of contact between people where they experience their strongest and most intimate involvements. In doing so it identifies intimacy as the primary site for addictive processes, the site at which the destructiveness of addictive relationships is most active[2]: the place where the action happens. However, before proceeding into this zone, a conceptual framework is required in order to talk sensibly about the relationship between addiction and intimacy. This chapter establishes a simple set of concepts that can be used to understand how addictive relationships and intimacies interact.

Living in Relationships

Part I concentrated on relationships from an outside vantage point. From above, the individual is seen as a central connecting point with a series of lines radiating out to other people and other objects. This

P.J. Adams, Fragmented Intimacy: Addiction in a Social World
© Springer 2008

representation has helped conceptualize overall patterns and the ways in which different objects connect together, but the view from above provides only part of the picture. Similar to the way flying in a plane over a city enables the observer to discern the overall shape and layout below, so looking at relationships from above gives a sense of the overall patterns of interconnection. However, observing from this outside position risks missing out on much of the detail of what is really going on down below. The bird's-eye view misses out on the rhythm of people's daily routines, on the nuances in conversations, on the pace and pressure of involvements, on the noise and silences in between, and most of all it misses out what it really feels like to participate in that network of relationships. To appreciate these complexities observers would need to swoop down closer and closer until they become part of the dynamic interchange. Once on the ground observers can then attempt to approach even closer by trying to crawl inside what it means to live within this set of relationships.[3] Accordingly, Part II develops a closer and finer-grained understanding of the processes associated with addictive relationships and demonstrates why looking at the social dimensions of intimacy opens up new opportunities.

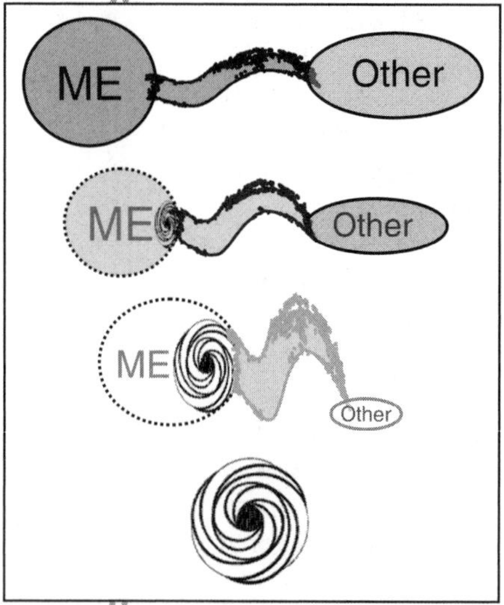

Figure 5.1 Turning inside

Intimacy is a special form of social relationship that can only fully be appreciated by moving from the world outside looking down to the world inside looking through. This critical shift in orientation is depicted in the figure in the inset box. It starts with the focus from Chapter 3 where a person, "me," is connected to an object (a person or thing, "other"). This is then turned progressively until the observer becomes the "me" who is looking in through the relationship itself. As the gaze changes, the self as an object gradually fades simultaneously with its connections, growing fainter until it reaches a point at which the gaze is totally focused on the internal detail of the relationship. The observer is now positioned internally looking as if through a pipe into the fabric of the relationship. The new orientation does not make the previous position any less meaningful, rather it provides an alternative vantage point from which to concentrate on the inner features of these social connections. It is a necessary move that enables the following discussion to explore some of the detail of what it means to live within intimate relationships.

Intimacy and the Four C's

What distinguishes intimacy from other types of relationships? How would one recognize when one is in an intimate relationship? What qualities could be used to define intimacy? These are tricky questions, and ones that previous writers on intimacy have typically tried to avoid.[4] The problem is that the closer the observer moves to the inner workings of experience, the more the subject matter becomes dynamic, diffuse, and ephemeral. The task is something akin to chasing shadows or pursuing the ends of rainbows; the more specific the language, the more exceptions get in the way, and the more general the language, the less it seems relevant. The later writings of Ludwig Wittgenstein[5] provide some guidance on how to approach such material. He argued that the way we use language is not built up out of discrete and definable categories; rather we build up meanings and concepts from recognition of sets of what he referred to as "family resemblances."

Many of the objects that we might refer to using the same words appear to share specific sets of resemblances or characteristics. For example, the category "table" can be seen to have characteristics such as "four legs," "a flat area to put things on," and "made of solid materials." Most tables have most of these resemblances; however, not all tables share all these characteristics. For instance a surgical table might have no legs and drawing tables might be sloped. In common use, it may be difficult to find tables that share all the main sets of characteristics because we tend to use categories in a flexible and fuzzy fashion.[6] Wittgenstein likened this loose-knitted way in which we use resemblances between objects to the strands that comprise a woolen thread or the strands in a bird's nest,[7] where the strength of the whole object is built up by each strand connecting with other strands. No one strand connects through the whole object, and some strands can be shorter than others, but together the combined strength of all their connections works together in providing sufficient integrity for the object to hang together as a whole.

This section unravels the four strands that run fibrously through the social connections that we tend to identify as intimacy, namely closeness, compassion, commitment, and accord (the four C's, see figure in the inset box). This set of strands has been identified specifically for the current discussion; it is not intended as an exhaustive description. Other arrangements and other sets of strands could be identified for other purposes. Nonetheless, these strands have been chosen because they provide a departure point for beginning a discussion on the complexities

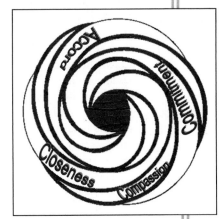

Figure 5.2 Strands of intimacy

associated with connecting to and disconnecting from intimate relationships, particularly as they apply to addictive relationships.

Closeness

Physical proximity plays a critical role in how we understand the nature of intimacy. Intimacy tends to emerge out of situations in which a person shares time and space with other persons or things. The space occupied together might take the form of sharing houses, sharing rooms, sharing offices, or sharing furniture. The time shared may vary from brief times together (sharing meals, entertainment, crises, and adventures) strung out over long periods, or, at another extreme, living almost continuously together over a lifetime.

Closeness in terms of time and space creates a sense of being close enough to touch or feel another's presence in a way that makes it more than just a presence; the closeness associated with intimacy involves a meaningful presence. The object of intimacy feels close in a way that typically incorporates layers of meaning and significance.

Another common meaning of "intimacy" involves being close in terms of connecting sexually. Sexual intimacy is a form of closeness that carries the sense of being in close proximity but adds the dimension of sexual arousal that typically includes physical attraction, physical caressing, genital contact, and orgasm. Perhaps because sexual intimacy involves very close forms of physical contact, it has in many circumstances come to be understood as what is meant by "being intimate." For example, in a court hearing, the question, "Have you been intimate with this woman?" refers clearly to whether or not the defendant has had sexual intercourse. This narrower understanding of the term excludes intimacy from many of the other forms of closeness such as that between siblings, between friends, and between parents and their children. For the purposes of this book, while accepting sexual intimacy as one of the forms of possible intimacy, the term *intimacy* is used in the wider sense of intimacy across a wide range of different ways of being close.

Intimacy is understood in the wider sense of relationships with caring others

The notion of intimacy as physical closeness is also commonly used in a more metaphorical sense of feeling in close psychological proximity to one another. This enables a sense of closeness to occur even though for most of the day the person is physically apart. For example, a woman might maintain her sense of psychological closeness to her lover by ensuring she thinks about him or her as often as possible. She might also carry objects with her such as jewelry, items of clothing, or photos that serve to remind her of this closeness. The use of such cues and reminders to help maintain a sense of psychological closeness can also function as indicators regarding whether a sense of intimacy is being reciprocated. Consistent indications that a partner is not thinking about or considering the other partner's feelings or needs casts doubt on whether the intimacy is truly reciprocal (see inset box). This expectation of mutuality comprises a key focus in later chapters.

Compassion

Another important dimension of closeness relates to the sharing of what is happening emotionally between intimates. To be intimate means to be able to project and interpret the emotional life of the person with whom one has chosen to become intimate. This capacity to reflect and respond to the emotional world of other people enables a sense of emotional connectedness that often provides the substance of what it means to be close. Admittedly a person cannot actually enter the experience of another person; we always remain separate. But from a base within one's own experience, people are able to construct from what they observe how they understand or imagine the other person is experiencing what is going on. It seems to operate a bit as though people reserve emotional spaces inside themselves with the assumption that the objects of their intimacy reserve a similar emotional space for them in return (see inset box). Key information is provided from subtle changes in expression, the manner of speaking, and the content in descriptions of events. From these sources, observers piece together a picture that they compare and contrast with their own experience and out of which they interpret likely emotional reactions.

The significance of this emotional receptivity to both the world of human relationships and the emergence of civil societies has been repeatedly emphasized by key writers and thinkers. For example, the German philosopher Martin Heidegger (1889–1976) used the term *care* (*Sorge*) to refer to this capacity as a key part of the nature of human existence and being. Similarly, Max Scheler

---

Jacinta/Wendy: Waning Intimacy

Wendy is speaking with her close friend, Sally, over a cup of coffee at Sally's house.

"I don't know about me and Jacinta anymore. We seem to be drifting apart."

"Huh? Surely not? You both seem so solid together."

"It might seem like that, but she never calls me at work during the day to see how I'm doing, not like James calls you. She doesn't seem to think of me at all. Last night I asked her whether she thought about me while I was at work. She looked confused, and said yes, but I could tell by the way she looked at me that she was lying, and that she doesn't think of me at all."

"Maybe she gets busy."

"She thinks of me briefly when I get home, then its dinner, going for a walk, then for me TV and bed, and for her it's going out to gamble. There's no real time for us to connect. For me it's no longer good enough and I keep wondering whether it would be better to split altogether."

Danny/Jack: Enduring Compassion

Julie is speaking to Danny's father, Jack, about their separation.

"Since Danny left it's been easier looking after the children. But for me personally it's been much harder."

"Harder? How?"

"Danny and I have spent years living closely together. Over time I feel I've learned to spot what he's thinking and how he's feeling. Now we've separated, and I can see by the way he acts that he is hurting bad."

"Are you thinking of getting back together?"

"No, that would do no good. But inside me, after living so closely with him for so long, to see him in pain, to see his life falling apart, it really bothers me."

"But you're no longer exposed to it."

"No, but inside there's a part of me that is always looking out for him, a part of me that senses what he's feeling."

(1874–1928) identified *sympathy* as the ground upon which all human meanings are held together. The psychologist Carl Rogers (1902–1987) identified *empathy* as a primary ingredient in communication, which has subsequently led to empathic reflection forming a cornerstone of modern counseling. These terms—*care, sympathy*, and *empathy*—and others terms, such as *concern, receptivity*, and *emotional responsiveness*, refer to a capacity that most people have to respond imaginatively to the emotional life of those around them. For our discussion of addictions, this capacity will be referred to as *compassion,* meaning the ability to identify and respond to the emotional world of other people. *Compassion* has been chosen over the other terms for two main reasons: First, the two parts of the word, *com-* and *passion,* convey a sense of parallel emotionality, a connecting to something with emotion. Second, in contrast to the other terms, *compassion* carries with it a stronger sense of responding or acting on emotions. For example, when feeling compassion for the poor, rather than concern or sympathy, one is more likely to act compassionately and perhaps donate money or provide other assistance. This sense of readiness to act is important in a social world because it is ultimately these actions that build up interconnections.

Commitment

Commitment, as the third strand, refers to the most active ingredient in forming intimate relationships. It is active because it requires a positive choice followed by a prescribed set of actions. The central action involves the giving of something, usually the giving over of a portion of one's life to a relationship. In a sense, commitment involves putting part of oneself on the line for another; it involves the handing over of a significant amount of time to a relationship with the understanding that time comprises a precious part of one's own limited being. Furthermore, in choosing to become intimate, the person is not only committing the time required to become close, but is also allocating other scarce resources such as space, affection, emotional energy, family resources, recreational resources, and money. This is why the values associated with commitment (values such as loyalty, solidarity, trust, reliability, and steadfastness) are so highly prized and monitored with regard to intimate relationships. They are of such importance that societies as a whole typically establish strong codes, rituals, and other social practices to monitor and support these investments. These include practices such as betrothals and marriage, friendship rituals, family celebrations, and anniversary gifting.

Commitment involves putting a meaningful part of one's life on the line in a relationship

The presence of commitment is identified through a variety of different tests of commitment. One test concerns whether or not a person demonstrates adequate interest, enthusiasm, or other positive emotions regarding the relationship. Unfortunately, it is common for people to display these emotions without remaining true to them, and given that intimacy involves the commitment of scarce personal resources, a more reliable test is often sought.

A second test concerns whether this positive regard is displayed consistently across different situations. Of particular interest is whether the person declaring commitment displays the same enthusiasm to others when one is not present. A person who disparages a friend behind the friend's back is hardly a friend. However, displays of emotion are fickle and may be motivated by ulterior motives such a money, sex, or control. A more reliable third test concerns whether the person sustains a commitment over long periods of time. The longer a relationship remains strong, the more it can be trusted and relied upon. Nonetheless, long-term relationships can evolve into low-value repetitive and automated involvements—habits of convenience: "I stay with you because I don't know how to leave."

Finally, an even stronger test of commitment focuses on whether the relationship will survive over a time of trial. For example, the friend who remains loyal through a period of extreme hardship (such as war, poverty, or illness) can surely be counted on as a true friend (see inset box). Yet these adversities involve challenges from outside sources; the strongest test of friendship involves times of trial that emerge from within the relationship itself. For example, an indicator of strong commitment would be when a relationship is sustained despite violations between members, such as when a married couple works through issues of an adulterous affair and succeed in restoring it back to positive intimacy.

Accord

The fourth strand refers to a more passive dimension of intimacy. Accord is less a matter of decision and action, and more something that emerges organically within the circumstances of ongoing compassionate and committed closeness. Accord is understood here as the sense of unity and connection that emerges within relationships. It refers, in a sense, to the final product of intimate togetherness. For wider networks, it is experienced as a sense of communality, cohesion, or transpersonal connectedness (see inset box). For example, in a sports team it might be referred to as "team spirit," or in a city as "brotherly love." In more

---

Cathy/Dion: Spotting True Friends

While Dion was driving his stepsister Shannon home from visiting a friend, she asks:

"How do you know if someone's a true friend?"

"Umm, well, my true friends stick by me, no matter what I go through."

"But say you did something really bad. Wouldn't they…"

"I guess there are some things that are unforgivable, like murder or terrorism. But mostly, even if I mucked up, my true friends would stick by me."

"Even if it was a bad muck-up?"

"Yeah. When you were younger, some time after my Dad disappeared, Mom was arrested and sent to jail. Everyone I knew read about it in the papers; it was really horrible, particularly at school. But you know what? I was really surprised by how many people kept away from me but even more surprised by how many stuck by me. It was pretty gruesome. The papers reported all sorts of bad things."

"I remember a bit. But see, those who stuck by you are your real friends."

"Yep, they sure are, but they're not always who you expect."

Jacinta/Wendy: Feeling at One

Later in her conversation with her friend Sally, Wendy says, "I know I've said I feel that Jacinta and I are drifting apart, but I'm still constantly surprised by the feelings that well up in me towards her. It happens unexpectedly, often in fleeting moments. It might be as we are walking together in a park; it might happen quickly in glances over dinner; it might happen in the middle of the night lying next to each other."

"Despite all the conflict?"

"We don't have conflict all the time. I still feel incredibly close to her. Sometimes I feel close during the day while I think of our happier times. They are all brief moments, but very important to me because they give me a sense of oneness and purpose."

intimate relationships its clearest form is experienced as love, oneness, and union. Indeed, at times it may really feel as if a "cord" is providing a primal connection between one person and another. This sense of accord is the subject of many songs and poems, but in plain prose it is difficult to describe other than to declare that it matters to those who experience it and that it is usually seen as the whole point of the intimacy.

Special Considerations

While intimacies between people comprise the most important form of connecting within a social world, human intimacy is highly flexible and dynamic and accordingly can take a wide variety of different forms. These forms share family resemblances involving different combinations of the four strands (four C's) discussed above. In addictive social systems where patterns of connection are disrupted, intimacy can take on a variety of alternative forms.

Intimacies with Nonhuman, Inanimate, or Absent Objects

The most familiar prototype of intimacy is that which occurs between two people. However, a sizable range of intimacies commonly occur with nonhuman or absent objects. Consideration of these will be important when later we examine the ways in which intimacies mutate within and around an addictive relationship. Here are five of these hybrid forms:

1. Cuddly toys: Intimacies can be formed with inanimate but lifelike objects such as dolls, teddy bears, and other cuddly toys. Closeness is strongly established, both in terms of time and proximity. A child might spend many hours physically holding on to the cuddly toy, walking with it, lying with it, stroking it, talking to it and so forth. Each of these establishes closeness with the object (see inset box). Commitment to the toy is often strong, with the toy accompanying the child when sleeping at friend's houses and despite the likelihood of peer humiliation, the child can express reluctance at abandoning the toy right into adolescence. Compassion can be observed in the ways the child talks to the toy, as if it has feelings and as if it is reacting emotionally to what is happening. Through these processes a

---

Jacinta/Wendy: Teddy

As part of Wendy explaining to Jacinta her loss of trust, she says, "When I was little, I always had my teddy bear with me to cuddle. I would lie with him in bed and tell him many of the hard things about the day."

"We do that too."

"Yeah, well, we used to. Now it's not so easy. With Teddy I would think about how he was reacting to problems. He was always there, listening and looking at me in a way that said, 'Don't worry, things will work out okay.'"

"But he was just a stuffed toy."

"But I could rely on him. He never played tricks on me."

sense of accord with the toy emerges that can lead to genuine grief should the toy be damaged or lost. Other more adult forms of intimacy with inanimate objects could involve special relationships with things such as a fancy car, a house, a garden, a gun, or a computer; each involving varying combinations of the four strands.

2. Pets: A person's close relationship with a pet can develop into a strong—perhaps for some their strongest—encounter with intimacy. The sense of closeness is usually built up by sharing physical proximity over large amounts of time. Typical activities include sitting with the pet, walking and playing together, stroking it, talking to it, and including it in a broad range of daily routines. Compassion is easier with pets than with inanimate objects because of the responsiveness and interactive quality of the relationship. For example, a dog's capacity to look happy or sad, relaxed or worried, and to look hurt when rebuked make it easier for the pet owner to identify with the emotional life of the dog (see inset box, above). The emergence of a strong sense of commitment is also highly likely. Some pet owners go to extraordinary lengths to ensure that the pet's needs and comforts are adequately addressed. This combination of closeness, compassion, and commitment, particularly for socially isolated people, can provide the basis for a strong sense of accord with the pet, an accord that can lead to a devastating sense of loss when the pet dies.

> ### Bert/Joan: Fiona's Dog
>
> Bert's daughter, Fiona, is telling her brother, Donald, what her dog, Toto, means to her.
>
> "Toto is my closest friend. When I come home she is always there looking up at me."
>
> "But you have other close friends."
>
> "I have friends, but none as close as her. She's always there for me. It doesn't matter what I do, or what happens to me that day, she always greets me, wiggles around, jumps up, tries to lick me. She's always happy that I'm home."
>
> "We don't get much of that from anywhere else."
>
> "Exactly, and it's because of her that I've been able to put up with all the negative stuff that happens in this house. No, really, she is my rock. I don't know how I would survive without her."

3. Deceased loved ones: The loss of loved ones through death, separation, or dislocation highlights two aspects of intimacy: first, that transitions in the formation and ending of intimacies happens at a slow pace, and, second, that an intimacy can be sustained long after the disappearance of the object of that intimacy. As discussed in Chapter 3, both of these processes contribute to the intensification of addictive relationships. When facing the loss of a partner, child, or parent, the experience of intimacy can persist long after the person has gone. For sudden losses, the bereaved may in the first few weeks continue to act as if the object of intimacy is still present; they set a place at the table, leave clothes in the wardrobe, and may even pretend to themselves in various ways that the missing person is still present. As illustrated in the inset box, above, this need for a process of adjustment can also happen with people who are familiar but not necessarily part of one's circle of intimates. As the reality of the loss sets in, people learn to live with the absence, but in many respects the intimacy remains. The bereaved still feel a strong sense of commitment to the relationship and spend hours

Cathy/Dion: Diana's Death

Cathy is chatting to Dion about people she has lost in her life:

"You know, when Diana [the Princess of Wales] died in that car crash in Paris, I was surprised by my reaction. I really felt genuine sadness. I thought I'd taken very little interest in her. How can I feel so much for someone who doesn't know me?"

"I guess it's because her image was everywhere, in magazines, on TV, in the news. Wherever you went you saw her pretty smiling face and read about her latest adventures."

"Yes, I guess. But I didn't realize how her constant presence had become such a part of me. It shocked me that I could feel so strongly about her dying."

thinking over the past in ways that stimulate their sense of accord. Their biggest challenge is the loss of proximal closeness, which in turn denies them access to the feedback and communication that enables them to feel compassion. To compensate for this they seek out objects linked to the deceased such as the grave, favorite utensils, photos, and other memorabilia. These indirect forms of closeness serve to trigger compassionate memories. Other forms of intimacy with absent objects can include intimates separated by war or migration, relationships with imaginary friends, and communicating through spiritualists or mediums.

4. Land: People can form intimate relationships with abstract or general objects such as with ideologies, ethnicities, and nationalities. One example of this type of intimacy concerns the bond people form with the land. Most people have a sense of identification with the land they inhabit, but this applies particularly for those who live and work close to the land, such as farmers, park rangers, environmentalists, and indigenous peoples. For these people their sense of identification often involves very profound feelings of being close and intimately connected to particular stretches of land (see inset box). In these situations, all four contributing strands of intimacy can be seen to be at play. For example, the farmer is in constant close physical proximity to his land and spends considerable lengths of time working it and walking close to its many forms and features. Out of this connection grows a profound sense of commitment and accord with the land, to such an extent that the farmer would vigorously defend that connection against any perceived threats. Compassion is more difficult to identify, except that for some people the land can become personified in such a way that the land is seen as suffering from the abuse of overexploitation or neglect or enjoying the benefits of good rainfall and drainage.

5. God: Another form of generalized intimacy occurs with objects of spiritual and religious significance. These can take many forms. In the monotheistic religions such as Judaism, Islam, and Christianity, a special

Danny/Jack: I Belong Here

Danny and Jack are talking as they walk across a paddock.

"Dad, I've always wanted to know… Why do you see this farm as so important?"

"Well, I inherited this farmland from my father, who inherited it from his father and so on.... I was born here and spent all my childhood playing all over it. I have worked over every bit of it clearing things, planting, looking after everything that grows."

"Yeah, but it's like any job."

"I walk over this land every day and I know all its nooks and crannies, every detail of how it changes each season. Everywhere I look I am reminded of things. That tree covered our picnics, that stream was where we swam in summer, and that hill always stands over us like a father."

"I remember those things, too."

"When I travel on business I feel an emptiness inside and I can't wait to return to walking over it again."

"I guess that's where we're different."

form of intimacy is understood to occur between the faithful and what they understand as God. For example, in Christian traditions the faithful establish a strongly personal relationship with God through his manifestation in the personhood of Jesus Christ. The relationship is established through reflection, prayer, and meditation. This proximal closeness is enhanced through the presence of statues, icons, and churches as venues that combine a wide range of religious imagery (e.g., using music, architecture, flowers, and incense). The relationship is further strengthened by the Christian liturgy that emphasizes the compassion of God and Christ, and the importance through faith of remaining committed to the relationships. Closeness, compassion, and commitment to God and Christ then combine synergistically into a strong sense of accord, leading to a sense that one's own puny individual existence is part of a greater order.

Unreciprocated Intimacy

As can be seen in these varieties of intimacy, particularly with the deceased and with inanimate and other objects, the relationships do not necessarily involve reciprocation. Many close intimacies are formed with objects that are either incapable of or unwilling to return the compassion and commitment they receive (as with dolls, dead relatives, and nationalities). This highlights the strongly flexible nature of how people experience intimacies and how the perception of intimacy adapts to circumstances. It is possible for a person to experience a very intense relationship when the object of affection is not even present. This is most clear when an intense relationship forms with an inanimate object or a missing or dead object. For example, in Charles Dickens's novel *Great Expectations*, Miss Havisham, a wealthy elderly woman, lives in the decaying environment of her wedding banquet, which has been left untouched since she was deserted by her husband-to-be on her wedding day over 30 years ago. She has continued to wear her wedding dress and has maintained her life as fixed at the moment of her wedding. She thereby maintains a primary connection to her future husband while for him it was a relationship that never was to be. Situations such as this, where the nature of intimacy between one party is different from the nature of intimacy with the other party, can be referred to as *asymmetrical intimacy*, meaning that the combinations and degree of

> **Danny/Jack: Unreciprocated Concern**
>
> Julie is confiding with a friend about her separation from Danny.
>
> "While I still have feelings for him, I don't think the same is happening for him. I think he stopped having feelings for me years ago."
>
> "Men don't speak openly about their feelings."
>
> "Hmm, that's true, and that's often what I told myself. So I carried on. I cared about him, listened to his problems, and stuck by him through thick and thin. But I could never see him really worrying about how I felt."
>
> "You can never tell. He's upset now, isn't he?"
>
> "He's upset because he's been forced out, not because he misses me. It's the same as before; everyone focuses on what he's feeling and forgets about me."

closeness, compassion, commitment, and accord experienced by one party are not matched by the combinations and degree experienced by the other party (see inset box, above).

The degree to which intimacies are asymmetrical varies both in extent and in type. For example, a form of intimacy that is clearly asymmetrical across a number of domains can be observed with someone experiencing unrequited romantic love. Here, while to the outside observer there is little chance of forming an equally balanced loving relationship, from inside the person nurtures the hope of reciprocated intimacy and may continue to pursue it even when there is little hope of success because the other person is married, unavailable, or uninterested. Although such a predicament is often difficult and upsetting, many facing it will still choose to continue building their personal lives around this hopelessly asymmetrical involvement.

A more subtle example of asymmetrical intimacy can be observed in the relationship formed between addiction counselors and their clients. Counselors help clients explore some the most intimate aspects of their

A counseling relationship involves a subtly asymmetrical intimacy

lives. These explorations entail the clients' disclosing details about the most private areas of their lives, details on their personal motives, fears, and insecurities, as well as details on the morality of their behavior and the behavior of those around them. Accordingly, clients begin to experience a close and specific intimate connection with the counselor, but this usually differs from the way the counselor may experience it. The commitment and compassion the counselor as a person brings into the therapeutic relationship has for some time been recognized as one of the most important features of this relationship.[8] But while developing concern for each client, it is difficult to reciprocate specific intimacy with each client when the counselor might work with over a hundred different clients in a year. What tends to happen is that the closeness with, compassion for, commitment to, and accord with clients is approached in a more general form. For example, the commitment to each client is driven more by a general commitment to the work rather than by the specific nature of that involvement. This means that therapeutic relationships tend to be subtly asymmetrical, and that this asymmetry needs to be managed carefully in helping clients move on to other more symmetrical opportunities.

A more problematic form of unreciprocated (asymmetrical) intimacy occurs when a relationship appears balanced and symmetrical, while in reality it functions asymmetrically. Intimate relationships of this type are *deceptively symmetrical*. These relationships pose all sorts of challenges, particularly when the deception becomes obvious. For example, when a young girl who idolizes a particular pop star discovers that he does not share any feelings or commitment to his fans, she is likely to feel outraged and to respond hostilely with acts such as burning his posters or breaking his recordings.[9] Similar outrage might occur when attacked by a special pet or betrayed by a close friend.

An even trickier form of asymmetry occurs when the deception is not generated by others but is constructed by oneself. Self-deception occurs when despite all signs to the contrary, a person still manages to pretend that the intimacy is symmetrical. For example, a father might continue to believe that his son is maintaining a committed and emotional connection to his family despite all evidence to the contrary. His son has not kept any contact and he has declared to others that he has disowned his family. Perhaps such rejection is just too difficult for the father to accept.

As will be examined in later chapters, in an addictive social system, the majority of relationships take asymmetrical forms. The addictive relationship involves asymmetry in terms of unreciprocated compassion and commitment. For other intimates surrounding the addictive relationship, their relationships are in a complex range of ways deceptively symmetrical. It is in the different ways of responding to this deceptive asymmetry that this book will explore options for intervention.

Quality Intimacy?

This section takes a brief look at a contentious question: Can one intimacy be considered of better quality than another? In other words, are some intimacies good and others bad, or are they just different and equally valid forms of the same process? This question is particularly important in a discussion of addiction. How one views the quality of life possible in an addictive system will determine the moral position adopted regarding the desirability of addictive relationships. Could an addictive relationship ever be considered a high-quality intimacy? It is tempting to evade this question, because indeed some addictive relationships could be viewed as of reasonable quality as they manifest reasonable levels of closeness, commitment, and accord.

Could an addictive relationship ever be considered high quality intimacy?

Binary Versus Continuum Perspectives

It is tempting to classify intimate relationships as belonging to one of two main types: high quality and low quality. As with other areas of health, this binary approach involves slotting key aspects of one's reality into category pairs: the weather is either fine or wet, people are either good or bad, clients are either compliant or disruptive (see inset box below). Thinking in binary categories is tempting and powerful. Their use helps organize a complex picture and facilitates decisive action such as when needing to know whom to trust in crisis situations. However, despite these benefits, their use also runs the risk of oversimplifying and stereotyping the subject material. For example, a common binary related to alcohol is the division of drinkers into "responsible" and "addicted." The distinction is useful in helping to identify people who require some form of assistance, but it also oversimplifies the diversity of possible relationships to alcohol and runs the risk of stigmatizing people in addictive relationships as weak and qualitatively different from those who drink in other ways. The consequent negative stigma discourages people from discussing pertinent issues and thereby making it less likely that they reflect and speak up about what concerns them.

Instead of dividing relationships into good intimacy and bad intimacy, an alternative approach involves positioning particular intimacies as points on a continuum of quality. A continuum interpretation involves looking at the world less in terms of fixed categories, and more in terms of gradations of intensity across a particular domain.[10] The shift from binaries to continua enables a more dynamic approach that is more responsive to the subtleties of time and place. It recognizes that over time relationships move through various stages, with the quality of each relationship varying as circumstances change. For example, over the course of a 30-year marriage, there will be multiple periods when the quality of the relationship between the partners will deteriorate and other times when the quality will peak. The shift to viewing the quality of intimacies as positions on a continuum also increases the legitimacy of reflecting and discussing the status of each relationship. When the quality is seen as either good or bad, the act of initiating a discussion about the relationship instantly implies that the relationship is bad; it becomes uncomfortable—and in some situations unsafe—to enter into such conversations. Alternatively, when the quality of intimacies is seen to vary dynamically over time, it reduces concerns about being lumped into the negative stigmatized category of low-quality intimacy. Consequently, reappraising the status of the relationship becomes a more relaxed, more comfortable, and perhaps a more normal activity.

Identifying Quality

If the experience of an intimacy is seen to vary across a continuum of quality, this then introduces the question of what criteria might be applied to identify and monitor these variations. Building on the ideas from this chapter, one important criterion for judging the quality of an intimacy is the degree of symmetry in the relationship between intimates, meaning by this the extent to which closeness, compassion, commitment, and accord are matched or reciprocated between members of a particular relationship.

Also, as discussed in this and earlier chapters, addictive relationships are not all-or-nothing events. The phases of initiation and intensification typically occur over long periods of time and, once formed, the strength and dominance of an addictive relationship will wax and wane as the people in the addictive system grapple with its various manifestations. Perhaps only in the very late stages of a well-formed addictive relationship have all vestiges of symmetrical and quality intimacy disappeared, and even then there can still be flickers of connectedness.

Consequently, across the trajectory of an addictive relationship it remains a sensible undertaking for surrounding intimates to reflect on the quality of intimacy, and the level of symmetry or reciprocation is the strongest indicator. This task of reflecting can then be viewed as an activity that is normal to undertake from time to time. For example in the inset box, above, Dion recognizes the chaos and disruption caused by his mother's addictive relationship, but at the same time claims that a certain degree of quality and reciprocity still survives—enough for him to retain some sense of accord. From the outside one might see him as fooling himself and buying into some form of deceptive symmetry. However, he has been in this situation since his childhood, and during this time he has developed a realistic appreciation of what his mother's addictive relationship entails. It is therefore reasonable for Dion to spend time considering the extent to which he has retained some strands of quality in his relationship to Cathy. Deceptive symmetry is more likely to creep in when this form of reflection is not occurring, and for those who are wary of self-deception, it still remains a fine judgment distinguishing a meaningful but waning intimacy from a deceptively symmetrical intimacy.

The following chapters adopt the position that the level to which an intimacy contributes to personal and collective well-being varies in quality but not in an either/or fashion and more in the form of a continuum of intensity. It will be argued that the processes of social fragmentation in addictive social systems lead to asymmetry in the relationships that result, on balance, in lower quality intimacy—hence the need to do something about them. At the same time, this exploration also acknowledges the possibility that some levels of quality intimacy can be achieved in addictive systems.

Cathy/Dion: Remaining Close

Lying in bed one night Dion is speaking to his partner, Lisa, about his relationship to Cathy.

"You know, despite everything that goes wrong around Mom's drug use, I still feel incredibly close to her."

"Does that mean you accept that she's not going to change?"

"No, I really think things would be different if she quit. Much better. But even so, if she keeps using, I still think we can be close."

"Maybe your support just makes it easier for her to keep using?"

"Maybe, but you know I've stopped trying to make it easier for her. No, it's something else. Despite everything, we still have moments when we feel close and when we know what's happening with each other on the inside."

Chapter 6

Intimacies in Addictive Contexts

"What are you crying for, Helen? What the deuce is the matter now?"
"I'm crying for you Arthur," I replied, speedily drying my tears; and starting up,
I threw myself on my knees before him, and, clasping his nerveless hand between
my own, continued. "Don't you know that you are a part of myself? And do
you think you can injure and degrade yourself, and I not feel it?"
"Degrade myself, Helen?"
"Yes, degrade! What have you been doing all this time?"
"You'd better not ask," said he with a faint smile.
"And you had better not tell—but you cannot deny that you have degraded yourself
miserably. You have shamefully wronged yourself, body and soul—and me too, and I
can't endure it quietly—and I won't."

(Anne Brontë, "The Tenant of Wildfell Hall")[1]

In previous chapters, addictive relationships (those connecting a person with an addictive substance/process) were viewed from above, looking down on connecting objects. As signaled by the passage from Anne Brontë's book, this chapter delves more into the intricacies and dynamics faced with intimacies in addictive contexts. It takes the analysis of intimacy developed in the previous chapter and applies it in detail to addictive systems. Since the lived experience of such systems differ for those who are in an addictive relationship and for those who live around them, this chapter approaches intimacy from two separate angles: first, from the point of view of inside the addictive relationship, that is, between the person and the addictive substance/process; and second, from the point of view of other intimates, that is, between other people in the immediate social system with the person in the addictive relationship.

Intimacy Within Addictive Relationships

This book contends that an addictive relationship is a hybrid form of intimacy and one that by its very nature is asymmetrical. This section examines this asymmetry across the four strands of intimacy (closeness, compassion, commitment, and accord).

P.J. Adams, Fragmented Intimacy: Addiction in a Social World
© Springer 2008

Intoxicated Closeness

Intoxication involves episodes of closeness with an addictive substance/ process that are psychologically transformative. This closeness is not just with a neutral object (a bottle or a pill); on the contrary, the connection is charged with meaning and psychological potency. For example, by injecting heroin or gambling in a casino, people experience their immediate reality in a significantly different way than when they are not intoxicated. This close- ness happens in several different forms. The obvious form involves sharing time and space and directly consuming and interacting with the addictive substance/process. A sense of close- ness is built up through the many hours devoted to planning, preparing, obtaining, and consum- ing the product. Another form of closeness is the sense that the addictive substance/process is ready at hand for use when needed. Naturally with the product close by this also means that intoxication too is ready-at-hand. As illustrated in the inset box, the product does not need to be consumed; by staying linked to the product, by carrying the quarter tablet in a pocket, the mere availability of the product for consumption can maintain a strong sense of connection. Closeness is derived less from use and more from its readiness for use. Other examples of similar closeness occur in anticipation of getting drunk at the end of the week and creating a drug stash for access during lean times. A third form of closeness is derived from associations with the things, sensations, and events that surround consumption. These associations carry an indirect sense of proximity. For example, a sense of closeness can result from carrying the paraphernalia of injecting, wearing clothing associated with drink- ing, or on a regular basis reading up on track betting.

> **Jacinta/Wendy: Tranquilizers My Friend**
>
> During one of their long evening conversations Jacinta says to Wendy, "You talk about my gam- bling; what about your pills?"
>
> "I took tranquilizers to keep from getting uptight at work. They really helped me relax in running meetings and making presentations. But unlike your gambling, I never liked taking them."
>
> "But you do take them and I don't see them as different than my time on the slots."
>
> "I've cut down to practically nothing. I may still need to carry a quarter of a tablet around in my pocket. I never used it, but if I don't have it..."
>
> "Don't you feel a bit silly walking around with that?"
>
> "But without it I feel nervous about meetings and presenting and this makes me mess things up and I only get more nervous. Knowing the pill is there if I need it gives me confidence."

The psychological dimensions of closeness to an addictive substance/ process go in one direction—from the product to the person. It is difficult to conceive of a way that these products might feel close since inanimate fluids and substances lack consciousness. Furthermore, this one-way close- ness tends not to focus on specific objects, and tends to occur more with classes of products. For instance, a sense of closeness is unlikely to emerge with one tablet of amphetamine on its own; closeness is felt toward that class of drugs as a whole. In terms of how intimacy was discussed in the last chapter, this positions the closeness experienced in addictive relationships as somewhere in between a relationship with a significant inanimate object (such as a car, a picture, or a house) and a relationship with a significant gen- eralized object (such as the land or a particular ideology). The close proximity of specific objects provides the sense of physical closeness, while the link to a general category of product enables the closeness to be experienced across many periods of time and different contexts.

Passionate Embrace

While addictive relationships are low in compassion, from the point of view of the person in the addictive relationship, it is still a very passionate relationship.[2] These passions occur in both positive and negative forms. On the positive side, through many episodes of intoxication the relationship brings to the person considerable joy, playfulness, camaraderie, and excitement, and the person might recall with strong affection the many associated events and adventures. It also provides periods of feeling normal, relaxed, and accepted. On the negative side, troubles with the outside world lead to a wide range of unwelcome feelings. These feelings permeate the person's experience resulting in significant and common states of mind. To capture these states of mind, the following discussion identifies four varieties: low threshold frustrations, a sense of impending disaster, a sense of inner malfunction, and a sense of not belonging.[3] Each of these states of mind interacts with negative feelings that gather, form, and condense into a set of strong generalized emotions.

Low-Threshold Frustrations

People in the outside world gaze at the person in the addictive relationship and see a talented, capable individual—admittedly with a few problems to sort out—but a person with a clear capacity for responsible and loving social involvements. Inside the relationship it is a different story. The world appears a severe, hostile place (see inset box). As the addictive relationship intensifies it becomes increasingly less compatible with maintaining other involvements in the world. Tension emerges for the person between the wish to maintain the addictive relationship and the ongoing desire to stay connected elsewhere. As the tension progresses it feels as if the task of maintaining the addictive relationship is constantly being challenged by others.[4] Outsiders question, they challenge, and they appear to be trying to make things more difficult. This is further complicated by the harm that occurs during periods of intoxication.

> **Bert/Joan: Endless Frustration**
>
> In a rare moment of closeness Joan asks, "Bert, why do you change moods so quickly?"
>
> "I guess most people see me as calm, reasonable, polite... I'm friendly, I got a great sense of humour."
>
> "Yeah, well, maybe at work you're like that."
>
> "But it's a facade. Underneath I'm a boiling pot of anger, just waiting to erupt."
>
> "I see it, but you seldom show it outside the home."
>
> "I was driving in heavy traffic yesterday and some jerk pulled out in front of me without indicating. I felt this immediate and intense rage rise from my stomach into my chest then exploding in my head. I thought, 'Get him, get him, he's the enemy; he's the reason things go bad every day.' I had this sense that I had to do something to get back at him. So just to piss him off I chased him and tailgated him all the way home."

Events, such as an insult, a slap, or a minor betrayal, increase the likelihood of challenges from others, and at times these appear to come from all directions: family members, the police, a bank officer, and friends. Wishes and expectations are constantly frustrated, often leading on to the perception of being trapped in a fortress where even small upsets become symbolic of wider unease.

Impending Disaster

Again, from the outside there appears more that could go right than wrong; the capacity is there, opportunities abound, goodwill and support are available, and although some major problems exist, these are not insurmountable. This view is not shared by the person inside the addictive relationship. The intensifying relationship with the addictive substance/process and the consequent deteriorations in other relationships leads to a sense of being on a roller-coaster that is heading blindly toward unknown disasters.[5] Nonetheless, the addicted person does not jump off; rather, this constant sense of foreboding promotes stronger attachment to the addictive substance/process. Disasters could happen in any place at any time. The weather might be fine and everything is going well, but just around the corner lurks a catastrophe yet to be encountered (see inset box, above). When nothing disastrous occurs this does not necessarily lead to any decrease in foreboding. One fear connects with other possibilities and one reprieve only means future catastrophes will be worse. The addictive relationship seems the only reliable source available for protection.

Inner Malfunction

For some, rather than the world outside generating the sense of threat, the menace appears to come from within. While outwardly everything seems resolvable, inside a different reality emerges (see inset box, above). Rather than seeing the perceived negativity as

---

Danny/Jack: Just Around the Corner

Jack can see Danny is feeling low.

"How's it going, Dan?"

"I wake up in the morning, the sun is shining, the birds are chirping, I have no pressures or hassles for the day, and everyone is fine. But inside I feel really bad."

"Some days are just like that."

"No, this happens a lot. Even though I can't see anything bad, it feels like just around the corner hangs a thick black cloud and that the moment I turn the corner everything will turn bad."

"But it doesn't, does it?"

"No. But it's a feeling I can't shake off. At first it was only there a little, but now I feel like this most the time. Sometimes it's stronger than other times, but it's definitely there, and it scares me when I think of the future."

Jacinta/Wendy: A Screw's Loose

In a quiet moment late one night, Wendy remarks, "Jac, sometimes I sense a great sadness in you."

"Yeah, deep within I feel there's something wrong. I don't know what it is, except I know it's there."

"Oh, not knowing what it is, that must be hard."

"I dunno. Sometimes it worries me that perhaps something really bad and unthinkably unpleasant happened to me in my childhood. Perhaps deep within my mind there's a loose screw that needs tightening, but it's buried so deep that it's unreachable. Perhaps I'm fundamentally handicapped, or insane, or even evil."

"You know it's not like that."

"Whatever it is, something seems seriously wrong inside, and I'm constantly drained by having to keep up appearances while everything inside feels it's about to crumble."

the result of an addictive process, the ongoing troubles are identified with some vital internal part of the psyche. The exaggerated attachment to the addictive substance/process and the deteriorating connections with the world are attributed to a nonspecific inner malfunction. For some, this malfunction may have a specific focus (such as those relating to losses or abuse in the past) but for most the malfunction is nonspecific: something is going wrong inside but it is buried too deep to identify. This unpleasant position of living with a malfunction that nothing can be done about leads to a constant and generalized sense of inadequacy, a sense of not being good enough because unlike other people something very wrong is happening inside. The sense of inadequacy further reinforces the attractiveness of the addictive relationship over other attachments.

Not Belonging

Another state of mind that emerges out of efforts to protect the addictive relationship is a sense of being alien, of not fitting in, of being somehow once removed from the rest of what is going on. It can feel as though other people belong to an inner circle to which one has been excluded. As Cathy tries to explain to Dion in the inset box, while people perceive her as confident and socially connected, inside she feels separate, different, and not belonging. Cathy finds this sense of alienation is relieved periodically during intoxication, but as the addictive relationship strengthens, these periods lengthen. As a consequence other people increase their disdain for the addictive relationship, thereby further compounding the sense of being the outsider. Gradually the specific experiences of not belonging merge into a general sense of alienation leading to a constant sense of unwanted isolation.

> **Cathy/Dion: Displacement**
>
> Cathy, following a period of sickness and depression discloses to Dion:
>
> "My whole life has been a grand mistake."
>
> "Oh mum, you don't need to say that."
>
> "No, no. It really feels like I was born from the wrong womb, at the wrong time, in the wrong century, in the wrong place in the wrong city, to incorrect parents and into the wrong environment. I just don't fit in."
>
> "But you're always great at mixing people."
>
> "No, it's not how I look, it's how I feel. It's like when I was at elementary school and the class is asked to pair off. Everyone else manages to find a partner but I'm the one left-over. As an adult, I have continued to feel like the one left-over."
>
> "It's not how you appear."
>
> "Put it this way. At times I feel like a goldfish staring out of a bowl, somehow in the place, but not really participating. I console myself by thinking that one day people from my true origins will discover me and transport me through time to the place I truly belong."

Fear, Resentment, and Shame

As indicated above, these four states of mind productively interact with three generalized negative emotions in a way that for many characterize the experience of living in an addictive relationship.[6] First, a generalized fearfulness accumulates in partnership with all four states of mind. This fear is typically experienced as a strong but nonspecific fear of something that is vaguely wrong with the world, wrong with oneself, or wrong with one's place in the world. At times, it may take a specific focus (such as a fear of discovery or fear of dismissal), but more often than not these specific instances are absorbed into an ongoing amorphous fearfulness. The second generalized emotion is resentment. Resentments consist of accumulated and unresolved anger that result from episodes of real or perceived harm and violation. For example, a person might feel initial anger and outrage in response to a colleague's public insult, but should these feelings be left unresolved the anger can turn in time into an ongoing sense of resentment. Resentment generated by violations can happen both before and during an addictive relationship. Intoxication often serves to block the resolution of prior violations, such as parental neglect or sexual abuse, thereby enshrining resentment as a founding element in the addictive relationship. As the addictive relationship intensifies, violations occur as a natural consequence of challenges from the outside world

> **Bert/Joan: It's a Mess**
> Bert is feeling low and begins confiding in a friend while having a beer after work:
> "Y'know, at home, well, it's all a terrible mess."
> "I'm sorry to hear that, Bert."
> "I feel really bad every time I walk in the door. I don't know where it all comes from. I know some pieces of it: I'm angry that the children don't speak to me anymore, I feel bad about the rotten things I do to Joan, I'm sorry I don't earn more for them... But it's worse than all these things."
> "Maybe you need a break."
> "Oh, I tell you, that's what I need, a break; a break from all my hassles. But that'll never happen. No, I'm stuck with this mess. And you know what? For some strange reason I'm also really worried all the time; I'm worried about what Joan might be saying to her sister; I'm worried about what she's telling the children, I'm very worried about what might happen if anything changes; I'm worried about anything and everything. That's why I spend so much time here."
> "You're just one big scaredy-cat."
> "Yeah, I guess so. Want another beer?"

(e.g., marital conflict, court orders). This leads to additional perceived grievances that pile further layers onto the generalized sense of resentment. The third generalized emotion, shame, occurs as the flip side of resentment. Shame accumulates from several sources: shame for letting negative things happen in the past, shame from ongoing violations in current intimacies, and shame at being in an addictive relationship. As with fear and resentment, over time the contributing specific foci of shame blur into a generalized what sense of shame. In the inset box, above Bert makes a half-hearted attempt to convey what some of this complex of feelings means to him (although his capacity to reflect on it is limited).

The four states of mind and associated emotions are not unique to what people experience in addictive relationships. Most people experience some of these from time to time. For instance, it is not uncommon to have periods of feeling like an outsider or that an unforeseen disaster is about to happen. But these feelings are experienced more acutely and continuously by people in addictive relationships. The addictive social system acts like a magnifying glass that concentrates into its focus a range of common negative emotions that take on an exaggerated form. The difference is not in the type of emotions but in their extent. The demands of living in an addictive relationship plus the effects of intoxication prevent normal processes of resolution from occurring. What in normal circumstances would be addressed and resolved in addictive contexts accumulates into one tangled unmanageable block that hangs deep within and obstructs movement in alternative directions.

Unshakable Commitment

As discussed in earlier chapters, the strongest and most perplexing aspect of an addictive relationship is the extent to which the person in it will go to ensure its survival. The commitment appears to override all other instincts, and loyalty to it can eclipse interests associated with the personal well-being as well as concerns about the well-being of the family and the community. From the vantage point of looking through the strands of intimacy, the question that comes into focus is: How can intimacy with an addictive substance/process override all other intimacies? What might explain such unshakable loyalty?

At least part of an answer can be identified in the way consumption of an addictive substance/process interacts with negative emotions and states of mind. In the early years of engaging in the intoxicating effects of an addictive relationship, the negative emotions associated with the four states of mind appear to diminish because intoxication provides periods of reprieve. For example, in the early years of his marriage Danny had recognized that after about three glasses of wine, instead of experiencing his normal range of feelings, such as specific frustrations, worries, and regrets, he found that these emotions dissipated and he began to feel relaxed and strongly connected to the social context in which he drank. As he continued to drink it seemed less of a worry that Julie would be angry with him for coming home late, it seemed less important that his boss was annoyed with him, and it was no longer a big deal that his traffic fines were mounting up. As he indulged more in this form of reprieve, he found that it also affected his general state of mind. He began to feel less general frustration; any sense of an impending disaster was replaced with a sense that he was able to handle any situation, and he no longer felt displaced and left out; on the contrary, he felt he was vitally connected to his fellow drinkers in a way that felt normal. Thus intoxication became an antidote to the poison of his accumulated negative emotions.

Intoxication can become the antidote to the poison of accumulated negative emotions

As the addictive relationship intensifies and social fragmentation and other deteriorating circumstances accrue, the affected person may attempt to break the commitment and to step outside the relationship. But, with some surprise, the person finds that stepping away is more complicated than it seems. For example, in earlier years when Cathy's two children were young, social workers had threatened to remove the children because of the squalid conditions in which they were being raised. In response, Cathy entered a detoxification unit vowing to the social workers that for the sake of the children she was going to stop using. Her family and friends responded immediately by praising her and celebrating the change. No more threats of overdose, no more police, no more living in substandard flats or uncertainty about whether the children would be fed; at last everything is going to sort itself out. Indeed, in stopping her use things outside did begin to improve.

She experienced fewer problems and she began to restore some of her relationships. However, as she moved beyond the initial improvements, the absence of periods of intoxication led her to experience the world very differently from those around her. As she later describes it to Dion in the inset box, below, being drug-free meant there was now no reprieve from her negative states of mind and associated emotions. At times she faced unrelenting feelings of frustration, anxiety, resentment, and alienation. Everyone around her was happy with her progress, but she was deeply unhappy and yearned to be back in a space where her feelings no longer mattered. She soon returned to using and, unfortunately, the period of going straight had only served to strengthen her commitment to the addictive relationship.

Both of the above examples (Danny and Cathy) illustrate some of the processes that entice and engage people into entering and committing themselves to addictive relationships. Once committed, they then find themselves caught in a dilemma between two undesirable positions: on one side is the intoxicated world of feeling normal but enduring the consequences; on the other side, is the bleak world of ongoing frustration, inadequacy, and alienation, but one that meets the approval of others. The more relief intoxication provides from these negative states of mind, the more social relationships deteriorate and fragment, and consequently the stronger the generalized negative feelings grow, reinforcing the need for further intoxication. People in addictive relationships find themselves trapped in an oscillating pattern of involvement, flip-flopping between drinking and abstaining, using and

> **Cathy/Dion: When I Stop...**
> Cathy is trying to describe to Dion what life would be like for her without drugs:
> "In the past, whenever I stopped using, the world outside celebrated. But inside... inside my inner self despairs."
> "But that's just the initial adjustment."
> "No. I have tried to live without drugs from time to time, but it never seems to last long. When people find out I've stopped, they are happy, they congratulate me and they open up more with me. To them the problem is solved... but for me it is anything but solved."
> "Well, surely things get better."
> "Maybe on the outside, but inside I feel awkward and exposed, strong feelings come up that I don't know what to do with and their expectations of me to be normal only confuse and frighten me more."

stopping, overindulging and cutting down; but throughout all these oscillations, commitment to the addictive relationship keeps managing to intensify and consolidate.

Ambivalent Accord

For people in addictive relationships, accord is very problematic and is the source of much internal conflict. On the one hand, the strengthening relationship to an addictive substance/process is transposed onto a circle of connections that are already well formed and that typically include relationships to partners, parents, children, and close friends. On the other hand they find themselves drawn ever closer and becoming more committed to the addictive relationship. Since the needs of both often clash, the accord—

already formed with their intimates—conflicts with the commitment forming with the addictive substance/process. They are now confronted with the challenge of shifting their commitment from real people to unfeeling objects as inert as alcohol. From the outside the likely winner is obvious, for surely the sense of unity between people is more potent than accord with things. What could be stronger than a husband's bond to his wife or a daughter's bond with her mother? Sadly this expectation is not likely to be met when it comes to addictive relationships. Commitment and identification with the addictive substance/process has the capacity to override all other bonds, no matter how strong. As discussed in earlier chapters, it is not just the immediate connection between the person and addictive substance/process that forms the connecting bond. The bond is built up via a reorganization of a person's whole framework of connections to form many layers of linkage to the addictive substance/process (see Chapter 3). This multilayered connection is what provides it with potency, and its combined strength tends in the long term to override the immediate sense of identification in person-to-person intimacies.

In the meantime, while the reorganization of connectedness is getting under way, this does not mean that people in addictive relationships simply switch off the accord they have built up with their intimates over many years. At many points they are likely to find themselves caught between the multilinked strength of the emerging addictive relationship and the solidly compassionate person-to-person accord, and this ambivalence can provide an important opportunity for intervention in the early and middle phases of an addictive relationship. For example, as described in the inset box, despite his gathering connectedness to his alcohol and drug use, Danny still retains a very strong sense of accord with his two children. He has made some half-hearted attempts at change, but it is not until his involvement with his children is threatened that he considers any serious efforts at change. In many similar circumstances, threats to person-to-person accord can provide sufficient incentive for people to at least question their allegiance to addictive relationships. As will be explored in later chapters, such incentives can also provide the basis for collective action.

> **Danny/Jack: Disruptive Visits**
>
> Julie has decided to put her foot down regarding Danny's visits with the children.
>
> "Look," Julie says looking straight into Danny's eyes, "I do not want you visiting us anymore here. I've asked you not to come here plastered, and every time you visit you stink of alcohol."
>
> "Julie, I'm having a difficult time at the moment. You know how much Adrienne and Luke mean to me."
>
> "Last weekend I left you with them and came home and you'd just left them watching videos while you were zonked out in the back room. They have so many things to do, and what's the point when you don't even talk to them."
>
> "I know, I know," pleads Danny. "I know it's not right. I need to change, and I will. I've booked myself into rehab and this time I know I have to change. I know it's my last chance. Please, please don't stop me coming. It means so much to me."

To summarize, this discussion has identified how in addictive relationships the four strands of intimacy form asymmetrical links between the person affected and the addictive substance/process. Furthermore, as the addictive relationship intensifies, the strands of connectedness with other intimates begin to change. The next section switches from the addictive relationship to examining the changes in intimacy for people in surrounding relationships.

Intimacies for Others

The main characteristic of intimacy for other people attached to an addictive social system is its asymmetry and its potential for deceptive symmetry. For the person in the addictive relationship, connection to the addictive substance/process gradually takes on more and more importance to a point where this hybrid intimacy gains priority over other connections. Relationships with other people fit into this system as long as they do not threaten the addictive relationship and as long as they serve some purpose for its survival. For others, particularly close family members, the reduced status of their relationships creates a priority imbalance, with aspects of their relationship—their feelings, needs, and resources—becoming of secondary concern. For long periods they might behave as if the priority of their relationships has not been downgraded; either they have not realized it yet or they pretend. As the addictive relationship intensifies and the priority imbalance becomes more obvious, they are eventually compelled to recognize the secondary nature of their relationships within the addictive social system. Curiously, once the imbalance is fully appreciated, a large proportion of intimates will still choose to remain in the system, bravely putting up with their reduced status. With their own needs and access to resources given significantly lower priority, the question now arises: how is it possible when the intimacy is so one-sided that membership of an addictive social system can still be so binding?

Why do intimates remain attached to these asymmetrical & unrewarding relationships?

This section explores the asymmetrical experience of intimacy for people closely connected to an addictive relationship, and discusses the one-sided nature of each of the four strands of intimacy: closeness, compassion, commitment, and accord.

Spasmodic Closeness

As people in addictive relationships devote more energy to obtaining and consuming their addictive substance/process, closeness in other relationships diminishes both in terms of proximity (space and time) and in terms of mental and emotional involvement. Intimates resist this shift with strategies involving pressure and surveillance, but the slide away seems unstoppable. Yet, there still remain moments of meaningful connection, times together where the person seems genuinely focused on the needs of the relationship and when both parties appear to connect and communicate with respect and affection. As these times become less common, they also become more important. Such moments signal the potential for the relationship to become

Danny/Jack: It's My Fault

Julie, while putting her son Luke to bed, is asked:

"Mom, why does Dad get so grumpy?"

"Since we separated he's been going through a hard time."

"Okay, but he used to get just as grumpy when he lived at home. Sometimes he's great. We go out and kick a ball around and have fun. But other times he just sits in the chair snapping at me if I make too much noise. I never know whether he's going to be fun or grumpy."

"He's been going through a hard time for a long while. I know he doesn't really want to be like that."

"Sometimes I think it's because of me he's grumpy. I then try hard to please him, not to make noise, not to nag him or anything."

"Oh, Luke, your dad really cares for you. It's not you he's mad with; he's more mad with the whole world, or himself, I dunno… but certainly not mad with you."

(or return to) a quality intimacy. In between patterns of roving presence and absence, sobriety and intoxication, and calmness and tension, these moments of closeness provide fleeting glimpses of the hope of symmetrical intimacy that almost cruelly serve to strengthen the resolve to keep striving.

The uncertainty and unpredictability of closeness is a potent process in itself. The irregularity is difficult to manage because it complicates the extent to which a person is willing to be in a relationship. For example, when it is uncertain whether or not employees are going to turn up for work, even if other aspects of their performance are adequate, for the employer the unpredictable absences outweighs all other considerations. Similarly, with intimacy, a person who is only unpredictably and episodically close provokes for the other party high levels of anxiety, often high enough to place the whole relationship at risk. For example, as illustrated in the inset box, above, Julie and Danny's ten-year-old son Luke has been feeling the effects of his father's unpredictable closeness for a long time. Before his parents separated he can remember some good times, and occasionally when his father came home from work they would talk and have fun together in a good way. However, at other times when Danny came home drunk, Luke can remember him being hugged, talked to, and laughed at in ways that made him feel uncomfortable. This unpredictability then extended into the separation. Now, sometimes when Danny visits he is sober but very irritable and Luke copes by shutting himself away in his room. At other times he arrives intoxicated and perhaps in a deeply black mood. Over time Luke has managed to adjust to each version of his father and knows which way to handle him best. The trouble is he never knows ahead of time which of these various versions of his father will walk through the door. In anticipation, he spends each day wondering and worrying about the next contact. His anxiety can rise to a point that he has difficulty enjoying the few times they are genuinely close. He finds that it works better when he reduces the uncertainty by maintaining a constant distance and not anticipating any closeness.

Unreciprocated Compassion

Unreciprocated compassion is the fountainhead out of which addictive relationships can cause boundless emotional pain to other intimates. People who have fallen in love with someone who does not love them in return will appreciate to some extent how this kind of asymmetry can lead to severe pain and hurt. To experience passionate feelings toward another person and the person remains emotionally unavailable is a special kind of torture. At one level the intimate feels repeatedly bruised and humiliated in their attempts at giving and sharing that in return are coldly dismissed and brushed aside. At another level the person experiences intense feelings of vulnerability, rejection, and worthlessness. At yet another level, the intimate is taunted by the uncertainty of potential symmetry: "Maybe I haven't tried hard enough"; "Maybe if I loved her more"; "Maybe it's safer not to try." These experiences of unreciprocated compassion over long periods of time can gradually corrode the capacity and the willingness to seek intimacy and further disempower intimates from forming other close relationships. To examine these processes further, two types of asymmetry need to be distinguished: *deceptive symmetry*, where the intimate is unaware that compassion will not be reciprocated; and *recognized asymmetry*, where the intimate understands what is going on.

The false belief that a relationship is emotionally symmetrical when in reality it is asymmetrical places intimates in very emotionally vulnerable positions. The person in the addictive relationship might actively pursue the false impression through strategies such as feigning emotional disclosures, promising changes, and occasional displays of affection. These may provide sufficient evidence for the intimate to carry on believing that their emotional worlds are synchronous. Alternatively, in situations with poor evidence of reciprocation, intimates might fabricate their own evidence through strategies such as interpreting episodic presences as highly significant, by pretending the troubles are only temporary or by dwelling on memories of the past. For example, Jacinta is spending more and more evenings playing on electronic gambling machines at the local bar. Wendy sometimes accompanies her, but Jacinta seems happier when she can sit at the machines by herself. This leaves Wendy spending many hours at home alone, and on evenings when Jacinta does stay at home, they often end up arguing about her absences and the drain on their finances (see inset box). While in her heart Wendy can feel their relationship slipping away, in her head she thinks of it as simply a phase Jacinta is going through and that she is still number one in her life. If she stands by her and keeps on loving her, their intimacy will eventually be revived to the same levels of closeness they had experienced in the past.

The brutal dimension of a deceptively symmetrical intimacy is the unexpected shock of direct encounters with this absence of compassion. Here the person in the addictive relationship appears to act in an unrecognizably cold-hearted fashion and seems desensitized

> **Jacinta/Wendy: Staying Out**
>
> Wendy challenges Jacinta when she comes home one night.
>
> "You said you were only going to spend a couple of hours on the slot machines in the bar. I waited and waited. It's been six hours."
>
> "Don't you want me to have some fun? I work hard all week at the supermarket and looking after Elliott. I just need some time to unwind."
>
> "But this keeps happening over and over. You never seem to think of the effect it is having on me."
>
> "Yeah, yeah. I've heard it all before."
>
> "I feel really lonely here by myself all the time. Can't we spend more time together?"
>
> "Look, I don't need this at the moment. I'm going to bed."
>
> "Hey, stop," Wendy yells as she marches to the door. "Come back and talk. Don't slam the…"

to the feelings of surrounding intimates. For those new to addictive systems, this is an unfamiliar world. The principles by which normal intimacies operate seem no longer to apply. The expectations and responsibilities that define roles in normal systems of intimacy—that of parents, children, lovers, friends—have been flipped over, and instead of compassion, the person encounters instances of deception, disloyalty, duplicity, heartlessness, and even violence and abuse. Perhaps driven by memories of how close the rela-

Expectations that define roles in normal contexts are flipped on their heads

tionship was in the past or perhaps unwilling to face the consequences of accepting this asymmetry or perhaps fearful of thinking otherwise, many intimates remain optimistically attached to addictive relationships despite continuing to encounter shocks and disappointments. Nonetheless, as the intensity of the addictive relationship builds and intimates are forced more and more into subservient support roles, acceptance of the asymmetry increases in probability.

Intimates who have come to realize the asymmetrical nature of such relationships are in a better position to manage and protect themselves from shock and disappointment. This adoption of *recognized asymmetry* is more realistic and enables them to adjust their expectations according to the varying emotional capacities of the person in the addictive relationship. This position can still involve intimacy, but not the symmetrical intimacies that occur between two people in normal circumstances. The intimacy can be thought of as resembling relationships that occur with nonhuman or inanimate objects (such as pets or cuddly toys), relationships in which it is unrealistic to expect compassion to be reciprocated. However, even in situations where an intimate fully appreciates that feelings are unlikely to be reciprocated, and even when the reasons for this lack of reciprocation are fully understood, it does not diminish the pain that results from unreciprocated love. The dismissal of anyone's emotional inner world is hurtful whether it is intentional or a product of other forces; such dismissals cuts to the core of being human.

To return to the previous example, over time Wendy is able to accept that Jacinta's gambling has become central in her life and that their relationship is a secondary concern. She achieves this by thinking of her as having something like a medical condition that prevents her from behaving consistently and considerately in close relationships. This understanding frees Wendy from expectations that she will behave any other way, and it enables her to stop feeling angry and focus more on what she can control in her own life. However, whenever Jacinta is in close physical proximity, Wendy still feels overwhelming sadness at losing the closeness and compassion they once had.

One-Sided Commitment

A person typically enters an addictive relationship with a range of intimacy commitments already well formed. These might include an ongoing connection to parents, a marriage, a responsibility for dependent children, and perhaps a commitment to a close circle of friends. As the addictive relationship asserts priority over these other intimacies, commitment to them begins to wane. Less time is shared with them and interactions occur unpredictably. Their relationships shift from having value in themselves to having value for other purposes; for instance, they are treated more as sources of money or as mechanisms for covering up misdemeanors (see inset box). Whenever these shifts are contested, new elements are introduced into the relationships in order to contain matters. These might involve strategies such as violence and deception that aim to control, distort, and distract intimates from effective challenge. For these intimates, it steadily becomes clearer that they are now connected into relationships in which the other party has little commitment to its quality. Whatever the strength of the relationship in the past, intimates now find it is their energy which is maintaining the relationship with little hope of meaningful reciprocation. What is surprising here is how many intimates in these situations choose to maintain their commitment and maintain it for large portions of their lives.[7] The following looks at several factors that might account for why intimates remain committed to these one-sided and predominantly low-quality relationships.

> **Bert/Joan: Disloyalty**
> At a party at work, Joan has a chance to speak with William, who was a close colleague of Bert's.
> "William, how come you and Bert don't get together much anymore?"
> "That's a long story... you sure you want to hear it? Well, Bert and I had lot of hard times together. We fought side by side for the union, we dealt with difficult people, and we made changes to the system. Through all this Bert and I grew closer and closer. We relied on each other and backed each other up."
> "Yeah, he's always spoken highly of you."
> "Umm, but over the years I knew he was drinking more and more. Sure, he confined his drinking till after work and made sure it didn't interfere with our activities, but I could tell he was handling things differently. But then we hit a very major crisis that threatened both our jobs, and he suddenly turned on me. He blamed me for the crisis and accused me of being disloyal."
> "I know what that can be like."
> "I couldn't understand how he could be so cold and heartless. He refused to speak with me and it seemed as if all our time together had come to nothing. I tell you this in confidence and because I respect you... In hindsight it felt to me that all along our relationship had been based on how useful I was to him, and then when I was no longer useful, I was cast aside like a worn out pair of shoes."

One important factor is the inertia created by broader involvements. People in addictive social systems, including people in the addictive relationship, maintain a network of other connections around them. For example, a child is typically connected to school, to friends, to sports interests, and to neighborhood play. To abandon commitment to a parent in an addictive relationship by, for instance, running away from home, has the potential to disrupt all these other involvements. Each relationship occurs within a system or network of other connections, and disrupting one is likely to lead to disruptions in others. Accordingly, it makes sense to put up with the negative impacts of the addictive relationship for the sake of maintaining all the other connections. For example, for Joan, Bert's drinking has transformed the home environment negatively, with her life and the lives of their children exposed to his erratic behavior and episodes of chaos and abuse. She often thinks of leaving, but she recognizes that leaving would disrupt all they have worked toward during the last twenty years; she has invested so much time and money into the building and design of their home and their beautiful garden, they contribute significantly to the local community and the school, and all her friends live close by and most of them have involvements with

Bert/Joan: Frogs

Joan and her sister Mary are sitting in a café discussing the troubles Joan is experiencing in her marriage. Mary says, "I can't understand why you've stayed with him for so long."

"Yes, looking back it's a bit weird."

"In other parts of your life you are so strong. I've always admired that in you."

"Mmm, I never thought I would let that sort of thing happen and end up in this sort of marriage." Joan pauses and stares at a glass of water. "I guess, I make sense of it... I make sense of it by thinking of myself like a frog."

"What?"

"Well, when a frog is put in a pot of boiling water, it instantly knows it's in peril and it jumps out. But when a frog is placed in a pot of cold water and the pot is heated gradually, the frog gets accustomed to it and stays put until it's too late, and it's boiled to death."

"Nice one."

"This is what happened to me."

"You got boiled to death?"

"No." They both laugh. "When Bert and I first got married we were very close. We shared everything."

"Yes, I remember, two little lovebirds."

"He didn't change suddenly into the drunken oaf he is today. It happened gradually, bit by bit. I kept making allowances for him and remembering the good times. By the time it was obvious, it was too late; I was too immersed in children and home, and too afraid to challenge the status quo, so I just gave in and let it roll on."

Bert too. "No, leaving would spoil all this," and she concludes that it is worth putting up with other unpleasantness.

Another factor for remaining committed is the typically slow and disguised way in which addictive relationships tend to emerge (see inset box). For many intimates, the person in the addictive relationship is more than someone who treats loved ones poorly; he or she once reciprocated high levels of closeness, compassion, and love. Memories of these times plus momentary glimpses every now and then are often sufficient to keep the embers of hope alive. Intimates might rationalize their one-sided commitment by telling themselves that the other person's commitment still lurks there somewhere underneath. Joan might tell herself, "This isn't his true self"; "I still see the little boy in him"; "He is still the same person I married." The contrast between memories of what the person was and how the person now presents is blurred and difficult to see, which consequently poses difficulties in reviewing the ongoing commitment.

Other factors also contribute to the ongoing commitment. For example, intimates may be genuinely afraid to disconnect due to violence, intimidation, and other controlling behaviors (the focus of the next chapter). Also, these and other negative impacts can lead to reduced self-esteem, and intimates may gradually lose confidence in their ability to make decisions and act, two key ingredients when looking at change. This is often compounded by levels of guilt and self-blame where intimates see themselves as responsible for deteriorations in relationships, which leads them to increase rather than decrease their level of commitment. Furthermore, the social expectations associated with particular roles (such as being a partner or a parent) exert a strong influence: "I made a vow of commitment to her 'through sickness and in health' at our wedding." Children are expected to remain devoted to their parents, parents to their children, spouses to their partners, employees to their workers, and best friends to each other. Knowledge of what these roles and associated expectations of loyalty and commitment mean is a common resource within the broader social networks. These expectations can act as discouragers of change, particularly when those outside have little evidence that things are amiss within the relationship.[8] These factors (some of which have been discussed in preceding chapters) individually and collective provide pressure on intimates to retain ongoing commitment to the addicted social system.

Unilateral Accord

The sense of accord for intimates toward the person in the addictive relationship tends to diminish earlier than commitment. As the addictive relationship intensifies, intimates compete with it for opportunities for closeness, but, despite their best efforts, they find progressively less compassion is reciprocated. Any residual sense of accord or unity progressively fades like flowers without sun, leaving commitment as the main binding force. However, accord can still play a part, particularly in the early and middle stages of an addictive system. Intimates retain and sometimes cherish a sense of accord even while their circumstances are in crisis. Furthermore, the type of accord varies according to the role intimates play within the addictive system. The child experiences accord differently than a parent does, and the partner differently than a friend does. The following discussion briefly reviews some of these differences, leaving it to Chapter 8 to expand on these roles more fully.

For young children, their relationship with their parents is usually their first experience of intimacy, and attachment here acts as the blueprint for the intimate attachments to come.[9] As a child's parent becomes increasingly preoccupied by an addictive relationship, the extent and regularity of connection is reduced, but this relationship is important as the child's first exposure to intimacy, which means it typically persists as it a special relationship. As children mature, they learn to stay physically close but emotionally distant. This protects them from the unpredictability and other negative features of the relationship. Nonetheless, the sense of being linked to a parent despite damaging behavior can persist throughout and into adolescence (see inset box, below). Similarly, for parents, the task of bringing children into the world, rearing them, caring for them, and guiding their development creates a sense of connection that can endure many of the disturbing episodes of intoxication, associated risk, and episodes of abuse that typically occur with adolescent addictive relationships. Despite repeated disappointments and ongoing hurtfulness, parents often perceive a fundamental level of connection that persists throughout the most trying of circumstances. For partners and lovers, the sense of unity and accord has evolved out of many years of close contact and shared experience. As discussed earlier, despite ongoing transgressions, remnants of accord can persist fueled by memories of past togetherness or by unpredictable moments of closeness. Similarly for close friends, depending on the length and depth of previous closeness, the bond of friendship for many will endure for some time.

Jacinta/Wendy: I Want to Be with Her

During one of Jacinta's many evening absences, Wendy is chatting with their son, Elliott, when he says, "It's nice just the two of us; more quiet and calm. But I still miss Jacinta."

"But you see a lot of her during the day after school."

"Yes, but I'm busy doing homework and practicing piano and she's too busy to talk. It's now, when you get home, that we all should be together."

"But sometimes we argue."

"I know. That's nasty. But other times it's fine and I want to be with her so we can talk and laugh."

Systems of Intimate Connections

This chapter has examined the processes associated with intimacy in an addictive relationship and the surrounding close relationships. To reduce the complexities, attention has focused on intimacies as they occur one by one. In actuality they seldom occur in isolation and are typically entangled in a complex and multilayered network of relationships. For each member of this system, the circle of intimates surrounding one person overlaps and interlocks with the circles of intimates around other people. The strength of these interlocking circles then form into layers of increasing closeness around each person, and on the closest layer, the layer where there is the strongest overlap, that is where people identify as family. Consequently, for the purposes of this discussion, the term *family* refers to the layer of strongest interlocking intimacy around a person. This understanding is intentionally broad and recognizes both the traditional meaning of family as a group of people connected by blood or marriage as well as the looser understanding of a group without blood or marital links connected purely by varying degrees of closeness, compassion, commitment, and accord. Secondary layers involving less connection and overlap are referred to as either extended families or friendship networks. Subsequent layers refer to related contexts such as neighborhoods, collegial networks, communities of concern, and other communities.

Family *refers to circles of interlocking intimacy*

A diverse body of literature focusing on families as social systems has been published. The notion of a *system* is particularly important for two reasons: First, a *system* involves complex interactions where one point in its networks is connected in multiple ways to other points. Between any two points, besides the direct links, there are also indirect links where one point links back to another point through a series of other links. This complex and dynamic network means that whatever happens at one point will have consequences for other points throughout the system. Second, systems behave differently than their component parts. For example, looking at the cooling system in a car, the radiator plays a role, but we cannot understand its role by looking only at the radiator. It needs to be observed relative to other parts before its characteristics begin to make sense.

The application of systems theory to families affected by addictive relationships has generated a range of approaches to intervention. For example, Peter Steinglass and his team in their book *The Alcoholic Family*[10] applied understandings from systems theory, as developed for use in family therapy, to addictive systems. They began by emphasizing the adaptive and resilient qualities of families:

> Aware of the existence of this multiplicity of internal and external stresses, the observer of family behavior cannot help but be impressed by the ability of the family to manage and control these challenges. Despite living in a constantly changing environment, and despite sudden and unpredictable encounters, the family is able to maintain a sense of balance, a coherence, a regularity to its life. It is quite

an impressive performance. To account for it, it seems that there must be powerful "built in" mechanisms that regulate family life by providing organizational structure and by helping to determine the rules that govern sequential behavioral processes.[11]

According to them, as any family does when responding to change, they adapt to the strengthening addictive relationship in their midst by striving to restore an optimal point of balance between what is happening outside the system and what is going on inside. This balance, or homeostasis, enables the family system to survive as a unit through periods of internal and external rupture and change. To explain these processes in more detail, Steinglass and his team adopted two psychological constructs: family temperament and family identity. Family temperament refers to the collective response styles that families take on in establishing routines and solving problems. Each family varies in how they might do this. Some respond with low energy and rigid boundaries and tend to exclude outsiders from what is going on. Other families respond with high energy, swapping roles as the need arises, and including others as often as they see fit.

As can be seen from their description, the family operates as a unit by principles and processes that are different from those of its members. The system has a life of its own. They extend this system by arguing that families also evolve identities of their own, and that the addictive family system will adopt its own special identity. The development of this family identity involves the gradual emergence of major regulatory principles for family life. When an addictive relationship forms within a family, the family as a whole is challenged as to whether it adjusts and adapts or whether it excludes the addictive relationship and continues to function with the addictive relationship on the sideline (or working around it). In situations where families decide to adjust, they are then faced with the long task of reforming their identity with the addictive relationship as a vital part. This process of family adjustment occurs over a long period of time and can be broken into three phases: early, middle, and late. The early phase involves the formation of the alcoholic family identity. The middle phase entails the family system reaching an equilibrium or homeostasis, where the family establishes its own regulatory systems and temperament. The late phase involves adapting to changes brought on by unmanageable deteriorations in relationships and life circumstances. The early and late phases are about change and transition, whereas the middle phase is about stability and the maintenance of boundaries.[12]

Families respond as a whole by seeking ways to adapt to changing circumstances

In terms of a social paradigm, the approach developed by Steinglass and his colleagues is limited because it tends to apply particle psychology to social systems, a move that almost attributes human qualities to collections of people. For instance, this can be seen in the way they speak of family systems as having their own motivations and temperaments. Despite these reservations, for the purposes of the current analysis, their approach does highlight three salient points. First, their approach recognizes families (or overlapping circles of intimacy) as systems that operate in dynamic and interactive ways.

Strength of Strands Across Phases			
	Early	Middle	Late
Closeness	Irregular	Minimal	Absent
Compassion	Strong	Waning	Absent
Commitment	Strong	Strong	Challenged
Accord	Waning	Absent	Absent

Changes to one part of the system entail changes to another. Second, it recognizes how the social processes between people can work differently from those of the individual; the family has a life of its own. Third, its division of family responses into early, middle, and late phases recognizes the slow process of change associated with addictive relationships in families. The table in previous page takes these phases and lays out how they might apply to the four strands of intimacy. As discussed earlier, a sense of unity and accord is the first to be affected, with closeness and compassion phasing out simultaneously, leaving commitment as the last binding strand before it too is challenged in the late stages.

This chapter has explored the importance of asymmetry in intimacies within an addictive system. It has illustrated ways in which addictive relationships distort, fragment and rupture connections within overlapping circles of intimacy (the family) and how they generate low quality and asymmetrical or deceptively symmetrical intimacy. The next chapter examines the use of violence as the ultimate expression of asymmetrical processes within intimacy relationships.

Chapter 7

Intimacy and Power

By and by he [Huck's Pap] rolled out and jumped up onto his feet looking wild, and he see me and went for me. He chased me round and round the place with a clasp-knife, calling me the Angel of Death, and saying he would kill me, and then I couldn't come for him no more. I begged, and told him I was only Huck; but he laughed such a screechy laugh, and roared and cussed, and kept on chasing me up. Once when I turned short and dodged under his arm he made a grab and got me by the jacket between my shoulders, and I thought I was gone; but I slid out of the jacket quick as lightning, and saved myself. Pretty soon he was all tired out, and dropped down with his back against the door, and said he would rest a minute and then kill me. He put his knife under him, and said he would sleep and get strong, and then he would see who was who.

(Mark Twain, "Huckleberry Finn"[1])

The previous chapter surveyed the general ways in which fragmenting asymmetries evolve in addictive systems, but the observation that these asymmetries occur does not explain how they are achieved. Attention now shifts to the processes and techniques that make these asymmetries possible. The passage above describes a critical point in *Huckleberry Finn* where Huck's father (Pap), who is in an addictive relationship to alcohol, attempts to kill Huck. Huck responds by leaving town to pursue his life on the river. While this level of physical violence does not occur within every addictive system, abuse and other forms of controlling behavior are commonplace. Such controlling tactics vary in degree—from slaps to fatal stabbings—and in kind—from verbal threats to ongoing surveillance. What is common to all these strategies is that they involve an attempt of one person in a relationship to impose a level of power over the other person.

Power is a critical concept in making sense of how relationships operate. Every relationship involves differences in power, and these differences are often a necessary part of both orderly social functioning and the definition and maintenance of social roles. In some relationships one party is more powerful because they have access to skills and resources that the other party lacks. For example, the recognition of teachers and doctors as having superior understanding is a necessary part of entering into relationships for the purpose of learning or being cured. At other times this imbalance is reversed. For example, in the interactions between a brother and sister, the brother might access one type of power because he has a license and a car and can drive himself places whenever he wishes, but the sister may have more access to friends, so unlike her brother she has more

105

P.J. Adams, *Fragmented Intimacy: Addiction in a Social World*
© Springer 2008

choices in terms of access to social events. Their different access to these resources positions them at different times with strategically more power; he can negotiate around access to transportation while she can negotiate around access to social events.

Normal intimacies involve a dynamic seesawing of differences levels of power

In normal intimacies, this dynamic seesawing in positions of power is common. For example, in many necessary ways parents of young children operate with more power, which they use for their children's guidance and protection; as the children develop in their teenage years, this power is progressively challenged as a means for adolescents to establish zones of their own powerfulness.

In a social world, and particularly within intimate relationships, power is utilized in two importantly different ways: power to and power over. The use of power in the sense of *power to*, is characterized by a willingness by one party to accept a degree of powerlessness in order to be able to achieve a greater purpose, as in power to learn, power to win, power to heal, and, importantly for this book, power to become intimate. *Power over* involves an explicit asymmetrical use of power in which the willingness of the less powerful is not considered. For example, when Stalin inflicted his purges on the people of the Soviet Union, he imposed his intent without consideration of the will of his people; he made use of *power over* because the secret police had created sufficient fear for people not to resist. Similarly in intimate relationships *power over* involves the imposition of one person's will over the wishes and willingness of another person. This is usually achieved by means of a series of controlling tactics that create a platform of fear and deception upon which it is then easy for one person to impose power over another. For those who become overwhelmed by this use of *power over*, they soon find themselves behaving, thinking, and feeling according to the needs of that other person and either subjugate or lose sight of their own needs.

This chapter explores how controlling tactics are used to achieve asymmetrical positions of *power over* within addictive relationships. It focuses on how violence and other person-controlling behaviors are used to preserve the addictive social system from threats of discovery, challenge, and coordinated opposition.

Controlling Tactics

It is tempting for those outside looking in on an intimacy where violence is occurring to become preoccupied with the horror of seeing the outcome of one particular beating, but the effect of this one act pales in comparison with the cumulative effects of multiple beatings and repeated episodes of intimidation, humiliation, and other terror provoking tactics.

The potency of violent behavior only makes sense when placed within the context of an integrated program of other abusive acts. A slap, an insult, a lie, a threat, a broken promise—each act, as an isolated incident, may not appear to have major significance, but when taken together the effect of each act functions interactively, contributing cumulatively to a complex fabric that serves to enmesh the recipient (see common examples in inset box, on side). For example, a minor criticism of a partner's appearance, when placed in context with repeated messages of inadequacy and backed up by physical intimidation, can have a major impact on the partner's level of self-esteem. Similarly, the timing and mode of delivery can amplify the effects of the abuse. For example, a man who adopts strategies of occasional and unpredictable violence toward his partner can effectively promote sustained periods of fearfulness; his partner can never be sure when to expect the next round of abuse, and thus she is caught in a constant state of anxious vigilance. In this way the effects of the brief and infrequent episodes of violence gradually permeate the longer periods containing no obvious violence.

Besides the systematic and programmatic use of controlling tactics, from the point of view of a person receiving the abuse, their effects are cumulative and global. Unpredictable physical violence at one point in a relationship triggers ongoing vigilance regarding whether it will happen again. As described in the inset box, the recipient is constantly monitoring for signs that might indicate upcoming abuse. This vigilance enables the man to promote fear using signals and prompts. It may only take a slight change in intonation or the raising of an eyebrow for him to prompt her terror and guarantee her compliance. Episodes of stronger abuse may be required from time to time to restrengthen the link, but in the longer term this becomes less necessary and the prompts are usually all that is required. In this way the cumulative association between violence and other behaviors enables the effects

---

Common Controlling Tactics

Physical, sexual, and emotional abuse
• Hitting, punching, shoving, stabbing
• Sexual coercion, sexual ridicule, rape
• Mind games, put downs, humiliation

Intimidation
• Strong-arm tactics, blocking doors
• Shouting, posturing, breaking objects
• Hinting at violent potential

Restricting freedoms
• Controlling money, credit, transportation
• Denying access to information and mail
• Controlling access to alcohol and drugs

Surveillance systems
• Watching, following, spying, stalking
• Questioning, interrogating, torturing
• Confining into monitorable spaces

Controlling other people
• Restricting access to friends, children, pets
• Lying, implying false judgment, deceiving
• Imposing one's own version of events

Imposing fragmentation
• Interfering and splitting up other relationships
• Isolating from social involvement or activities
• Imposing silence regarding important issues

Bert/Joan: Ongoing Fear

Joan is visiting her physician because of a black eye.

"Joan, this isn't the first time he's hit you."

"No, it's happened before." She pauses, quietly staring at the floor. "I'm frightened of him now most of the time. At first I thought he hit me because he was drunk and couldn't help himself. But now he hits me whether he's drunk or not."

"Joan, you don't deserve to be treated like this."

"What's worse, I don't know when it's going to happen. Sometimes when major things go wrong he is very understanding but at other times, even over very small things, he just explodes and I know I'm in for it."

"That must be really scary."

"Sometimes he doesn't hit me; he just glowers, or stares at me, or stands across the doorway. But the effect is the same… it's just as scary. I instantly remember all the other times he has hurt me and I feel just as terrified whether he hits me or not." She looks up. "Look, I'm sorry, I shouldn't be talking to you about this. Please, don't tell him or anybody else. It would destroy our home."

of violence to spread into every corner of victim's lives.[2] It affects them physically, mentally, emotionally, and socially.

The use of violence and other controlling tactics is common in addictive social systems, and their co-occurrence can be observed from several different angles.[3] Practitioners and community professionals regularly encounter the consequences of alcohol and drug use and violence.[4] For example, family physicians may hear accounts of violence from the partners of heavy alcohol- and drug-using patients. Similarly, professionals working in law enforcement and other justice agencies (police, courts, prisons, probation) are confronted on a daily basis with the association of violence with the use of addictive substances/processes.[5] This is not only obvious in assaults and other violent crime, but it can also emerge as a part in custody disputes, theft and fraud. For example, controlling tactics may emerge as a means of forcing family members into handing over their savings to support an addictive relationship to gambling. Those working with people affected by violence through shelters, women's programs, and men's stopping violence programs tend to find that alcohol and drug intoxication is a factor in as many as half of their clientele, with a sizable portion (perhaps as high as a fifth to a quarter of clients) affected by addictive relationships.[6] From another angle, controlling tactics are also commonly present with clients presenting to addiction services.[7] This becomes more obvious when practitioners and services have fostered an awareness of violence issues and when information is actively sought from other family members.

Violence & other controlling tactics are commonplace in addictive systems

A major challenge here involves untangling the effects of intoxication within an addictive social system from the effects of intoxication alone. All addictive relationships involve intoxication at some level, but not all intoxication occurs with people in addictive relationships. People choose to become intoxicated to addictive substance/processes for a wide variety of reasons. An adolescent may seek to get drunk as a socially approved way of being accepted into a peer group or of signaling one's entry into adulthood. For others intoxication is used to boost confidence, to provide entertainment, and to lubricate social events. Often in the course of such usage, violence and other antisocial behaviors occur, thereby reinforcing the impression that intoxication is the main driver for interpersonal violence. However, in many situations, the presence of intoxication may mask the contribution of addictive processes. Unfortunately, from outside an addictive social system it is seldom clear whether a person's intoxication is driven by addictive processes or by some other intent. When addictive relationships are present, there also tends to be elaborate systems in place to conceal information about what is really going on from the gaze of outsiders. While outsiders (such as neighbors or work colleagues) may have some inkling that the person is upset, the information is fragmentary and leaves them in doubt as to what is really going on. This doubt encourages them to conservatively assume that it is intoxication rather than addiction that is the active ingredient.

The Myth of Disinhibition

In the description in the inset box, Joan is assaulted by her intoxicated husband. It happens on an irregular basis but frequent enough for Joan to experience high levels of anxiety most of the time. As a result of the violence she feels as if she is constantly walking on egg shells, worrying about saying or doing the wrong thing, worrying that he is watching her and will find out what she is thinking and doing, worrying what will happen each evening: Will he hurt her physically? Will he pursue a long session of interrogation and humiliation? The outcome of her various worries is that she remains constantly terrified by the prospect of his violence. She is also concerned about the effects on their two young children; they must have seen or heard things, but they have said nothing. Fear pursues her all day and drives out other emotions. She does not talk to friends because she is afraid of the consequences of Bert finding out and because she is embarrassed by her weakness. She feels isolated and lacks confidence, and her head is full of thoughts about the way Bert looks at the world.

> ### Bert/Joan: Bert's Homecoming
>
> Lying awake in bed at 2 a.m., Joan has spent the last two anxious hours waiting for Bert to return. The car is coming now; she can see the lights through the curtain. The sight fills her with dread. She hears the car door slam. Is he in a good or a bad mood? She hears him trip on the steps, cursing loudly at the darkness, and continuing to curse as he wrestles with the key in the front door. She recognizes that he's not in a good mood tonight.
>
> He staggers into the room, glaring at her in the bed. "So what's this I hear about you wanting to visit your mother's?"
>
> "She's been sick."
>
> "Thought you could go without me finding out?" He continues to glare at her. "Fuck, she's a useless old cow. Filling your head with nonsense about you doing your own thing. The bitch never liked me."
>
> He lurches suddenly across to the bed and grabs at Joan. She is quick to move away but with one hand he manages to grab her nightgown and with the other he hits her hard across her chest. She yells from the pain and the shock.
>
> "You are not going to see that bitch." He continues to hit her. "She's done nothing for us but gripe and complain…"

The role alcohol plays in Bert's behavior could be understood in several ways. It could be that Bert, normally a quiet and polite man, tends to lose his inhibitions when he drinks. Just as people when drunk are more likely to say things they regret, so when he drinks the feelings he normally suppresses come blurting out in an uncontrolled fashion, and every now and then this spills over into violent outrages. A second way of looking at this is to view Bert as someone who is highly concerned that his behavior is understandable and defensible, particularly in the eyes of his male work colleagues. In his own eyes, punishment is a necessary process for maintaining order in the home, so he needs to use it. But he also knows he has to be careful because not everyone would agree with him. For this reason he reserves his violence for a time that most of his friends would appreciate as being understandable: when he is intoxicated. After all, everyone knows that intoxicated people lose control, hence in his male social circle this drunken violent behavior will appear fairly natural.

Another way to look at Bert's abuse is to widen the gaze and to view his actions as very much under his control and that the violence is there intentionally in order to maintain a position of power. Several aspects of the scenario indicate a managed event: it occurs at home late at night when few people are likely to hear; he hits Joan across her chest and other parts of her central trunk where she is normally clothed and thereby reduces later chances of detection, and he is unpredictably violent thereby maximizing her fearfulness. Furthermore, the target of his outrage, her contact with her mother, is important as a challenge to his control. He knows his power over her will weaken if she is able to find other sources of support and to hear from them messages that might challenge his authority.

Still another way to look at his behavior concurs with the previous view that the violence is a controlled event aimed at minimizing threats, but the reason is less to preserve his role as a man in charge at home, but to minimize threats to his addictive relationship to alcohol. Within his circle of intimates Joan stands out as having the capacity to mount a major challenge to his drinking. It is important to keep her weak and subordinate in order to prevent her from ever effectively challenging his commitment to the addictive relationship.

Particle Explanations

As discussed in Chapter 2, theories from within a particle paradigm draw on biological or psychological understandings that explain events in terms of attributes and processes associated with people as discrete individuals (or particles). Social and other contextual processes are acknowledged but are usually attached peripherally to the individual. When it comes to making sense of the strong relationship between violence and addictive substances/processes, various attempts have been made to apply *Particle* particle-derived explanations. Most of these have focused on alcohol and *explanations* tend to explain its relationship to violence in terms of its disinhibiting *focus on the* effects.[8] The two main variants are biology-oriented and psychology-*disinhibiting* oriented particle explanations, both of which emphasize processes occurring *effects of* within the person.
intoxication Biology-oriented particle explanations focus primarily on mechanisms in the brain, and alcohol has attracted the most attention to date.[9] Alcohol acts essentially as a central nervous system depressant and is transported by blood into the brain and progressively depresses activity across the large outer folds of the brain called the cerebral cortex. In the early stages of drinking it initially affects the blood's main entry point in the middle part of the cortex, which controls motor coordination; the drinker begins to make mistakes in their muscle movements. From there its action spreads backward to affect vision and forward to affect judgment and behavior control. As its action spreads, it depresses brain activity in two ways: it first depresses activity that restricts and inhibits behavior, which leads the drinker to do and say things that they would normally avoid; it later depresses brain activity that stimulates behavior leading to effects such as lethargy and drowsiness. It is alcohol's action at the very front of the brain in the first disinhibitory stage that is of most interest in understanding its relationship to violence. This has led to an

interest in the role certain neurotransmitters,[10] particularly in reducing the levels of serotonin in the brain, which animal studies have shown moderates aggressive behavior.[11] This work has also led onto genetic studies looking at how variations in serotonin levels might explain why some people are more prone to being aggressive when intoxicated than others.

Psychology-oriented particle explanations build on biological notions of disinhibition and use a variety of brain-behavior models (or "mental models") to explain the association. For example, in the inset box, above, Bert's explanation to his friend makes use of the simplest and perhaps most common model which links the concept of pressure to the reasons for violent outbursts. In this model the mind is viewed as a closed container that, as it fills, builds up tension and pressure, leading inevitably to a collapse or explosion. It is much like filling a tank placed on flimsy supports, eventually something gives and the whole structure comes tumbling down and "I just lose it." The inset box below lists examples of the use of other common mental models linking mental processes to violence. For each one, alcohol is the final trigger of aggressive behavior for psychological processes that are already well established. For example, in the coiled-spring model, past trauma and resentments accumulate into ongoing rage. This rage could emerge at any time but is more likely to be expressed when intoxicated. In this way, intoxication is viewed less as a driver for violent outbursts and more as a catalyst for behaviors that are likely to emerge in some form eventually. Furthermore, notice how in each example the source of violence is located within the psyche without considering the influence of social and other contextual issues.

> **Bert/Joan: "I Just Lose It"**
> During his morning coffee break, Bert is sitting outside the back of the store chatting to a close work colleague, William. Bert looks up and says, "When I'm pushed enough, when people hassle me, when they go on and on at me about this and that, I feel this pressure building up inside, to a point where I feel I'm going to snap."
> "Shit, everyone has their breaking point, man." They pause, and look at the windows of the building next door.
> "And that point usually comes when I've had a few too many drinks. When I drink it's like all the pressure built up earlier that has nowhere to go, now is primed and ready for release. I'm ready to go, and it only takes one person to say the wrong thing and I just lose it."
> "Yeah, and it all comes tumbling out. Sure, that's normal. Everyone loses it a bit when they're drunk... say and do things they later regret."
> "Yeah, and last night I yelled at the kids."

> **Mental Models of Disinhibition**
> *Hydraulic pressure*:
> "Pressure just builds and builds in me over time like water in a blocked pipe until I can't stand it anymore and I just burst, and it tends to happen when I've been drinking."
> *Coiled spring*:
> "The events of my childhood, the poverty and abuse from my father, have wound me up so much that it only takes a small insult for all this inner pain and resentment to pour out, making some poor unsuspecting person a target for all my inner rage."
> *Personality change*:
> "When I've been drinking something happens in my head that causes my personality to change. Things that don't normally annoy me get to me and I'm ready to take anyone on."
> *Skills deficit*:
> "When I feel a strong emotion, I lack the ability to both control how I react, and how I express my feelings so that when I'm angry and I drink it all tumbles out in an ugly mess."

Problems with Particles

Particle models focusing on disinhibition are the major explanatory resource used in relationships, in therapy, and in research to account for the link between violence and addictive relationships. Despite widespread use, their application is questionable on a number of fronts.[12] For example, research on affected populations indicates that chronic abuse of alcohol is a more important factor than disinhibition; in other words having an overall intense relationship to alcohol matters more than being drunk at the time.[13] Of even more pressing concern is that on closer inspection the notion of disinhibition does not fit with many of the features of intoxicated violence in families.

Here are four such inconsistencies:

1. Violence also occurs outside intoxication. Family members often report that, while they acknowledge episodes of severe abuse happen during intoxication, violence is not reserved exclusively to these times; the full array of controlling tactics are just as likely to happen when the person is sober or straight.[14] Some of the more subtle tactics, such as mind games and surveillance strategies, are more likely to happen when the person is not intoxicated. For instance, when Bert is drunk his controlling tactics consist of shouting and other forms of intimidation. When he is sober he resorts to putting intimates down and restricting their access to money and mobility. But these are not set in concrete; Bert from time to time uses scare tactics when sober and surveillance and restricting freedoms when intoxicated. If disinhibition were really the key driver, then virtually none of these controlling tactics would happen outside of his being intoxicated; for most intimates caught in an addictive social system, this is clearly not the case.

2. Violence happens with other addictive substances/processes. Violence and other controlling tactics are also surprisingly commonplace in addictive relationships to other drugs, even drugs with an apparently calming effect such as cannabis or minor tranquilizers.[15] Furthermore, similar patterns of violence can be observed with addictive relationships to things other than substances such as gambling, sex, and work.[16] For example, in the inset box, Julie describes how Danny could be just as abusive to her whether he was intoxicated to alcohol or cannabis. It could be argued that similar brain pathways are activated for each of these substances and processes in ways that lead to similar disinhibition. But this would be stretching the argument somewhat. If a range of brain mechanisms are involved, leading to very similar effects, it seems highly unlikely that they would converge on common pathways.

3. The delivery is highly crafted. Violence and other controlling tactics in addictive systems are not deployed in a disorganized and random fashion. The tactics are typically used in skillfully

---

Danny/Jack: Cannabis

Julie is talking to Jack, trying to explain her reasons for leaving his son, Danny.

"One thing that confused me was his smoking weed… I thought cannabis was meant to make a person calmer and mellower."

"Yeah, I thought it was better than grog."

"Well, one time Danny came home from work and he'd only been smoking cannabis, a lot of cannabis, I could tell because his eyes were all bloodshot and he didn't smell of booze. For some reason he was hopping mad. Maybe things had gone bad at work, maybe they'd noticed his condition, too."

"His boss did talk to me a couple of times about that."

"Anyway, he launched into me about fancying another guy or something. He ranted and raved for ages. He didn't hit me, but he threw things, kicked a hole in the wall, and his yelling was very loud. I was really scared and I could see the children were terrified."

"I'm sorry you went through that."

"It's not your fault but I knew then that we couldn't go on like this."

managed and coordinated ways that suggest the user is practiced and familiar with how the tactics operate and their likely effects. The combination of tactics can include episodic physical abuse, regular put-downs and humiliation, and elaborate strategies aimed at isolating family from potential supports. In contrast to intoxication where multiple use of strategies are likely to be affected by poor judgments and rash decisions, in addictive systems violence is employed in ways that influence the behavior of everyone in that system. As can be seen by the earlier example of Bert's homecoming (see earlier inset box), intoxicated intimate partner violence can and does involve a range of fine grade judgments that ensure the violence is not detected and that its impact will generate maximal fear. This coordinated use of power over is not consistent with other examples of intoxicated behavior (such as drunk socializing or drunk driving) where judgments are affected and behaviors are poorly managed.

4. The control is effective over long periods. Besides being an organized event, the combination of controlling tactics tends to be deployed in a highly effective fashion. The tactics are not only effective with one person, but also typically maintain deep and sustained levels of fear for everyone in the addictive system. Furthermore, it is not unusual for people who reflect back on their childhoods within an addictive system to comment on how fearful they had been over a long period of time, perhaps well into their later lives[17] (see inset box). Again, this use of tactics of interpersonal control with many people and over long periods of time is not consistent with intoxication. It would be expected that inconsistencies and misjudgments during intoxication would lead to periods of poor control in which family members would gather strength to leave or implement changes. These opportunities seldom happen spontaneously.

> **Danny/Jack: Parents**
> Jack is erecting fences with a farm assistant he has worked with for many years.
> "How's your son doing, Jack?"
> "Not so good at the moment… He's taken to the bottle since he split with Julie."
> "That's rough. I've never told you this before but my dad was an alcoholic. He hit the bottle all his life and we reckon that's what killed him in the end."
> "I never knew that! My mom was alcoholic too! She drank at home all the time, we always had to pretend and hide it. It was terrible for all of us, that's why I'm so worried for Danny and his children…. We've worked together for so long and I never knew…. You know, you're the first person outside the family I ever talked to about this."
> "Me, too. Feels strange, huh? Although I left home 35 years ago I still can't talk about it. I still feel scared, like he's still watching me, waiting for a chance to hurt me."
> "I have this sense that our conversation is like a betrayal—a betrayal of family secrets to outsiders that someday I'll be punished for."

Violence as Communication

What is missing in particle approaches is recognition of violence as essentially an expressive act. Family violence is seldom a disconnected series of discrete abusive behaviors. It more typically carries important messages. A series of violent acts essentially states to the victim, "You deserve to be abused!" and

Danny/Jack: Last Hurt

Jack continues to describe his experiences to his work colleague as they erect fences.

"When I was young, my mother used to smack us with sticks until we bled. It could be for anything, but her smacking was particularly hard when she thought we had been talking to people about things at home."

"My dad used to punish us like that, too."

"When she was drunk it was usually a bit easier because we could usually get away from her. But she would go on and on about how useless we were and how her life was ruined when she had us."

"Yeah, and you never knew when it was coming."

"I used to think, how can a mother who says she loves me do these things? The thought that someone who loved you could hurt you was more emotionally distressing and more painful that the actual episodes of hitting."

"Yeah, and even as an adult I still feel hurt just thinking about it."

by implication, "You are worthless!" In this way violence can be seen as more than a product of cognitive and behavioral processes; it is an expressive vehicle in itself. For example, male partner abusers frequently choose to damage household objects in ways that appear more than arbitrary or out of control. On closer inspection their choice of what to damage appears purposely designed to convey strong messages; they might choose objects with emotional significance—a special present, a memento of past happiness—or they might choose symbols of safety or freedom—breaking a door, destroying a car or telephone—or they may even choose to hurt pets. In having expressive function, violent behavior can be seen to share many of the linguistic properties of verbal behavior; it has its own syntax, semantics and rhetoric. For example, a punch could be seen as one basic unit of a sentence, occupying a position much like a noun; the pauses and spaces between abusive episodes serve to punctuate and emphasize the next impending episode; the resulting fear and pain carry the meaning and significance of the action, and the various techniques of delivery—their context and associations—contribute to the rhetoric of its application (see inset box, above).

Violence as a Social Event

The switch to viewing violence as communicative or expressive sits uncomfortably with particle interpretations. It serves little purpose for people to communicate violently with themselves. Language and communication operate in the realm of interactions between individuals. Consequently this switch requires a rethinking of violence into a social paradigm where the significance of violence is not interpreted in terms of individual and psychological processes but in terms of the effects violence has within a system of social interconnections. Violence is seen as a means of communicating between individuals in order to influence how a system of relationships operates.

Social Expectations

A natural outcome of the widespread acceptance of the disinhibition myth has been the emergence of a common understanding that disinhibited behavior, including violence, is a normal and understandable outcome of intoxication. Ironically, the strength of this belief provides the base for its role in social interactions. In their book, *Drunken Comportment: A Social Explanation*,[18] MacAndrew and Edgerton argue that the way people behave during intoxication is in large part determined by social factors and codes of behavior.

> Rather than viewing drunken comportment as a function of toxically disinhibited brains operating in impulse-driven bodies, what is fundamentally at issue are the learned relationships that exist among men living together in a society. More specifically, we have contended that the way people comport themselves when they are drunk is determined not by alcohol's toxic assault upon the seat of moral judgment, conscience, or the like, but by what their society makes of and imparts to them concerning the state of drunkenness.[19]

The spirit of their position has been explored in a variety of studies on the social and cultural dimensions of intoxication.[20] For example, in an anthropological study of Cajun Mardi Gras, Rocky Sexton explored how while drunkenness at these events appears to be chaotic, it follows an idealized script with participants conforming to common understandings of intoxicated behavior:

During intoxication people often conform to common understandings of expected behavior

> The celebration involves a ritualization of disinhibition in which alcohol's role is overemphasized.... Thus, much of the perceived drunkenness in Mardi Gras is better viewed as a form of ritualized inebriation that is facilitated by drinking, the very act of which confers a degree of immunity on participants regardless of the amount consumed.[21]

Violence at such events can be viewed as occurring because intoxication is a socially sanctioned space for participants to act out old grudges, jealousies, and other motives.

Applying this to interpersonal violence, if it is understood—maybe even viewed as acceptable—to exhibit violence during episodes of intoxication, then it follows that reserving violent behavior for those episodes is an ideal way of making the violence seem more socially justifiable and of hiding its underlying intent. For example, a young man recently married has reached the conclusion that some forms of violence or controlling tactics are going to be required to control his wife in order to reduce his feelings of insecurity and jealousy. He knows that people will disapprove of blatant use of these tactics, so he looks for ways at making them less blatant and more acceptable. He soon realizes that if he reserves his controlling abuse to the end of the week when he returns home after being out drinking with his friends, he can easily dismiss the abuse by claiming it was a product of his drunkenness. This use of intoxication as justification works well with other men, particularly with men who are regularly intoxicated. They all understand that violence flows naturally from disinhibition associated with intoxication, so they are able to minimize the impact of controlling tactics with comments such as, "Oh, I was drunk at the time"; "You can't help yourself when you are out of it on drugs"; or "My mind was so possessed by gambling I didn't care about anyone else." Accordingly, intoxication becomes a convenient platform upon which to discharge messages that on the surface appear chaotic but on closer inspection can serve a broad range of social functions.

Feminist Social Theory

The feminist literature has addressed violence in intimate relationships, particularly male violence against female intimates and to a lesser extent toward children.[22] Its interpretation of violence is grounded firmly in a social rather than particle paradigm, ignoring theories that attribute violence to stress, poor skills, or troubled backgrounds. Instead, it focuses on the ways a man's violence toward his intimates serves specific social purposes. He chooses to be violent because he gains from it: he gains control of how his partner behaves, he gains protection from her legitimate complaints or criticisms, and he secures a position for himself in the home where male dominance and one-sided male privilege continues unchallenged.[23] Men are able to achieve these gains primarily because of a socially sanctioned inequality of power between men and women. Men have greater access to physical, economic, and social support, and this enables both more opportunities and more potent opportunities to apply power over their partners.

Feminist perspectives focus on the gains achieved through violent behavior

Efforts to reduce the incidence of male violence in the home also require addressing the social infrastructure that supports that violence, in particular the widely held beliefs that justify and minimize the violence and oppression of women. These include the following beliefs: men have greater entitlement to power than women, women are just as violent as men, and domestic violence is not as bad as street violence. Such beliefs help the abuser justify continued violence as well as encouraging those in contact with the abusers (friends, family, professionals, and institutions) to refrain from confronting the abuser.[24] From a feminist perspective, violence is seen as being used to protect perceived entitlements. Just as nations use their military forces to protect claims to land, and violent revolutions help the poor reclaim entitlements to resources dominated by the rich, feminist approaches seek to redress the power imbalance that women have in their entitlement to political, economic, and social equality. To redress this imbalance, women and men need to strive for positions of equality and respect where there is no place for men to behave violently toward women. Accordingly, effective responses to violence include the following: inviting men to take responsibility for their part in safety of those they live with; challenging the beliefs that support violence; and, on a broader front, holding institutions and professionals responsible for actions that may further endanger intimates at risk.[25]

Feminist understandings of intimate violence based on male privilege evolved from women's experiences and as such differ from the imported particle models (such as psychodynamic or behavioral approaches) and therefore they provide a more appropriate reference base for working with male partner abusers.[26] Nonetheless, the picture is more confused when it comes to violence in addictive systems. In the first place, since men are more involved with addictive substances/processes than are women, they are significantly more likely than women to enter addictive relationships, which gives the misleading impression that violence and addictive relationships are driven by issues associated with masculinity. In the second place, it is not only men, but also women, children, parents, and friends in addictive relationship who are capable of pursuing programs of control with their loved ones.[27] The beliefs about male privilege provide more opportunities for men to use controlling tactics to ensure the compliance of intimates. Finally, the reasons for men to exploit male privilege in maintaining positions of power can vary; for some it is the natural superiority of men; for others it reinforces a social order they believe to be correct in the home; and for others it protects their vulnerable inner world from scrutiny and challenge. However, for men in addictive relationships, maintaining male privilege is not a goal in itself, more an opportunity to achieve a specific purpose—that of protecting and preserving the addictive relationship itself.

Managed Intimacy

Violence and other controlling tactics can be used to achieve many of the same effects as addictive substances/processes. For example, Bert, who is in an addictive relationship to alcohol, admits to himself that one of the reasons he gets drunk is to avoid facing problems in his life and to preclude talking about issues that upset him. But he cannot sustain drunkenness all the time; he still has to spend much of his time in the bleak world of sobriety. As the addictive relationship intensifies, other intimacies need to be managed in order to prevent them from threatening the primacy of the addictive relationship. As discussed in earlier chapters, these threats can take many forms: intimates (such as Joan and the children) might question or challenge his use of alcohol, they might withdraw support for his lifestyle, and they might join forces to make his current lifestyle untenable. Over time he finds that violence and other controlling tactics provide a useful complement in that he can reinforce and sometimes achieve some of the same effects as his drunkenness, particularly with intimates: when people at home are frightened of him they do not initiate any conversations he might find unpalatable and thus he hears no complaints about his drinking; no one mentions his long absences or the perilous state of their finances or their lack of affection and closeness. Family members tiptoe around compliantly, trying hard to avoid any actions that might upset him. He only needs to shout now and then or to throw things around or perhaps to strike someone for their obedience to be assured. It does not really matter if he is violent when he is sober or drunk,

Controlling tactics are used to protect the primacy of the addictive relationship

the important outcome is to keep them fearful and thereby to contain any threat and maintain their compliance.

Tactics of Control

What differentiates violence toward intimates in addictive systems from other intimate violence is not the range of controlling tactics—very similar strategies are used—but the overriding purpose for which the tactics are being employed. Violence in other nonaddictive social contexts can occur for purposes such as maintaining male privilege, pursuing desires (e.g., sexual abuse), and responding to rage regarding negative parenting. Violence in addictive social contexts is used primarily to protect and maintain the core intimacy: the relationship with the addictive substance/process. While this is achieved in a variety of different ways, the following are several of the main forms:

1. Tactics for dominance: The ability to manage intimacies in ways that ensure the survival of the addictive relationship relies on achieving a position of sufficient dominance to activate *power over* processes. The simplest and most direct way to do this is by creating an environment of fear; when intimates are sufficiently afraid, their wills are more easily subjugated. These tactics can include the use of physical violence, threatening behavior, sexual coercion, and emotional put downs. As discussed earlier, such fear tactics can be enhanced by adding in confusion and uncertainty because fear is amplified when a person is unsure of what happens next. Besides these direct strategies, tactics for maintaining dominance can take many other forms: they can involve control of resources (such as money, transportation, and space), as well as control over the children; they might involve restricting access to sources of support (such as alienating relatives through drunken behavior at special events); they can entail elaborate mental maneuvers that place favored explanations over others (such as retelling past events in ways that make the other person look bad). One interesting and reasonably common example with illicit drug use is by one intimate controlling access of drugs for another. As described in the inset box, above, both Cathy and her previous partner Robert are in addictive relationships to opiates, but her partner maintained dominance and compliance by actively ensuring control over supply.

> **Cathy/Dion: Access to Drugs**
>
> Cathy is describing to Dion what it was like living with his father, Robert, before his disappearance.
>
> "There was a time after you were born that I wanted to change the way we were living."
>
> "Did you talk to him about it?"
>
> "Every time I question things he said he's going to block me from getting hold of drugs."
>
> "Why didn't you get them yourself? Then you could have been independent."
>
> "I didn't dare. He had all the connections and only he knew what to do. I once tried to score on my own and he found out and he knew the people and told them not to sell to me, and then he shouted at me for what seemed like hours. It just wasn't worth it."
>
> "But, getting it from him... he was always in charge."
>
> "I know, I know, but what else could I do? I couldn't risk not getting the drugs."

2. Tactics for information control: An important set of tactics involves maintaining control of information. The most common way to manipulate information is through various forms of deception. For example, in the above inset box, Jacinta makes sure that Wendy is not in a position to challenge her access to money by using tactics that prevent her from accessing their accounts. As her addictive relationship intensifies the deceptions become increasingly elaborate. She starts managing the accounts in such a complicated manner that only she can decipher them. Later, when suspicions seem inevitable, she resorts to creating diversions that distract attention from their finances. Other forms of control of information can involve collecting intelligence on intimates, such as where they are, who they are with, what they are saying, and then using this information to monitor potential threats and to devise counterstrategies. For example, Jacinta could use friends to keep track of the level to which Wendy is suspicious of her spending and then use this information to tailor her explanations accordingly.

3. Tactics for camouflage: Soldiers wear camouflage to blend into surroundings and to appear as a normal part of the environment, thus avoiding detection and deceiving the enemy. The camouflage of an addictive social system performs a similar function in blocking threats from others. If the family seems normal there is little reason for others to question or challenge the family relationships. To maintain the pretense of cordial relationships, violence and other *power over* strategies are employed to ensure the cooperation of other intimates. In the example in the inset box above, 16-year-old Fiona tells her teacher about the effects of her father's drinking, but when her parents find out, she is severely punished. Punishment for speaking out can include severe physical and emotional abuse, humiliation, and restricted access to closeness and compassion. The child learns these consequences

---

Jacinta/Wendy: Money Control

Wendy is talking to her friend Sally about her partner, Jacinta's, gambling.

"Looking back I made the mistake of letting her control all our finances. She made sure she managed all the bank accounts and kept feeding me false information on what state they were in."

"Couldn't you have checked them yourself?"

"When I tried to access them myself, she would accuse me of not trusting her, of being miserly and suspicious. It just wasn't worth the hassle. Besides she kept so many bank accounts and transferred money in complicated ways that I could never get an idea of the whole picture."

"You must have been suspicious later when creditors started threatening legal action."

"Oh yeah, but she created all sorts of diversions; she picked fights with family members, argued with people at work, then changed jobs. The money problems then seemed like a minor affair."

Bert/Joan: Childhood Dilemmas

One evening, alone by themselves, Bert's daughter, Fiona, is speaking to her brother, Donald.

"I know I shouldn't have, but last year I spoke to my teacher about the chaos at home. I didn't mean to, but after a sleepless night listening to them yelling, the teacher said I looked terrible and she asked me what's wrong. I finally broke down."

"I didn't know you'd done that."

"Yeah, and you know what, the teacher then talked to the principal and they asked to speak with Mom and Dad."

"Oh boy, that's asking for it."

"Yep, sure was. And when they got home both of them lectured me for ages about not airing our dirty linen in public. On and on about its none of their business and how could I shame the family like this."

"I can imagine."

"They stopped speaking to me for several days. I was also grounded. And about a week later, Dad came home drunk, woke me up, and started shouting at me about being ungrateful and disloyal. I was really scared. Too scared to talk to anyone."

"I guess you're not going to talk like that to anyone again."

and recognizes that it is dangerous to speak or behave in any other way than appearing to be a normal happy family. The child and other intimates thus find themselves engaging in regular routines of play-acting and pretense that then serve to distance their family from further scrutiny. In a similar fashion, other camouflage routines that are enforced include minimal contact with neighbors, keeping the house tidy and dressing well, quickly cleaning up any damage, using standard minimizing phrases ("we had fun and games last night", "she occasionally gets a bit merry"), and acting like a happy family at family gatherings.

4. Tactics for silencing: Silencing differs from camouflage and secrecy in that it relies less on deception and more on force. People avoid speaking out when they calculate that the disadvantages of speaking outweigh the advantages. Silence can be the goal of many controlling tactics. For example, threats of physical abuse can serve to frighten intimates into not talking about certain topics both within and outside the family.[28] However, probably the most effective and commonly used tactic to achieve both silence and compliance is the measured use of surveillance strategies. Examples of how the behavior of intimates can be monitored vary enormously and include following or tailing them on outings, interrogating them when they return, asking for information from friends or work colleagues, seeking information from children, tracking back the sources of concerning messages, and reviewing bank and credit card statements. Even though monitoring is episodic, intimates can never be sure when it is occurring, and this creates the impression that they are being constantly observed. As described in the inset box below, Joan begins to see it as too hazardous to speak about issues with anyone, and since she is often unsure when she is being observed, she maintains this silence.[29]

5. Tactics for bargaining: The opportunities for bargaining flow from the asymmetrical nature of the relationships the person in the addictive relationship has with other intimates. When people feel less closeness, less compassion, less commitment, and less accord than do their partners in an intimate relationship, this places them in a powerful position and provides a wide range of possibilities for control. The partner, who experiences greater attachment to the relationship, is vulnerable to the possibility of losing this connection. With less attachment people in the addictive relationship can use the connecting strands of intimacy as leverage for other purposes. Most importantly, they can influence how other their intimates behave toward the addictive relationship. In the inset box below, Wendy describes how Jacinta uses Wendy's desire for closeness and affection as leverage to prevent discussions about her gambling. For Wendy these moments

---

Bert/Joan: Mobile Surveillance

Joan is talking to her sister, Mary, about Bert.

"He insists that I carry this damn cell phone everywhere. He calls me during the day and asks what I'm doing and who I'm with. I tell him and he hangs up."

"That must be annoying."

"More than annoying. I never know when he will call; it can be first thing in the morning or even when I'm out late at night. He might go several days without calling but I still have to carry it. If I don't answer the phone, when I get home he interrogates me for ages until I tell him every detail of what I was doing. Sometimes he even checks it out."

"So you're never sure when he'll be checking on you?"

"Exactly. I hate the phone now. It seems like an eye peering at me all the time, making sure I don't do anything or talk to anyone that might give the show away."

of dwindling affection are very precious and the strategy introduces a painful dilemma: she feels caught between either addressing the issues or forfeiting highly valued but fleeting moments of closeness. Other similar strategies could involve staying away longer from home after a challenge, threatening to leave if certain topics continue to be raised, and having sex with other people in response to scrutiny.

6. Tactics for co-opting: Another range of strategies emerge from the fragmentation that is maintained within an addictive social system. Intimates feel isolated, and consequently they are less likely to be exposed to other people's ways of looking at events and more likely to accept perspectives provided to them by the person in the addictive relationship. Consequently, if an intimate looks as though she might challenge the addictive relationship, the other intimate can be co-opted to isolate, impede, or block any initiatives. In the inset box Donald's attempt to engage his mother in challenging his father's drinking is thwarted by his mother's unwillingness to upset the current arrangements. Perhaps she is too fearful of the consequences of confrontation; perhaps she feels guilty about his condition or the effects on her children, or maybe she still clings to the hope that in time Bert will change and the home will return to a loving environment. What Donald may not fully appreciate is that behind the scenes Bert has made use of a combination of controlling strategies, such as threats of leaving, threats of violence and humiliation, and promises of reform, that have effectively prevented Joan from challenging his relationship to alcohol. Consequently, Donald's first attempt to enlist his mother's support is stalled by her reluctance. His efforts fall apart and he is left feeling even more isolated and overpowered by the effects of the addictive relationship.

> **Jacinta/Wendy: The Cold Shoulder**
> Wendy is having morning coffee with her friend, Sally.
> "Whenever I question Jacinta about her gambling, we argue. While I do get upset, I can usually handle that. But what I can't handle is what happens later. She goes all quiet, keeps her distance, and doesn't talk to me for several days. I really hate that, and she knows it."
> "That must be awful." Sally pauses for a moment. "But isn't she like that a lot anyway?"
> "No. I've learned if I don't talk to her about her gambling and ask no questions when she comes home, she gives me lots of cuddles and is very affectionate."
> "I can see that's nice, given the current circumstances."
> "We're having so many difficulties now, my heart aches for those close times. I don't want to risk those moments of closeness by spoiling them by talking about problems."
> "So she's kind of sending a message that she will be close to you on the condition that you don't interfere with her gambling?"

> **Bert/Joan: Don't Say Anything**
> Donald is trying to persuade his mother, Joan, to take a stronger line with Bert.
> "Look, I don't want to leave with you and Fiona stuck in this crazy house. He'll kill you one day, Mom. We have to speak with him. Get him to see somebody or something."
> "Donald, your father has devoted his life to this family. He's going through a hard time now, ever since he didn't get promoted."
> "Oh don't make light of things. Fiona and I hear what goes on at night."
> "Please don't say anything. Please. It won't do any good. He'll only get mad and it'll be us who suffer."
> "But you can't let it go on any further."
> "I've gone this far. I've stuck with him through thick and thin and you have grown up as good children. I don't want that upset now."

The three chapters of Part II have addressed the dynamics of intimacy and explored how the asymmetrical relationships in addictive social systems generate a world of fragmentation and disconnection for those who inhabit them. This leads to Part III, which addresses the opportunities for change.

Part III
Families and Communities

Chapter 8

Fragmented Lives

Mam is sitting by the fireplace with Alphie in her arms. She shakes her
head. He went to the pub, didn't he?
He did.
I want ye to go back down to that pub and read him out of it. I want ye to stand
in the middle of the pub and tell every man your father is drinking the money
for the baby. Ye are to tell the world there isn't a scrap of food in this house,
not a lump of coal to start the fire, not a drop of milk for the baby's bottle.

(Frank McCourt, "Angela's Ashes'")

Frank McCourt's memoir of his early years in New York and Ireland
provides a heart-wrenching account of the consequences to a family of a
father's unrelenting commitment to a relationship with alcohol. It is hard to
read the book and not feel some frustration, some anger, perhaps even
some resentment at the father's ongoing allegiance to his drinking. If he had
stopped, all would have been different; he would have found employment,
the family would have had money for food and clothing, more of the
children would have survived, and the family may have stayed together. But
his relationship to alcohol continued on, uninterrupted by the chaos and the
fragmentation it was creating. The remainder of the family found themselves progressively isolated from each other and distanced from the world
around them.

Part III discusses in more specific detail the processes of fragmentation
within addictive systems, with the purpose of seeking opportunities for
change. The focus of this discussion encompasses the outsider perspectives
of Part I and the insider perspectives of Part II. This combination of perspectives helps build a rich description of the interactions between addictive
relationships and surrounding social networks.

Fragmenting Environments

As discussed in Chapter 6, addictive relationships (namely, those between
the person and an addictive substance/process) thrive in environments
where intimacies are fragmented, and, in a reflexive manner, such fragmentation
thrives wherever addictive systems form. The intensification of an addictive
relationship restructures the social environment in ways that reshape the lives
of all those involved. Intimates find themselves living within the rigidity of

P.J. Adams, *Fragmented Intimacy: Addiction in a Social World*
© Springer 2008

one dominant relationship from which a wide range of asymmetries are generated. The disruption happens in two directions: first, fragmentation leads to deteriorating relationships, splitting, and separations; and second, fragmentation leads in the other direction toward a binding but unloving closeness. The distortions that this fragmentation creates in turn influence the social connectedness within social networks as a whole. Disruptions to intimate connectedness seep out and infect the cohesion of families, neighborhoods, and communities. This then ultimately leads to decreases in the strength and resilience that a social system requires to respond to negative impacts.

Fragmented intimacies infect the cohesion of neighborhoods & communities

Research into the effects of addictive relationships on intimacy is at an early rudimentary phase. When compared with the effort put into understanding the effects on the individual person in an addictive relationship, few studies have focused specifically on trying to understand the effects on intimates.[2] Those that have looked closely at intimates have mostly focused on them as individual particles rather than looking at the dynamics in their relationships. For example, in a typical study of effects on families, Sher and colleagues collected information on 253 college students who had been brought up in addictive home environments and compared them to another group who had not been exposed. They found that across a number of measures those exposed to addictive environments were significantly more likely to develop their own problems with alcohol and drug use than those who were not exposed.[3] While this finding is important to confirm, it sheds little light on the social dynamics between childhood contexts and adult responses to intimacy. The methods adopted in such studies assume that each research participant is an isolated individual counted as a discrete unit. They thereby focus on the participant as a person-as-particle rather than a person-in-relationships and in this way miss out on the reflexive nature of relationships between individuals in their contexts. These methods have also led to an emphasis on measuring the qualities and attributes of individuals (personality issues, mental health concerns, and problems communicating). For example, as part of a large survey, by Mathew and colleagues found adults who were brought up in addictive contexts were more likely to report antisocial symptoms and anxiety disorders.[4]

Despite the paucity of social research into addictive relationships, two important observations have emerged relatively consistently across the research efforts to date: the first major finding is that people respond to addictive environments in very different and diverse ways, and the second major finding is that negative impacts are more likely in contexts involving violence and other controlling tactics.

To turn first to the diversity of responses, alcohol and other drug research has highlighted a wide range of ways in which close family members respond both at the time and later in their lives to exposure to an addictive home environment. There is some evidence that adults who were exposed as children to addictive environments go on to experience relationship difficulties in the marriage and as parents.[5] However, the research here is poorly developed, and it remains unclear how frequently or how strongly people will be affected.[6] Studies have found intimates can experience higher rates of depression and anxiety, lower self-esteem, higher incidence of antisocial or impulsive behaviors, problems with intimacy, generalized distress or maladjustment, and a greater risk of future involvement in addictive systems.[7] Nonetheless, these results indicate only overall tendencies, which are insufficient in predicting whether or not intimates will be negatively affected in such ways. While for some people living in an addictive system has major impact, for others it may have few observable lasting effects.[8] What will have profound effects on one person may minimally affect others, and what serves as a good approach for one situation can lead to poor outcomes in other circumstances. Some family members may even choose to see the addictive relationship in more positive ways over time.[9] So, all we can say at this point is that people respond to addictive systems in widely varying ways, which has helped stimulate interest in factors that might predict strength and resiliency in such contexts.[10]

People respond to addictive systems in a widely varying ways

To turn now to considering the effects of violence and other controlling tactics, investigators are increasingly finding that the combined exposure to addictive relationships and abuse are more likely to lead to ongoing problems for intimates than exposure to addictive relationships alone.[11] As explored in the previous chapter, when controlling tactics are minimally present, intimates have more freedom to pursue a balanced life around the addictive relationship and are more likely to build up their own systems of social connectedness. However, when faced with the orchestrated use of controlling tactics and other intimacy management strategies, relationships become both more strongly asymmetrical and more oriented around the addictive relationship. This enables the person in the addictive relationship to acquire increasing dominance within the social system and thereby to impede the formation of other connections beyond his or her influence. The outcome of living in this fragmented social environment is a weakened capacity to build up other sources of strength and a reduced ability to protect or moderate the negative effects.[12]

How Intimates Respond

The intensification of an addictive relationship has impact on the quality of other surrounding relationships in diverse ways. The effects are partly a question of timing, partly a question of social role, and partly a question of wider circumstances. For example, the impact on a child might vary depending on the child's age when the parent entered into the addictive relationship, whether the parent's role was important to the child, and whether the child has access to a range of other supports.[13] The extent of this diversity can be illustrated through a closer examination of the range of ways different people in different roles respond to the asymmetries. The following six subsections explore this diversity by scanning common ways in which partners, children, adolescents, parents, close friends, and other associates respond to the fragmenting effects of exposure to an addictive system.[14] The descriptions are supplemented with vignettes relating to our four sample addictive systems (Bert/Joan, Danny/Jack, Cathy/Dion. and Jacinta/Wendy).

Partner Intimacies

Partner intimacies take many different forms: a man and a woman commit to each other through the legal institution of marriage, other couples unite in private declarations of commitment, and same-sex partners mark their commitment with vows and ceremonies. The central purpose of the partnership can vary from romance to child rearing, from interfamily accords to financial agreements, and from sexual union to companionship. Furthermore, as time moves on these multicomplexities overlap, shift, and change. Addictive systems commonly emerge from within the complexity of these arrangements, and as a result partner responses to addictive relationships can vary markedly both in how they are experienced and how partners respond.

As fleshed out in the previous three chapters, the key challenge for partners is the emerging asymmetrical nature of their intimacy; people are dismayed when they encounter how their love and devotion is decreasingly reciprocated. In many circumstances partners are tempted to create the illusion of symmetry by forcing themselves to believe and behave as though their closeness, compassion, commitment, and accord are being reciprocated. This can be achieved either through the deceptive and controlling tactics of their partners or by active self-deception. For example, controlling and violent behaviors by the person in the addictive relationship might discourage any questioning of changes in the relationship, or the partner might simply choose to pretend that everything is the same as it always has been. As the addictive relationship intensifies, this position becomes increasingly unsustainable. Despite prolonged periods of feeling sorrow, or rage, or disappointment at their partner's unresponsiveness, they now face the prospect of their partnership being a relationship of secondary priority. The challenge that now confronts them concerns how and under what terms they will maintain intimacy with their partners who are increasingly focused on their addictive relationships. The following subsections discuss some common responses from a wide range of options. It assumes that since the closeness, compassion, and accord have progressively

Partners grapple with their relationships becoming secondary priorities

diminished in the relationship, it is commitment that functions most actively as the connecting strand.

Partners' Compassionate Commitment

Once partners have accepted with resignation the asymmetrical nature of an intimacy, which entails accepting that for at least the foreseeable future there is unlikely to be any genuine reciprocation, one option is to view the person in the addictive relationship as incapable of being anything else. There are various ways of thinking about this. Some might consider their partner as helplessly dependent and in need of caring supervision, like a wayward child or someone with a debilitating handicap. Others might see the lack of reciprocation as a temporary phase, a period of trial, but one that will ultimately lead to a passionate reunion. However, by far the majority opt to see their partners as suffering from a specific sickness or disease, one that lasts a lifetime and prevents them ever having a casual relationship with their addictive substance/process (see inset box, above). This interpretation enables partners to accept the ongoing intensification of the addictive relationship while avoiding tearing themselves apart with expectations of a balanced relationship. It also results in their feeling less anger and uncertainty within the relationship. The switch is often experienced as highly liberating because it frees partners from the chaos associated with investing in the relationship as reciprocated intimacy.

> **Jacinta/Wendy: She Can't Help It**
>
> Wendy is talking on the phone to her friend, Sally, about Jacinta's gambling:
>
> "I used to get so angry when she went gambling. I tried everything to get her to stop; I'd block her access to money, I'd hide her credit cards, I would plead for hours with her not to go."
>
> "Yeah, I remember what you went through."
>
> "So when she kept gambling I felt so betrayed. I looked at her as weak and immoral; I wouldn't talk to her for days, I'd threaten to leave her, and I'd pester her about treatment."
>
> "It didn't really make any difference, did it?"
>
> "Absolutely none. It was all a waste of time, she just kept doing it. But about a year ago I began to see her as suffering from an illness, the illness of problem gambling. This has made a huge difference. I no longer see her as weak, I don't try to control things, and I no longer have these intense feelings of anger."

Partners' Resolute Commitment

As the asymmetrical nature of relationships becomes more apparent, any feelings of compassion toward a partner in an addictive relationship become increasingly difficult to sustain. This is especially the case in contexts with low levels of closeness, where compassion is seldom reciprocated and where any remaining sense of accord soon fades. In these circumstances, an emotionally charged commitment is often replaced by

> **Bert/Joan: Through Thick and Thin**
>
> One morning Joan is talking with her son, Donald, about her relationship to Bert.
>
> Donald says, "Mom, he's never home much anymore and when he is here he mistreats you. You might as well be living without him."
>
> "I know, I know. He's hardly here anymore. But the day we married, I made a vow to your father, and before all my friends and family I promised that I would stick by him through thick and thin."
>
> "He doesn't care anymore, Mom. When he is here, he just puts you down all the time."
>
> "Look, Donald, Bert has a sickness, a terrible sickness. You don't walk away from people when they're sick."
>
> "But, but, whether you're around or not doesn't make any difference and..."
>
> "It does make a difference. I look after him in so many ways. He'd be in an awful state if I didn't look after things."

a commitment based on a sense of obligation and little else. As described in the inset box, above, Joan is having less and less to do with her husband, but she remains resolute in retaining her loyalty to their marriage. The drivers for such solidarity occur at many levels. At a personal level Joan avoids change because she does not wish to confront the issues associated with changing her commitment, issues such as admitting failure and facing shame. At a family level she recognizes that change would disrupt so many other aspects of their life, such as their income, their residence, and their friendships. At an extended family level she has concerns that changing her commitment would be perceived as unreasonable; from the outside Bert is seen as a decent person, he provides for his family, he has remained loyal to her, and he is well liked. At a societal level, by marrying Bert, she has made a fundamental commitment, and good spouses remain true to their partners no matter what happens.

Partners' Disengaged Commitment

One major option for partners involves remaining committed to the presence of the partnership but maintaining this commitment in a semi-detached fashion. The commitment here moves from the person in the addictive relationship to a commitment to the social system as a whole. The focus is on maintaining the relationships within the family while letting the addictive relationship take its own course. Life is built as much as possible around the addictive relationship without seeking or supporting any form of involvement. As illustrated in the inset box, Julie found she was better able to manage her busy life of bringing up two children with an episodically present father by becoming progressively less engaged and less emotionally available to Danny. She opted as much as possible to focus her efforts on herself and the children. They gradually spent increasing amounts of time with each other or with friends and less with Danny. While she remained committed to continuing the relationship and would support Danny if he needed help, she invested less time and energy in the relationship. She would help him clean up his messes and crises, but she put most of her energy into building up other relationships.

> **Danny/Jack: Julie Disengages**
>
> Julie, Danny's wife, is talking with Jack, Danny's father, about their early years of marriage.
>
> "When we were first together and it became clear he was going to stay out late, I blamed myself. I tried hard to make it attractive for him to come home. I kept the house clean and tidy, always had meals for him, talked to him nicely, and made everything pleasant."
>
> "Oh, I don't think that would have made much difference."
>
> "Yeah, you're right. So the next couple of years I switched to giving him a hard time: on his case when he got home, demanding he do jobs, locking him out—that sort of thing."
>
> "I bet that didn't work either."
>
> "Right. What did work was to begin living as if he wasn't part of what's going on. I never had any expectations, so I was never disappointed. I stopped worrying or caring about him or what he was doing, and focused all my energy on me and the kids."

Partners' Ambivalent Commitment

Ambivalence and uncertainty about continuing the commitment can occur at any stage of the fragmentation process and is particularly strong following a crisis. For example, in the inset box, following an argument Wendy is conflicted about whether to continue in her relationship with Jacinta. One part of her wants to believe the intimacy is still real and that they will experience periods of high intensity again, but another part of her recognizes that this is also very unlikely. She continually debates with herself the pros and cons of staying with Jacinta, who is still the woman she fell in love with but who has becomes decreasingly accessible. Since this type of ambivalence is for most people highly unpleasant, the drive to resolve it can provide a critical impetus for change. It could, for example, provoke Wendy into talking with other people, maybe to attend counseling, and perhaps to begin setting conditions on her continuing involvement.

> ### Jacinta/Wendy: An Ongoing Dilemma
>
> In the silence of the night Wendy writes in her personal journal:
>
> "I have loved her so deeply. But now I'm not so sure. In the early years we were very close; we shared everything and it felt like our lives naturally blended together. Now that time seems like long ago. Lately we share little together and I find her distance and her harsh words are slowly killing whatever is left inside me.
>
> "I know we could still rekindle the old feelings. She is the same person and I feel deep down she still wants to be close. But as time moves on and we share less together, it looks more and more unlikely that she will ever reciprocate my love.
>
> "What do I do? Continue to wait with the diminishing hope of a change? Or cut my losses and start a new life."

Partners' Separation

With separation, a decision has been made to withdraw commitment, and since commitment is likely to be the most active connecting strand, this withdrawal entails a severing of the relationship. In the partner's eyes, the asymmetrical nature of their intimacy has reached a point where the probability of quality intimacy is so low that it is no longer worthy of further investment. The decision to end one's commitment to a relationship takes different forms depending on the intensity of the addictive relationship. In the early periods, when the addictive relationship is less developed, the move to separate requires a strong and active decision. This is because much of the social system is still intact and separation involves disentangling from many other connections. The partner needs to work through strategies that reduce the levels of closeness, compassion and commitment, and, as with Julie in the inset box above, parents also need to attend to their children

> ### Danny/Jack: Why Julie Left
>
> Julie, Danny's wife, is explaining to their daughter, Adrienne, why she had decided they should leave.
>
> "I want to talk to you a bit more about why we're living in this house rather than the other. You remember how your father's drinking led to many problems between us?"
>
> "But Mommy, it wasn't that bad. Why couldn't you just carry on as before?"
>
> "Well, Adrienne, it was getting harder and harder to carry on that way. When he was, he was moody and grumpy, and I was really worried about the bad effects this might be having on you and your brother and sister."

and to negotiate their way through the issues their children face during the transition. At later stages, when the addictive relationship has intensified at the cost of many other connections, the decision to separate is less complex and can proceed more naturally. The closeness and compassion have long gone, the remaining commitment is wavering, and the lack of other connections make it easy to end the relationship without many consequences.

Children

Children growing up in an addictive system are exposed to the cycles of sobriety and intoxication as well as those of fragmentation and crisis. These experiences have profound impacts on them from an early age in terms of how they form and interpret their social connections with the world.[15] Children are born into social environments where the surrounding relationships are by necessity asymmetrical. They depend on these relationships for nourishment, safety, hygiene, and learning how to engage in a social world. Their helplessness contrasts with the levels of access their parents (and other adults) have to positions of power. Parents can dictate most aspects of their social environment; they can determine who they meet, and when and where. With this power comes the responsibility of ensuring that children are in a position to gradually

The asymmetries in addictive systems work against a child's drive towards independence acquire the skills and resources needed to build up their own power base. The key task for the child is to make use of these opportunities to reduce parent–child asymmetries and thereby function in an increasingly independent manner. While all four connecting strands of intimacy play a role in enabling this to happen, the critical strand for a child is proximal and emotional closeness. Under normal circumstances, parental compassion, commitment, and accord with their child remain strong (and asymmetrical) throughout childhood. These to some extent are givens. However, from an early age, children experiment with varying the levels to which they are physically and emotionally close to others. For example, they experiment with their own capacity to initiate and terminate closeness and they try out different ways of adapting to varying periods of parental absence. Correspondingly, as the presence of addictive relationships cuts across and distorts family connections, children commonly experiment with these disruptions in a variety of ways.

Children's Conditional Closeness

Children's natural exploration of closeness provides them with a range of ways to cope with exposure to addictive social processes. The parent in the addictive relationship appears close at times, then is distant and hostile, and then returns to show affection. Children cope with this variable and at times hurtful involvement by using distancing strategies, such as visiting their friends to get out of the house, or withdrawing to their room to play computer games (see inset box). They can subsequently reappear and join in with interactions when tension, conflict, and intoxication look less likely. As time goes by they use more advanced strategies, such as doing homework or household chores or playing sports, all of which are societally approved ways for children to spend their time and that help to reduce the tension at home. The advantage of conditional closeness is the ability to control the level of exposure to damaging effects, but the disadvantage is the early introduction to controlling tactics, a pattern that may recycle into future relationships.

> ### Bert/Joan: Havens
> The two children, Donald and Fiona, are comparing what they remember of the different ways they coped as children with trouble at home.
> Donald says, "Whenever I thought there was going to be fights, I used to go to my room and practice my clarinet and do my homework. I could stay locked away for hours."
> "You geek; I did it differently. You remember the McKenzies next door? I didn't really like their children that much, but I spent as much time with them as I could, because it helped me stay away from home. Their mom was always warm and open and she encouraged me to come whenever I liked."
> "How come I never got to know them?"
> "Oh, I never invited them to our house. I was always too ashamed and scared they might see something of the way we lived."

Children's Inappropriate Closeness

In environments with relatively little use of controlling tactics and little closeness, some children establish strong alliances with the parent who is not in the addictive relationship. With parents unpredictably available, normal parent–child boundaries are disrupted and children seek other ways of being connected,[16] such as adopting adult and co-parenting roles, caring for younger siblings, becoming a supportive confidant to perturbed adults, and even engaging in or seeking sexualized relationships with adults. As illustrated in the inset box, 12-year-old Adrienne responds by taking on an adult caring role. She interprets her responsibilities as both caring for her younger brother and sister and supporting her distressed mother. In doing so she prematurely takes on the responsibilities of an adult, a move that could potentially hinder her development as a child.[17]

> ### Danny/Jack: The Child Parent
> Danny and Julie's eldest child, Adrienne, is talking with a friend about how she could help with her parent's difficulties.
> "I need to be strong to keep things going. You know with my dad, well, when we were all together, he was mostly not around, and now that they've separated we see him even less."
> "That must be hard."
> "It's no good relying on him. Mom just sits around on the couch and frets. She worries about whether she should have left, how little money we have, and whether she should allow him access, and so on and so on."
> She pauses for a moment, and then switches to considering her own situation. "I just need to keep my head down, keep strong, keep the house going, and make sure things go okay for my younger brother and sister. If I don't stay strong, then no one will keep on top of things and we're all likely to go under."

Children's Volatile Closeness

In home environments in which intimates are close and make little use of controlling tactics, children can still encounter high levels of emotional uncertainty. Whereas on one occasion they might find their parents are fully and lovingly available, on another occasion their parents are preoccupied with their own issues. As depicted in the inset box, the main problem for children is not knowing what level of availability will greet them on each occasion. To manage this uncertainty, children typically develop a variety of responses to protect themselves from potential disappointment and hurt. One option involves reacting to the unpredictable availability of their parents with similar emotional volatility and perhaps hostility.[18] This may involve acting out either in the home, such as shouting, picking arguments, and breaking things, or outside the home, such as getting into trouble at school or fighting on the streets. These behaviors give the child some level of control over parental attention and can draw them away from preoccupations with their own issues.

> **Cathy/Dion: Two Homes in One**
>
> Cathy's daughter, Shannon, is describing to her older brother, Dion, how Cathy's heroin use affects her.
>
> "When I come home from school I never know what state Mom will be in. It's like I have two homes. In one home she kisses me, asks me about my day, and feeds me. The other home is chaos. I come home and she is stoned on the couch, either totally out of it, or yelling at us and crying about how hard life has been to her."
>
> "Yeah, I know, I went through all that too."
>
> "The trouble is, as I open the front door, I never know which of these two homes I'm about to walk into. If I did know I would have time to prepare myself. Instead, each time I walk home I become worried as I near the house."
>
> "It affects me less now, but I do remember how tense and worried it made me feel most of the time."

Children's Pretend Closeness

In environments of high volatility and considerable closeness, pretend closeness is often used to increase safety in a potentially damaging home environment. The child learns that pretending to be close reduces the chance of becoming a target of counterreactions stemming from threats to the addictive relationship and earns positive regard for helping to camouflage the family from outside scrutiny. The pretense can take many forms, but it typically involves sharing proximity with parents and expressing appropriate emotions, while internally not feeling any genuine closeness or compassion. Children who appear close and affectionate can assist in defusing otherwise hostile situations; they can reduce the chance that they will be the target of abuse and they give the impression of compliance and thereby reduce threats to the addictive relationship (see inset box, above). The ability to appear close while internally remaining distant could be useful in adulthood in dealing with relationships at work or in the community, but in nonaddictive intimacies could create future difficulties with communication and trust.

> **Danny/Jack: Diversionary Tactics**
>
> Danny and Julie's second child, Luke, is describing to his sister how he has handled tension at home.
>
> "Adrienne, I hate it when they both argue."
>
> "You don't seem that worried. You don't run out of the room like I do."
>
> "I know. But can't you tell I'm not me."
>
> "No, you seem to get quite involved."
>
> "I'm just pretending. When Mom starts up with Dad I'll crack a joke or bring up another topic or I'll show them some school work—anything that gets them onto something else."
>
> "Yeah, and sometimes you act all cute, and sit next to Mom and cuddle her. C'mon, I've seen you."
>
> "Maybe. Sometimes I wish I could be like a referee and blow a whistle and the match would be over."

Children's Social Isolation

One option for children, particularly in situations where closeness also entails strong use of controlling tactics, is to withdraw from intimacy altogether. This position of social isolation protects them from the pain and disappointment associated with unpredictable availability and abuse. To children, it is a reasonable option because relationships with their parents are their first experience of intimacy and they may conclude that all intimacies carry these negative experiences. Ways of withdrawing may take many forms. It may involve developing a quiet, polite, and shy demeanor that people gradually learn to accept as fixed (see inset box). It may involve spending long periods alone, pursuing hobbies in their bedroom, avoiding social events, and not engaging in conversation with others living in the home. It may even entail total noninvolvement, not making eye contact or speaking with anyone. The long-term implications of this withdrawal depend on such factors as how long it lasts, the severity of exposure to violence and other intimacy management strategies, and the extent to which it arrests the child's social development.[19]

> **Jacinta/Wendy: The Invisible Child**
>
> Wendy is speaking to her friend, Sally, about her 8-year-old son, Elliott.
>
> "Sally, I'm really worried about how withdrawn Elliott has become. He spends his time in his room on his computer, mostly playing games."
>
> "That's normal for boys his age."
>
> "No, no, he spends *all* his time there. Whenever he comes to dinner he says absolutely nothing. And if I ask him anything, all I get is yes, no, and grunts."
>
> "What does Jacinta think?"
>
> "She just says he's a shy boy and that's fine. I think it's something more. He used to be more outgoing, but as things in our relationship have got worse, I've noticed him engaging less and less."

Adolescents

Adolescents emerging from an addictive social system and about to enter their own social worlds face considerable challenges. Responses depend on a range of factors, but those who have been in long-term, highly fragmented environments are most likely to experience ongoing problems.[20] Conversely those who enter adolescence with stronger connections are less likely to experience overwhelming problems.[21] However, most adolescents in such environments will encounter some difficulties particularly with regard to their emerging capacity for compassion. The following outlines a few of the common responses.

Adolescents' Passionate Engagement

In environments involving less use of violence and other controlling strategies, many adolescents remain passionately and compassionately interested in connecting with their own parents, but their parents' availability is frequently interrupted with absences and intoxication as well as by their own

---

Danny/Jack: I Hate Her

One evening when Danny is visiting Julie, their son, Luke, sneaks into his sister Adrienne's bedroom while their parents can be heard arguing in kitchen.

"It's not nice to listen to, is it?"

"I hate her for all this," Luke says.

"You hate her? It's dad who's always plastered!"

"I hate *her* for staying involved with him. Dad really can't help himself. She's the one who lived with him all these years and now they're apart, she's making us go through all this stuff."

"Yeah, but she's trying to do her best by all of us"

"Huh? Her best? I tried to talk to her about Dad's drinking and she just says he's going through a rough time and that we need to be supportive. Supportive? She makes me feel bad for even raising it. Meanwhile things just get worse and worse."

---

preoccupations with the negative effects of fragmentation. On the whole adolescents react to these confusing connections with a broad range of strong negative emotions that include expressions of anger, resentment, and defiance. As depicted in the inset box, these feelings can be directed to either parent and can involve angry outbursts, brooding resentments, generalized shame, and overwhelming frustration. For some these feelings may manifest themselves externally in antisocial behaviors such as violent and disruptive behavior outside the home, regular alcohol and drug intoxication, and premature sexual activity with the risk of unplanned pregnancies.

Adolescents' Dispassionate Presence

In environments involving more frequent violence and other controlling strategies, adolescents opt for strategies that enable them to appear to be present and connected but in actuality engaging as little as possible emotionally with the parents. This can be achieved by a variety of means. As they may have done as children, some adolescents develop a world of close involvements outside the home (sports, school, visiting friends), others withdraw into their bedrooms, and others learn simply to disengage from those around them. One commonly effective way is through the use of addictive substances/processes. For example, in the inset box, Fiona is finding the emotionally volatility of home life increasingly intolerable but has learned that any attempts at being physical absent are severely punished. She then realizes that she can ameliorate home tensions by secretly and regularly smoking cannabis; she is physically there but psychologically detached. Other responses could involve feigned emotions, strategic sharing, and conflict management strategies. While these responses are adaptive in normal home environments, in the addictive environment they can create problems for intimacy in future circumstances. For example, the use of intoxication to cope with interpersonal tension could contribute in later years to the adolescent entering into an addictive relationship.

Bert/Joan: Present and Not Present

One night while their parents are out, Donald says to his sister, "Fiona, I'm really worried about all the dope you're smoking. I see the stuff lying around and I smell you smoking it."

"What's it to you? You haven't told Mom and Dad, have you?"

"No, they have no idea. So what are you doing?"

"It's so hard at home, all that tension and fighting. But if I stay away I get into trouble. The dope helps me chill out."

"Yeah, but there are other ways, you know."

"I'm not super-responsible like you, Donny. My way of coping is to be here and not here at the same time. With dope I can be at home and nothing worries me, so everything is sweet."

Adolescents' Dispassionate Responsibility

Adolescents who as children had adopted either inappropriately close or adult roles within the family can find themselves grappling with the same roles well into their adolescence. Their devotion is often driven by a strong sense of obligation toward the parents, which seems to bind them dispassionately but honorably to the home. As depicted in the inset box, Dion's sense of responsibility for his mother Cathy's welfare has persisted well into his twenties. All through his adolescent years, his mother's neediness has formed a core part of his social world. While other people (particularly Lisa) are encouraging him to explore new worlds, his sense of obligation discourages him from leaving. In this way, he compromises his capacity to form other relationships, thereby delaying the formation of his own independent circle of intimates.

> ### Cathy/Dion: She Needs Me
> Late one evening, Dion is speaking with his partner, Lisa, about the trip they're planning.
> "I can't see how Mom would survive if I left right at the moment."
> "Oh, come on. You're over 20, with plenty of money, and she can manage fine."
> "Yeah, but she has long periods of depression and I need to take care of the house and keep an eye on my little sister."
> "But Shannon is nearly 14 now. She's old enough."
> "Also, when Mom has had a heavy session, sometimes she passes out. I need to be around to make sure she is cleaned up and gets to bed. I'm worried that one day she will overdose. No, without me she is in danger and I could never live with it should something bad happen to her."

Adolescents' Clean Break

In contrast with dispassionate responsibility, another option is for the adolescent to leave the situation altogether. This can be particularly attractive to adolescents in home environments of considerable violence and volatility. In early adolescence a response to traumatic incidents might be running away and living on the streets, with all the vulnerabilities that entails. For middle to late adolescence it is more likely to involve a unilateral but planned exit with enough distance and anonymity to ensure that a separate social world can emerge. This for some adolescents can be a positive move, freeing them from the negative emotional impacts of addictive social systems, but for others the separation may interrupt developmental processes and leave a trail of unresolved issues regarding their parents.

Parents

The connection between parents and their children is established from when the child is first conceived and normally intensifies throughout childhood. The experience of unity and accord—represented literally as "a cord" in the womb—is reinforced by constant physical contact as an infant, by continual closeness as a small child, and by sharing all the emotional ups and downs involved in maturing during middle and late childhood. This close connection is normally further reinforced through unbounded compassion and high levels of commitment. Consequently the accord a parent feels for a child is of a high magnitude and one that for most lasts a lifetime. When a child enters an addictive relationship, all connecting strands of intimacy are tested, but this applies especially to accord. The key challenge for parents is managing their sense of unity and accord with the child while at the same time preventing themselves from being drawn destructively into the crisis and fragmentation that surrounds the addictive relationship. The following are some common responses:

Danny/Jack: Stepping Out of Line

While Danny was living with his father, Jack, one day he picked up enough courage to confront him with some home truths:

"Do you have any idea what it was like for your mother—God rest her soul—and me during your years of drinking?"

"You're not going to…"

"We used to wait up wondering if you would get home safely. I reassured her. 'He'll be all right, Rose, it's only a phase.' But it wasn't a phase. Your drinking got worse and worse. Then there were the calls from the police, the injuries and hospital stays, the job losses. Each one we experienced as a bitter disappointment."

"I'm sorry I was such a disappointment," Danny replies in a sarcastic tone.

"I'm sorry too. When your mother became frail we decided we could no longer expose ourselves anymore to your problems and that was when I told you to leave home. It was the hardest thing I ever had to do."

Parental Bruising Accord

The normal and understandable response to a child in trouble is to stay connected and tough out the hard times no matter what transpires. At a societal level this is what good parents are expected to do, but the entry of an adolescent or an adult child into an addictive relationship severely distorts these expectations (see inset box, above). For children the addictive relationship becomes of increasing priority and they act increasingly as if their parent's commitment is of little value. They become less reliable (e.g., not keeping appointments), more deceitful (e.g., telling lies and stealing), colder and more ruthless, and, what is most distressing, they dismiss the sense of accord cherished by their parents. This is no longer the child they raised and loved; this is somebody else. But at the same time it is the same person; the parents cannot possibly pull away because of their strong sense of union. The more intense their sense of accord they have built up over the years, the deeper the penetration of feelings of pain and rejection. Each rejection, each crisis, is felt as though they are receiving repeated blows; blows to which they have no defense. The pain and hurt is sustained as long as they maintain contact, but the contact itself comes at a significant cost to their own well-being.

Cathy/Dion: Stepping Out of Line

Cathy is speaking with her son, Dion, over dinner.

"When your grandparents first found out I was using drugs they came down on me like a ton of bricks. Not that it did any good. I had discovered the pleasures of heroin and nothing was going to get in my way."

"But you must have known how much it scared them."

"Yeah. In the early days I did try to clean up, and they tried hard to help me. But then I got into it again."

"How did they respond?"

"Well, I remember them both asking me to leave home. That was sad. As I left they looked so crumpled. Then they kept in contact from time to time, but only when I expressed an interest in changing. I guess anything more was too painful. Of course, I never seriously considered changing."

Parental Conditional Accord

Parents can also moderate the pain of rejection by remaining connected but varying their closeness, compassion, and commitment depending on the levels to which they are reciprocated (see inset box, above). When their child behaves in ways that are respectful of their relationship, the parents allow themselves to get closer. As disrespectful and controlling behaviors occur, the parents distance themselves. This may affect decisions regarding whether or not the child could live at home, how much a parent tries to communicate, and how much they are willing to invest money and support. This approach is not easy to pursue and has a limited duration. The use of strategies involving pretense and deception make it difficult to know whether the intimacy is real or not, and as the addictive relationship intensifies, genuine reciprocation becomes less likely, leading to fewer opportunities for accord.

> **Danny/Jack: All My Fault**
> While visiting his grandchildren, Danny's dad, Jack, sits down with Julie and starts reflecting on what went wrong.
> "When he started drinking heavily, Rose and I had no idea it would lead to this."
> "I suppose all his friends did the same."
> "But as parents, where did we go wrong? We brought him into the world and loved him all through his childhood. I remember him as always full of energy but always affectionate. I would never have expected things to turn out this way."
> "You did nothing wrong, Jack."
> "Did we love him too much, or too little? Did we ignore him when we went through rough patches?"
> "I don't think so."
> "I worried so much about that bad group he got in with before leaving school. I wish we'd controlled that more."
> "Maybe, but how could you? By that stage he was already in charge of his own life and unlikely to take your advice."

Parental Inappropriate Accord

An alternative way for parents to remain strongly linked is by adopting roles that fall outside normal patterns of parental behavior. This enables parents to maintain connection with the child but in ways that avoid exposing them to the punishing responsibilities of parenting. Shame for the parent is also an important driver. The parents who watch their child's connections with the world deteriorate are haunted by questions of their own responsibility: Was there something they did that promoted the addictive relationship? Do other people consider them responsible for the state of their child? In the inset box above, Jack expresses the shame and rejection he felt as his son's addictive relationship to alcohol consolidated. For some parents, this can be further complicated by not only feeling shame themselves but also feeling shameful on behalf of the whole family. Out of this sense of shame some parents find themselves seeking to stay connected in the hope that they might play a part in rectifying the situation. For example, Jack already recognizes that having a close parental relationship with Danny is hazardous, and instead he might attempt to strike up other roles such as becoming a work colleague (by offering him work), or pursuing common interests, or even becoming a confidante (by sharing his problems). This way he stays connected with his son but in ways that entail minimal conflict, hurt, and shame.

Parental Distant Accord

Another way for parents to maintain a sense of connection but to protect themselves from the pain of deception and rejection is by reducing their

Cathy/Dion: Keeping a Distance

Cathy's mother, Maureen, is talking with her son, Dion.

"I so much want to know how Cathy is doing; what she is feeling, what she is thinking, whom she is meeting."

"Well, you can find out just by visiting her."

"At times I sit by the phone and think about calling her; but I know from the past as soon as I make contact our lives will be turned upside down. She will be asking for money, involving me in hassles with boyfriends, courts, employers; she'll start picking fights with others in the family and eventually start shouting at us."

"I know. You're too old for that sort of thing."

"Dion, don't think I'm cold and cruel. It's because I love her so much that I needed to stop calling. When I know exactly what she is up to, I worry all day and stay awake all night wondering if she is safe."

proximal and emotional closeness. This can be achieved by pursuing as little contact with the child as possible. For instance, they might cease inquiring as to what the child is doing away from home, they might converse as little as possible, or they might encourage the child to live somewhere else. As can be seen in the inset box, these distancing strategies have the advantage that they enable a moderate quality of life while allowing the addictive relationship to take its course. It is a stance that is commonly recommended to parents and avoids the debilitating effects of bruising accord and the collusion associated with inappropriate accord.

Parental Disowning

The disowning of a child, the permanent disengagement from the child, is a radical response and likely to occur only after extended periods of distressful involvement. However, in situations where a parent's own well-being is at risk, this might be the only viable option, and as the child grows into adulthood, it is not unusual for parents to completely cut the child out of their lives.

Close Friends

Friends connect for all sorts of reasons. For some, friendship emerges from time spent in close proximity (as at work or because of shared hobbies), for others the connection emerges out of strong emotional and compassionate identifications (as with mentors and soul mates), and for others it emerges from a commitment to a common cause (as with campaigners and sports teammates). For whichever reason, reciprocated levels of commitment and accord normally result in a symmetrical connection valued by both parties. When they are strongly asymmetrical—one friend invests more in it than the other—friendships tend to wane. When the links are symmetrical and when they involve all four connecting strands, then friendships are experienced as strong and are likely to last a long time. However, different types of friendship tend to involve emphasis on different strands. For example intimate friendships at work are built on daily proximal closeness, while intimate friendships formed through traumatic events such as war and disasters are built on commitment and accord. For many of those in addictive relationships, connections to friends may comprise their main source of intimacy because, for reasons described above, connections with family members have deteriorated.

The following are common examples of responses by close friends, but depending on the intensity of the friendship, many of the responses discussed earlier with family members are also possibilities.

Friends' Precarious Closeness

A central dilemma for close friends is whether to openly address the strengthening addictive relationship. On their first attempt to speak out about it, they may find their friend interpreting the conversation as a direct threat. As described in Chapters 3 and 4, a considerable amount is at stake regarding the continuation of the addictive relationship, and open discussion could be interpreted as a challenge to its survival (see inset box). Possible counterreactions from the person in the addictive relationship are likely to include angry outbursts, silences, and the withdrawal of all contact, at least for a short period. Whatever the response, close friends are liable to feel severely punished for speaking out, and they then face the choice of whether to continue addressing the issue and face similar hostility, and most likely the loss of the friendship, or to keep quiet and continue in their friendship as it stands.

> **Jacinta/Wendy: Stepping Out of Line**
> Wendy's friend, Sally, is speaking with her about Jacinta's gambling.
> "When we first raised the topic of her gambling, she would simply ignore us or change the topic. So James took a more direct approach and stated to her straight out, 'Your gambling is a problem.'"
> "I bet she didn't like that," says Wendy.
> "Well, she went very quiet. Afterward she stopped talking to either of us and avoided meeting us."
> "Yeah, I remember. I'd come round but I couldn't get her to visit."
> "It only lasted a month or two but we had learned our lesson and we never brought it up with her again."

Friends' Volatile Compassion

As experienced by other intimates, close friends can find themselves connected to a person in an addictive relationship in dramatic and passionate ways. Their feelings often waver between intensely negative and intensely positive. At one moment the friend might feel outrage and abhorrence at the way the person is being treated. At another moment the feelings might be of intense sympathy for the emerging problems and isolation. For example, in the inset box, Sally at times feels angry with Jacinta, but at other times, because she is aware of Jacinta's many positive qualities, she also feels considerable sympathy. As a truly close friend she finds it hard to maintain a distance from the fragmentation processes in the addictive system. The more intimate a friend, the more important for the survival of the addictive relationship and accordingly the greater the need for this

> **Jacinta/Wendy: Anger and Sympathy**
> While sharing a coffee, Wendy's friend, Sally, says, "As Jacinta's gambling got worse, I started feeling very angry for the way she was treating you and the effects it was having on Elliott. She was causing you a lot of anguish."
> "I could see you were short with her at times."
> "Then on other days I would feel really sorry for her. She was ruining everything and would soon have nothing. That was terrible and she couldn't help herself."
> "Yeah, no one deserves that."

relationship to be managed. As other intimates experience, Sally finds herself caught between wanting to help and needing to protect herself.

Friends' Distant Commitment

Perhaps as a response to their own negative experiences or those observed in other people, close friends may adopt positions that involve continuing the connection but preventing any flow of strong emotions. This way they maintain a loyal and caring involvement with the person while protecting themselves from any negative or controlling impacts. As time goes by this position involves a fine balance that is difficult to maintain. By staying involved, the friend is forced to witness the progressive deterioration and fragmentation within the family system and accordingly emotional responses are difficult to suppress. As illustrated in the inset box, Mary keeps regular contact with Joan, and tries hard to avoid repetitive discussions and attempts at change that she knows are futile. In this conversation she defers to other professionals and tries changing the topic. On other occasions she has tried reassurance, distraction, and even walking out. She wants to support her sister, but Joan keeps drawing her into repetitive discussions and pointless analysis. While keeping her distance works to some extent, as time goes on and Bert and Joan's connections with family, friends, and work deteriorate, she finds it progressively more difficult to remain emotionally aloof and finds herself repeatedly dragged into many of the feelings of hopelessness that Joan experiences.

> **Bert/Joan: Keeping a Distance**
>
> Joan's sister, Mary, has in the past also been her closest confidante and friend.
>
> "Mary, he's carrying on just the same."
>
> "Joan, you know what I think. We've gone over it again and again. I can't really help you. He needs to see a therapist."
>
> "I'll never get him to see anybody."
>
> "I don't know how to help you. You can go and see someone yourself."
>
> "But Mary, I don't think I can go on like this much longer."

Friends' Waning Accord

Often close friends do not make a definitive decision to end a connection; rather, they find the relationship slowly dissipates of its own accord as the addictive relationship squeezes them out. For some, perhaps, it emerges as a means of emotional protection; the contacts become increasingly token and ritualistic, the conversations become increasingly stilted, and little attempt is made to connect with each other's inner life. Unlike those caught within an addictive system, the friend normally has the advantage of being part of another circle of intimates within which those connected to an addictive system form just one part. As contacts occur less frequently, these other relationships become stronger and more valued in that person's social world, and accordingly the links with the addictive system tend to fade away, thereby adding to the experience of fragmentation for those in the addictive system.

Colleagues, Neighbors, and Other Associates

Associate relationships are not, strictly speaking, intimate relationships because they are defined by role and function rather than by what they mean to those in them. However, the surrounding network of associates—work colleagues, neighbors, physicians, hairdressers, and the many other people that comprise a person's broader social environment—contribute significantly to the extent to which people perceive themselves as part of a social world. For this reason it is worth considering briefly some of their likely responses.

Associates' Conditional Closeness

Associates often find themselves living and working alongside people in addictive relationships. Over time they encounter the many unpleasant consequences of intoxication and observe the fragmentation occurring within other intimacies. In response they adopt strategies that enable them to function in their respective roles but to avoid, or at least manage, their level of personal involvement. For example, in the inset box, Cathy's neighbor has had previous negative involvements with drug users and prefers now to manage her degree of exposure by avoiding meeting with Cathy outside her own home.

> **Cathy/Dion: Neighborly Involvement**
>
> Over the last 2 years Cathy and Dion have developed a friendly relationship with an elderly woman in the apartment next door. Over a cup of coffee one day Dion asks her, "Why don't you come over to our apartment some time?"
>
> "Well, you see dear, I'd like to, but I'm not sure what I'll find. Don't get me wrong, I like your mom, but she takes drugs, and I have lived next to other people who take drugs and I've found getting involved only leads to trouble."
>
> "But she might be different?"
>
> "Yes dear, she probably is, but I feel better if I keep to myself. I'll be friendly to your mom, but I can't be her friend, if you know what I mean."

Associates' Compassionate Challenge

Community and work associates are often in a good position to speak out and challenge the formation of an addictive relationship. For example, as realized in proactive employee assistance programs,[22] work colleagues are often well placed to lead or participate in challenges to an emerging addictive relationship. They have the advantage of being less affected by controlling tactics than are family intimates and less affected by likely counterreactions such as insults and threats of nonassociation. Furthermore, access to work and its associated benefits—such as wages and distribution networks—can play important roles in accessing the addictive substance/process and consequently

> **Danny/Jack: Work Colleague Challenge**
>
> Danny's boss decides to talk frankly with Danny over lunch.
>
> "You and I have relied on each other at work for several years."
>
> "Yep, we're a team."
>
> "I really respect you as a worker and I want to keep working with you but I really need to talk with you about something rather sensitive."
>
> "Well, okay."
>
> "This is difficult to say… I'm really concerned that when you turn up to work hungover from the night before, your work is affected."
>
> "I do my job okay."
>
> "No, you seem hungover most days, it makes you slow in the morning and uncoordinated, and I'm worried one day that one of us will get badly hurt."

threats to work can translate into threats to an addictive relationship and thereby create incentives for change. For example, in the inset box above, Danny's boss raises the topic of how his drinking is impacting his work performance. While his challenge is unlikely to impact on Danny's emerging addictive relationship, it does add more weight to the variety of other people and circumstances that are questioning this relationship.

Associates' Commitment Liability

A common dilemma for associates is that even though they might feel considerable compassion and closeness to people in an addictive system, the ongoing pursuit of the connection may create problems elsewhere. For some, the period of a crisis is the most likely time to get involved, but that is also the time that people are most likely to get hurt. Getting involved can prove enormously costly and associates soon learn to back away. Similarly, reversion is a hazardous period when associates are both likely to get involved and likely to experience collateral damage.[23] For example, in the inset box, Bert's friend had previously attempted to help his work colleague out during a time of crisis only to find his contribution rejected or exploited. He now recognizes that it is more sensible to keep his distance because further involvement is likely to impact negatively on the people in his immediate circle of initimates.

> **Bert/Joan: Getting Too Close**
>
> In the street one day Joan runs into a work colleague of Bert's whom he has worked next to for over ten years. During the conversation she asks, "How come you and Bert don't get together after work anymore?"
>
> "I really care about him and we work well together. But some years back I made the mistake of getting too involved with his life. Joan, you know how it is; I got so tangled up and confused and ended up worried all the time. And that began seriously affecting me and my own marriage."
>
> "But he really needs steady people like you."
>
> "I know, but while he keeps drinking I know that if I allow myself to get too close, I'll just end up upset again. I do care about him, but it's a question of priorities. I can't afford to let him affect my life."

Associates' Disassociation

As with any of the roles discussed above, associates can also resort to partial or complete disassociation. This could mean working alongside others and only interacting with them as much as is needed to get the job done. In more challenging circumstances it could involve moving to another neighborhood, changing jobs, or actively cutting off all forms of contact.

Broader Social Dynamics

While discussion here has focused on the action of addictive relationships on family systems, these processes also occur in the broader context of social structures and institutions. Here the concept of social fragmentation can be

usefully applied to deteriorations on a broader front. When an ice-flow fragments, the cracks forming between two masses have implications for the
integrity of the whole mass. The formation of one crack increases the likelihood of other cracks and, potentially over time, with cracks forming elsewhere, the mass as a whole slowly loses its core integrity and begins to
disintegrate. In a parallel way, fragmentation at a local level mirrors and
sometimes contributes to fragmentation in a broader context. For example,
the system of cocaine production in Colombia, besides elevating the number
of addictive relationships to cocaine, has facilitated reformation of social and
economic structures as a whole. Similarly countries with high per capita consumption of alcohol, such as Spain and France,[24] are forced to grapple with
its broader impacts on their health, justice, and welfare systems. To make
sense of these broader social dynamics, this study of addictive relationships
would need to examine interactions at the level of class, ideology, and econ-
omy. This broader focus is beyond the capacity of this book. Nonetheless, to
emphasize the importance of wider social structures, the following discussion briefly touches on three relevant zones of interaction: community, gender,
and culture.

Community Dynamics

The social fragmentation generated in families by addictive relationships
spills over and has a range of consequences for communities both at the level
of neighborhoods and at the level of larger multineighborhood aggregates.
Besides the sense of isolations these families experience within their communities, other fragmenting effects include the disruptions caused by marital
separations, the loss of involvement of people who could contribute to the
vibrancy of a community, the health and mental health consequences of
violence and other controlling tactics, the impact of associated crime on
police and justice facilities, the health care costs associated with injury and
illness, the impacts on the viability of businesses (particularly from gambling), and the mental anguish for people in neighborhoods, schools, and
workplaces from witnessing the deteriorating quality of life for people close
to them. Accordingly, communities are not in a position to stand back; they
are affected by addictive relationships in significant ways and have a duty to
their own well-being to seek ways of addressing these disruptions.

Communities have a duty to respond to the negative impacts of addictive systems

Different communities choose to respond in different ways: some communities ignore addictive relationships in their midst, others prefer taking a
punitive and blaming approach, some openly recognize their existence but
offer little in assistance, and others recognize them and actively try to assist
change. In communities that maintain low levels of recognition, the people
who come in contact with affected families will have difficulty knowing how
to respond: "Here is something big that nobody talks about, and what could

I possibly achieve by myself?" Exposed community members are uncertain about what they are encountering, uncertain about their role, and confused over whether to get involved. Such uncertainty encourages people to step back and keep their distance. A circle of noninvolvement is created around the family, which further increases the family's sense of alienation. At one level community members interact with these families as they do with any other family in the course of day-to-day activities. But at another level conversations are intentionally shallow, with few attempts to discuss intimacy issues and certainly no discussion of the addictive relationship. This distancing is also visible with professional involvements. For example, general practitioners are likely to view patients from families affected by addictive relationships as difficult to deal with, or to believe that addiction problems are beyond their purview.[25] Consequently, the stance of communities regarding addictive relationships plays an important role in the levels of social alienation and fragmentation experienced by families, and affects the opportunities for families to access support.

Gender Dynamics

Gender plays a significant role at all levels in the evolution of addictive relationships. In most countries men are significantly more likely than women to develop addictive relationships.[26] For children growing up in addictive home environments, boys tend to react differently than girls do. For example, research has commonly found a tendency for females exposed to addictive social systems to display more internalized effects (such as depression, low self-esteem) and males to exhibit more externalized behaviors (such as violence and conduct problems). These responses are in turn further moderated by whether the parent in the addictive relationship is the father or the mother.[27] Another important gender difference emerges when intimates reappraise their involvement with addictive families; husbands are more likely than wives to leave and to leave earlier, which means more women than men are left to grapple with the long-term effects of these fragmenting environments.[28] Furthermore, gender attitudes and social structures have an important contribution. For example, as explored in Chapter 7, the greater access men have to money and social influence enables them to use violence and controlling tactics more effectively than women can. This in turn enhances their capacity to minimize potential threats and to maintain their addictive systems on an ongoing basis. Later, when women either in addictive relationships or living with them attempt to reintegrate, the social processes and supports required often take a different form from those required for men. For example, rehabilitation (reintegration) programs specifically for women tend to place a stronger emphasis on opportunities for open and nonthreatening communications of emotions and relationship issues.[29]

Men respond differently than woman to the drivers of addictive relationships

The social processes contributing to these differences are complex and multilayered. In addition, the interrelationships are not fixed and vary considerably according to context. For example, the higher prevalence of men in addictive relationships to alcohol tends to vary according to consumption practices, which in turn are influenced by how alcohol is licensed and regulated, which then relates to how alcohol is sold, how much it costs, and how it is promoted.[30] This can also be seen in the way prevalence varies for women according to changes in their consumption patterns. For example, the rates of female problem gamblers have risen markedly in contexts where electronic gambling machines are placed in venues that are more accessible to women.[31] These observations suggest the social expectations and norms associated with being male and being female play a significant role in the way and extent to which people establish their relationships with addictive substances/processes.

Cultural Dynamics

Different cultural ways of looking at the world play an integral role in shaping the types of relationships people choose to establish with addictive substances/processes. For example, patterns of alcohol use are strongly intertwined with cultural beliefs and values, which have resulted in a fascinatingly wide range of customary practices associated with drinking. Through the use of anthropological methods, these differences have been studied in Jewish, Irish, Italian, and other European cultures, as well as in the cultures of Asia and the Americas.[32] Within each of these cultural contexts addictive relationships and associated patterns of social fragmentation have emerged in different ways, and accordingly each cultural context has devised different strategies for responding to them.[33]

The fragmentation associated with addictive systems often interacts with the dynamics of culture change in a variety of ways. Many recent emigrations have involved people from cultures that value collectivity moving into modern urban societies where individualism and personal success is more highly prized. For example, families from traditional Chinese cultural backgrounds emigrating to Western cities bring with them the collective capacity of their families to endure severe hardships. However, when people develop an addictive relationship to an addictive substance/process, such as to gambling, this family collectivity can serve to further isolate them from the resources of their host community. As the addictive relationship intensifies the well-being of the whole extended family can slowly deteriorate as family members collectively prop up their affected loved one for fear that others will find out that something is going wrong. As things get worse, the belief that the family should manage its own problems and the threat of loss of face (particularly in a new land) encourages them to turn more inward and fall back on their

Fragment-ation expresses itself in varying ways in different cultural contexts

own resources to manage the problem. This can then lead to a progressive draining of all the family's hard-earned resources (money in the case of gambling), which results in further alienation, often with tragic consequences.[34] A similar pattern can be observed with the emigration of people from small nations in the South Pacific.[35] For example, Vili Nosa studied how in their emigration from Niue to New Zealand, Niuean men for the first time were exposed to alcohol, which then resulted in alcohol slowly acquiring a role in processes that determined social status and social connectedness.[36] This intensified cultural linkage soon led to problems associated with intoxication, family conflict, and violence.

Perhaps the clearest and most perturbing examples of the negative interactions between cultural change and the fragmentation that accompanies addictive systems occurs in cultural contexts where social fragmentation is already established by other means. For example in indigenous cultures, such as the Australian Aboriginal and First Nation North Americans, the impacts of colonization lead to the confusing experience of being an outsider in one's own land.[37] Consequent deteriorations in social connectedness provide an ideal environment for addictive relationships to thrive because their intensification meets less resistance. Correspondingly, the imposition of addictive processes on top of the alienation already experienced with colonization leads to a doubling of fragmentation with crippling effects on affected families and communities. These same dynamics can be observed with immigrant populations, particularly in those immigrant communities that have difficulty in reforming their own connectedness or in connecting with the dominant culture.[38]

The interactions between fragmentation in addictive contexts and fragmentation within broader social systems are beyond the scope of this book, but they undoubtedly play a significant role in the patterns and trajectories of addictive relationships. These processes warrant further exploration in future projects and highlight another zone where theories within a social paradigm can make a strong contribution.

Chapter 9

Collective Opportunities

When I am here, or anywhere I like, and am busy, then drink's no fear at all and I'm well, terribly well, and gay, and unafraid and full of other nicer nonsenses, and altogether a dull, happy fellow only wanting to put into words, never into useless, haphazard, ugly, unhappy action, the ordered turbulence, the ubiquitous and rinsing grief, the unreasonable glory, of the world I know and don't know.

("*Dylan Thomas*"[1])

Earlier chapters have examined the various ways in which the intensifying strength of intimacy in an addictive relationship is paralleled by reducing levels of intensity in other intimacies. The emphasis on the strength of these processes risks giving the impression that addictive relationships become too strongly embedded to allow any change. But this impression is certainly not what is intended; people in addictive social systems can and do—through considerable effort—make changes to these systems. Since social processes have played a critical role in the emergence of addictive relationships, this book contends that social processes also offer opportunities for restoring people into an interconnected, nonaddictive social world. The big opportunity that will be explored in this and subsequent chapters concerns the potential of collective strength between people in counteracting and reversing the trend toward fragmentation. It proposes that groups of people associated with the addictive relationship can connect with each other in ways that override fragmentation processes. In a world of improving social relationships the addictive relationship becomes increasingly isolated; it has no real currency and spins by itself like an unattached cog. The person in the addictive relationship can no longer manage both worlds. He or she is confronted with having to choose between intimacy with the addictive substance/process or intimacy with people. Pursuit of both intimacies becomes increasingly less viable. Furthermore, even when the choice is made in favor of the addictive substance/process, improved social integration lessens the impact of the addictive relationship on other intimates, thereby freeing intimates to pursue their own pathways to improved well-being.

149

P.J. Adams, *Fragmented Intimacy: Addiction in a Social World*
© Springer 2008

Empowerment and Connectedness

What can individuals isolated in an addictive social system hope to achieve? Often attempts to address the situation are thwarted by unexpected countermoves that only lead to feeling more isolated. Each of these failures contributes to an increasing sense of helplessness out of which the addictive relationship seems to emerge even stronger. Other people become more preoccupied with their own issues—more silent, more reluctant, more avoidant, and perhaps more frightened about doing anything. Friends, work colleagues, and neighbors know that something is going on but they say nothing and when approached tend to back away, looking as though they do not wish to get involved in anything this messy. Where in this fragmented, split up, and isolated home environment is there any hope of change? Where are the resources capable of challenging the strength of the addictive relationship?

In situations where people feel totally disempowered, there are two important sources of strength that can be accessed for change: power within and social empowerment. *Power within* refers to an extraordinary inner reservoir of spiritual strength that people access when other sources of strength fail them. It is commonly accessed by people in addictive relationships as a key ingredient in attempting a reintegration process. This important source of strength is a domain of study in its own right,[2] but it is beyond the scope of this book. While acknowledging the importance of power within, the social orientation of this book means it is more focused on opportunities associated with *social empowerment*, that is, the power that emerges from people connecting with each other, the power of collective action. Fortunately, the notions of social empowerment and collective action have attracted considerable attention in social health research over the last 20 years and are increasingly recognized as critical ingredients in determining the health and well-being of a population.

Social empowerment emerges from people connecting with each other

Empowerment

The primary ingredient to collective action is empowerment.[3] As discussed in Chapter 7, the application of *power over* involves the imposition of the will of somebody in a more powerful position onto somebody less powerful. The direction for the application of power is from those with more power ("top") to those with less ("down"). In a home environment, this top-down application of power typically generates an atmosphere of silence, compliance, and sometimes fearfulness. Even when applied benevolently, top-down processes tend to result in emphasizing the power of the strong and de-emphasizing the power of the weak. For example, when a parent provides total guidance to a child, the child learns to rely on this guidance and can end up strongly dependent on the parent in the future. The same processes operate for small and large groups of people.[4] The application of top-down interventions on communities tend to empower the ideas, resources, and values of the elite and powerful, whereas bottom-up processes enable communities to realize their own strengths and capacities. This is a costly lesson that has had to be repeatedly learned and relearned by many communities. For example, when Western governments apply their solutions to poverty in African communities, these well-meant interventions have typically led to projects with a poor cultural fit that have not advanced community resilience and independence.[5]

Solutions that emerge bottom-up from amidst collectives of people are more likely to find ownership and durability. This happens for several reasons. First, social situations are generated from a broad range of influences that include factors related to geography, history, politics, culture, customs, economics, social structures, as well as local ways of thinking and behaving. People living within a social situation are more likely than outsiders to be familiar with all its complexities and subtleties and therefore to be in a better position to know what would fit the context. Second, ownership is a powerful process in itself and involves a special form of social connectedness. It functions similarly to when a person buys a house; the act of owning establishes from the outset a relationship of commitment, which in turn defines clearly a set of roles and responsibilities. The owner is expected to guide, protect, and look after that which is owned. Finally, in some ways the process of connecting matters more than the individual outcomes. In difficult circumstances, it is often solidarity with others nearby in similar positions that provides the strength for change rather than deriving strength from people outside. In the long term, binding with outsiders, particularly with those in safer and more powerful positions, contributes little to the ongoing sense of empowerment.

Solutions that emerge bottom-up more often find ownership and durability

Social Connectedness

Earlier chapters have examined the ways in which deterioration in social connectedness results in social environments that make people more vulnerable to the effects of addictive relationships. It can be seen as a vicious cycle in which loss of strength leads to increased fragmentation, which then leads to increases in vulnerability and so forth. The importance of social connectedness is not unique to addictive systems. Social health research is increasingly finding that levels of social connectedness play a critical role in determining vulnerability to a wide range of health and well-being issues. For example, adolescent health researchers are uncovering how weaker social connectedness makes adolescents more vulnerable to the negative effects of poverty, sexual abuse, racism, mental health concerns, and many other threats to well-being.[6] Furthermore, the effects they measure do not involve vague or ambiguous correlations; the relationships to social connectedness are typically strong and central in the results. In two studies in which I have played a role—one on sexual abuse and the other on gambling—we found that levels of social connectedness to home, friends, and school emerged consistently as the most important factors in predicting both risk and resiliency. Similarly, studies on addictive relationships have found that social connectedness acts both to make them less likely and to increase the likelihood of reintegration.[7]

These two processes, empowerment and social connectedness, operate together in building the capacity of a social system to withstand the fragmenting effects of addictive relationships and other distorting influences. Social capacity building[8] refers to activities that increase the potential for social connectedness to occur within particular environments. If addictive relationships are interpreted at a social rather than an individual level, then these processes become central in the opportunities for change, both in terms of preventing addictive environments and in terms of achieving change.

Reconnecting Intimates

As the addictive relationship intensifies, top-down intimacy management strategies continue to fragment relationships in the system and undermine points of resistance. The more family members feel isolated and alone with their concerns, the stronger their sense of helplessness. They begin to feel caught in a hopeless cycle of crisis and fragmentation from which they cannot find a way out. The following discussion examines the social interactions in addictive systems in order to find the best opportunities for collective empowerment.

Intimate Response Phases

Prior to forming an addictive relationship, family members and other associates are likely to experience their social worlds as roughly similar. As the processes of fragmentation spread their effects across an addictive system, they split the social world of those involved into two: the social reality of the person in the addictive relationship, and the social reality of other intimates. The two worlds are now on a different course (see inset box, below) that contrasts the different phases of what is likely to be experienced. The left side focuses on the person in the addictive relationship, and is the same as the diagram discussed in Chapter 4 (see Fig. 4.2). The right side focuses on the cycle of five main phases experienced by other surrounding intimates (partners, parents, children, and close friends).

The initiation and intensification of the addictive relationship remain in the domain of the addictive relationship. However, once the processes of fragmentation get properly underway, intimates are drawn into the pattern of fragmentation and

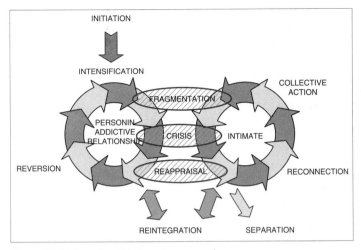

Figure 9.1 Twin cycles of intimacy response phases

crisis, which then initiates for them their own cyclical response to the situation. Both cycles share the experience of repeated fragmentation, crisis, and reappraisal, but the intimate cycle differs in its opportunities for reconnection and collective action. Furthermore, each cycle can rotate at different rates, and people on either side can find themselves caught in one phase for a long time. For example, it could initially take many years for fragmentation to run its course and lead to a crisis. This means that the faster these phases cycle, the more frequently those involved will enter phases of reappraisal, which then present them with the opportunity of considering reintegration. This is important because intimates often need to cycle around several times before collective action develops sufficient strength to generate a crisis that propels the person in the addictive relationship to consider change. The following discussion considers each phase of the intimate cycle.

Phase 1: Fragmentation

The problems for intimates tend not to emerge until the intensification of the addictive relationship is well underway. The early experiences of fragmentation occur directly between the intimate and the person in the addictive relationship. Later, as the fragmentation spreads to relationships with other intimates, the quality of the relationships between intimates themselves begin to deteriorate. For example, children might start resenting their mother's continued loyalty to and support for the father's addictive relationship. Further fragmentation occurs when nonintimate social connections also start to fray, such as when friends and colleagues are excluded from family life. As explored in previous chapters, the primary purpose of this fragmentation is to reduce any potential sources of threat to the primacy of the addictive relationship. As long as these threats are managed adequately, the fragmentation remains reasonably stable. When the person perceives an increase in threats, this triggers

---

Danny/Jack: Smooth Times

During one of Jack's visits to his grandchildren, he begins talking to Julie about the early days of her marriage to Danny.

"I suppose things were bad all the way through."

"No, funnily enough, in the early days, when we were really busy with the babies, I never really questioned his time away in the evenings. Then we sort of got on okay."

"He was drinking less then?"

"No, he was drinking heaps. It was just that I never challenged him. It wasn't until later, when the kids started school, that I started complaining about his absences and putting demands on him to get more involved. Then things started to get rough."

"He did things that frightened you?"

"No, he wouldn't hit me or anything. But he would shout or sulk, or he'd just stay away, almost like he was punishing me for something."

Jacinta/Wendy: Ongoing Crises

Wendy is reflecting with her close friend, Sally, about the various crises brought on by Jacinta's gambling.

"You know, that time I first discovered Jacinta had stolen money, it seemed like the end of the world for me."

"It was pretty bad."

"We ran around going to counselors, we paid people back, we talked and talked, and she kept promising she'd never do it again. But then these things just kept happening—lying, stealing, court cases... Now, it seems like we're in one constant state of chaos, and there are no good times."

Bert/Joan: Maybe It's Over?

Joan is talking with her sister, Mary, about how to move on from her latest crisis with Bert.

"It's just too hard, Mary. This last blow up—I feel he's hit me just one time too many."

"You have been very strong Joan. Really. I'm amazed at how many times you've tried to get him to change."

"I'm not sure if I have another attempt in me."

"What if I teamed up with you and your children and we all pulled together? Then he might listen?"

"Maybe, but this time something in me has clicked and I don't know if I really want to be with him. He has hurt me deeply. Mary, I'm beginning to think I'm now only in the relationship because I'm scared of doing anything else."

---

the need to increase fragmentation, which in turn leads to some form of crisis (see inset box).

Phase 2: Crisis

The experience of crisis is a social event because every intimate within the addictive social system is drawn in at some level. Crises range in form and intensity: they can erupt suddenly in interpersonal conflicts that may involve violence and the heavy use of other intimacy management strategies; they can occur when significant members in the family system decide to separate; they can be precipitated by external events such as court proceedings or hospital admissions; they can develop into more prolonged crises that result from ongoing money problems, marital disputes, and mental health issues such as anxiety and depression (see inset box). During each crisis those involved tend to focus their attention and effort on getting through it and finding a way to restore some level of normality. After the crisis settles and a restored or reorganized stability returns to the home, intimates then have the opportunity to reflect on the meaning of the crisis and to reappraise their participation in the social system.

Phase 3: Reappraisal

The postcrisis period of reappraisal is a critical point in the intimate cycle. It can occur at three levels. The first level relates to whether or not the intimate wishes to continue as a member of this addictive social system. The seriousness at which leaving is considered depends on levels of freedom; for example, male partners with greater access to money and mobility are perhaps more likely to consider leaving than female partners with fewer economic or occupational prospects.[9] But even for those with little choice, the possibility of leaving is an important consideration; for example, children often entertain postcrisis thoughts of running away from home (also see Joan's dilemma in the onset box above).

The second level of appraisal concerns the conditions and circumstances under which a person continues to participate in the addictive social system. The cycling repetitions of fragmentation and crisis can appear overtime as inevitable and fixed. The following questions need to be addressed: What can be done to make this more tolerable? How intense a relationship can the person tolerate with the addicted person? Can the person lead her own life, keeping the effect of the partner's addiction reasonably contained?

The third level of appraisal concerns the opportunities for intervening and changing the nature of the cycle itself: Could things be brought to a head leading onto a crisis that may result in significant change? Does the person have the power to change the system itself?

All three levels of appraisal—leaving, adapting, and changing—require strength and support, which moves intimates to the next phase of building strength through reconnection.

Phase 4: Reconnection

Intimates learn early on that individual action is unlikely to counter the strength of an addictive relationship, and usually results in further fragmentation and isolation. In a weakened position, individual challenges may even lack sufficient strength to trigger a crisis. For example, a spouse may have threatened to leave so often that it is no longer considered meaningful (see inset box). Genuine threats to the addictive relationship require strength, and strength is derived from within a network of social involvements. Action requires a platform of social connectedness before the options of leaving, adapting, or changing can be considered. Unfortunately, in addictive systems this is problematic, because the strength to make the change is missing. The intensification of the addictive relationship has led to fragmentation and disconnection all around. The primary task is that of reconnecting. Reconnection can occur at many levels: it can involve the person in the addictive relationship; it can occur with other intimates such siblings, parents, children, or close friends; it can occur with people outside the circle of intimates (other friends, interest groups, work colleagues); and it can occur with professional (physicians, counselors, or school teachers.

> **Cathy/Dion: Going It Alone**
>
> Cathy's 13-year-old daughter, Shannon, is confiding in Dion about her attempt to question their mother about her drug use.
>
> "Last time I talked straight with her, she just made lots of promises, said she wouldn't use and we'd spend more time together, and that she'd... well, so on and so on, but it didn't take long for her to get back into the same routine."
>
> "So you challenged her. Very brave. But I found doing things on my own didn't achieve much."
>
> "Yep, me too. The drugs are just too strong and whatever I try is pointless."
>
> "No, no. You did well. Maybe you underestimated the forces you were dealing with. You might need to look at coordinating efforts with others, like with me and Lisa."

Phase 5: Collective Action

Reconnection is in itself a form of action, and, as the strength of other networks gather momentum, reconnections themselves have the capacity to unsettle and disrupt the use of intimacy management strategies. The person in the addictive relationship will act in the interests of protecting the relationship by attempting to impede these reconnections. However, through intoxication, absences, and inattentiveness the person may be unaware of the extent to which intimates are reconnecting. As intimates strengthen connections with others separate from the addictive relationship, they begin sharing with one another the experiences they have in common, which leads them on naturally to consider options for change and perhaps to plan a collective action. In the example in the inset box, Donald and Fiona have already progressed in their reconnection. Their repeated discussions are now enabling them to formulate plans and to make progress in building up their collective base. Perhaps in time the broader group, including Joan, might be ready to challenge Bert's drinking by declaring an ultimatum regarding the consequences of his continued use. Such a challenge could be sufficient to prompt Bert to question his addictive involvement, but at this stage is probably more likely to lead Bert to make deceptive claims or promises or to disengaging further with his family. Either way, responding collectively improves the position of the intimates. At the very least it helps clarify the level of strength and commitment of the person to the addictive relationship, but more than that, it helps build the platform for later and more potent collective attempts at challenging the addictive relationship.

> **Bert/Joan: Getting Together**
>
> The teenage children, Donald and Fiona, are speaking more frequently about the chaos at home.
>
> "Donny, since we first started talking about Mom and Dad, I've also started to tell others about what we are going through."
>
> "So have I."
>
> "I've spoken with a teacher and she sent me to a school counselor. I'm speaking with one of my close friends. Each time I talk with someone I feel a little less frightened, less angry, less alone."
>
> "I wish we could get Mom on board."
>
> "Well, I think we may have a chance there. I've noticed a change in her lately. After that last fight she didn't bother to run around cleaning things up. She's gone all quiet, and I think she's looking at things differently."
>
> "What if we talked with Aunty Mary?"
>
> "Yes, I was wondering that too. She might know how to speak with Mom."
>
> "If we both went to talk with Aunty she might take us more seriously. Then we might all have a chance of speaking with Mom."

Responsibility for Change

After having identified the social opportunities for change, the next questions are: Who is responsible for taking these opportunities? Is it the individuals in the immediate addictive social system? Is it the circle of intimates as a whole? Do neighbors have a role? Do social institutions (such as health services and government) have some responsibility? In a social world all these levels interact, and determining responsibility is not a simple matter.

Particle Responsibility

In a particle paradigm, the origins and maintenance of addictive relationships are interpreted primarily in terms of psychological and biological processes that focus on the individual as an autonomous particle (see Chapter 2). Accordingly, responsibility for negative impacts is placed either on the individuals concerned or on the processes operating within them. For example, in identifying the pilot error as the cause of airplane accidents, responsibility is attributed to either the pilot as a person or on internal problems such as perceptual, attention, or emotional deficits. This also means that the responsibility for changing and fixing the problem rests primarily with individuals. Without reference to a social world, interpretations of freedom and choice, which are both complex concepts, are simplified to the level of behaving particles. Individuals rather than collectives are held accountable for their action (or inaction) because they are the primary reference point. For example, when a person has a toothache it is his or her responsibility to seek treatment; responsibility is then transferred to the dentist to provide a suitable remedy; after which responsibility is transferred back to the patient to comply with aftercare instructions. Similarly, with drug use, according to a particle orientation, it is up to drug users to determine whether or not they continue using, just as it is up to affected family members to make their own decisions for change when they are ready.[10]

> **Who Is Responsible?**
> - The mother for being too enmeshed
> - The father for being too absent
> - The drinker for being too selfish
> - The drug user for being diseased
> - The children for being too compliant, too rebellious, too withdrawn
> - The friends for being too judgmental
> - The work colleagues for being too uncaring

A fragmented social system is ripe for attributions of responsibility in a particle fashion. Isolated individuals lack social reference points and thus have little to protect them from taking on negative messages of responsibility such as those listed in the inset box. They find these messages difficult to resist because they lack the social involvements to form alternative positions to counter them. The reception of such messages further disempowers their already disempowering circumstances. The messages locate the primary causes in the individuals; therefore, people begin to see themselves as solely responsible for change. This is a heavy burden for both the person in the addictive relationship and the immediate intimates. They are at the hub of a fragmented system attempting to cope with their isolation. Messages that transfer the majority of responsibility back onto them serve only to increase their sense of helplessness and to reinforce feelings of stigma and shame. They also encourage others indirectly involved to back away from the situation, thereby further isolating the family system.

Particle-oriented treatment services have the potential to further compound these effects. Addiction practitioners meeting one-to-one with clients participate in a process that further reinforces the view that people within the addictive social system are wholly responsible both for the problem and for the decision to change. The focus for intervention is reduced to decontextualized individuals in decontextualized clinic environments. Watching with mixed feelings from a distance, intimates experience further fragmentation, as the preoccupations of their loved ones switch from the addictive relationship to this newly formed therapeutic relationship. In this way, they see themselves as being relegated to bystanders, further diminishing the priority of family connectedness. Furthermore, addiction practitioners, whose knowledge, training, and credentials place them in positions of power, risk imposing their preferred solutions on the client. This may not have been their intention, but their position of expert overlays and potentially devalues the solutions generated by family members.[11]

Responsibility in a Social World

As a social event, the origins of an addictive social system are multilayered and complex, and consequently responsibility for change does not rest on one or two individuals. In the inset box four layers of connectedness are identified: intimates, neighborhood, community, and society. At the layer of intimates, the addictive relationship can be seen to occur among relationships between other intimates. As the arrows indicate, an intimate can have relationships with the person in the addictive relationship as well as with the addictive substance/process (such as when a family member tries to restrict access to an addictive substance). The next layer, neighborhood, refers to the range of commonplace relationships that are available to intimates. These typically include neighbors, wider circles of friends, extended family members, close work colleagues, interest groups, and mentors. Thus a neighborhood is not necessarily defined by location. In modern urban societies relationships at hand tend to occur more in the form of a community of interests, where circles of work colleagues or common interests define involvement.[12] The next layer, community, refers to the groupings and social connections that com-

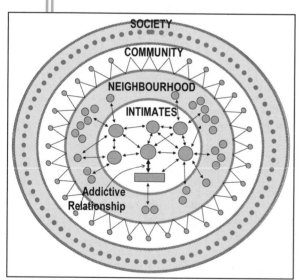

Figure 9.2 Layers of social connection

prise the broader social context. These connections include people associated through the local schools, local health services, local government, and through work and community organizations. The final layer, society, is nebulous and diffuse, but it is an important connection because it refers to broader membership of structures and processes that define how people think.

With a focus on relationships rather than particles and with this wider multilayered perspective, the question of responsibility becomes considerably more complex. To return to the example of responsibility for a toothache, both patient and dentist have some responsibility for actions that lead to healthier teeth, but they are only part of the picture: other intimates play a role in supporting the patient to initiate and maintain tooth-care practices; the community has a role in ensuring adequate and accessible services are in place; and the broader society has a role in promoting knowledge about and positive attitudes to dental hygiene. In moving across these different levels, a confined focus on particle responsibility emerges as merely one part of a more complex picture. The task of identifying responsibility moves from attribution to negotiation with an overriding sense that all people connected directly or indirectly, at whichever layer, have a role to play (see inset box, above).

> **Levels of Responsibility**
> - The individuals for engaging in collective action
> - The circle of intimates for developing the connections for collective action
> - The neighborhood for directly supporting responses by intimates
> - The community for building strengths that empower individuals and groups
> - The society for protecting people from threats to social connectedness

Socially Connecting Environments

In a social world, finding opportunities to connect is a cross-layered responsibility and the role of intimates is only part of a wider picture. The interconnections between people in neighborhoods, communities, and broader society can also contribute to the development of living environments that build strength through social connectedness. For people in socially fragmented addictive environments, increased connectedness brings them closer to a place that is at odds with addictive relationships and where intimacy management strategies are less likely to be effective. Furthermore, increased connectedness shifts those involved away from particle responsibility toward a sense of collective responsibility. While the role of nonintimate social connections will be explored in more detail in Chapter 12, the following discussion identifies some of the multilayered advantages of socially connecting environments.

People in socially connecting environments strive to strengthen the connecting strands between intimates. This responsibility applies particularly to members of a circle of intimates. While the addictive relationships promotes isolation between intimates, intimates remain independent beings capable of strengthening their connection with other intimates by engaging in activities that promote symmetrical closeness, compassion, commitment, and accord.

People in socially connecting environments make the most of their opportunities to connect. This responsibility applies particularly to the immediate but nonintimate circle of relationships referred to earlier as the neighborhood. Addictive relationships thrive in environments of social fragmentation, and vice versa. The stronger the surrounding relationships, the more difficult it becomes to pursue an addictive relationship. This means that the people near the addictive social system, such as friends, neighbors, and work colleagues, can play a role by encouraging social connection.

Socially connecting environments support open responses to addictive relationships

People in socially connecting environments support open discussion about addictive relationships. This responsibility applies particularly to the community layer. While all communities continue to encounter the negative effects of multiple addictive relationships in their midst, many choose to do nothing, which can be very disempowering for the people in the addictive system. It reinforces the strategies of silence and deception already active in the addictive system, and more importantly it discourages talking about addictive relationships. A socially connecting community would seek to increase the visibility of addictive relationships through open discussion in community forums and local media, by supporting the development of services and community initiatives, and by providing guidelines and other self-help materials.

People in socially connecting environments seek to reduce the shame and stigma associated with addictive social systems. This responsibility applies particularly at the societal layer. People at other layers find it difficult to pursue their opportunities and responsibilities when the people associated with addictive relationships are reviled. Common negative messages such as "addicts are weak and unworthy of care" and "the situation is hopeless" are immobilizing for all concerned. Broader social institutions (such as government departments, nongovernmental organizations, health services, and professional bodies) can play a role through public education and social marketing in changing these views.

Change Processes

The social opportunity for change has been located on the intimate cycle, and responsibility for change has been located across the various layers of connectedness to people both inside and outside the addictive system. As discussed earlier, the key social opportunity within the double intimacy cycle in an addictive social system is the phases in which intimates reconnect and move onto collective action. In a context where social connections serve primarily to maintain the status quo, this is the major site to launch a process of change.[13] In the fragmented world of an addictive social system, the four strands linking intimates (closeness, compassion, commitment, and accord) have all been weakened, and some may have disconnected (see Chapter 6).

The goal now is to explore how these components might be brought together in some form of collective action.

Building Reconnection Capacity

The primary task in building the capacity for change involves the restoration of these links. To start with, opportunities for closeness between intimates can be fostered by increasing the amount of time intimates share together, then using that time to share enjoyment and communicate more openly about feelings beginning with the emotions of the moment. As these connections become more, attempts can be made to talk generally about emotions such as worries, fears and insecurities. For example, in the inset box, Wendy has recognized that her preoccupation with Jacinta's gambling problems has diverted her from attending to the needs of her son. She too has begun noticing that he seems quieter and more isolated that usual. After her conversation with her friend Sally, she resolves to devote less of her time to worrying about Jacinta and more time to Elliott. She makes a point of going places with him and talking with him. Slowly, as closeness and communication improves, the capacity for compassion begins to emerge. He begins to indicate that he fears their arguments would lead to them separating; he signals his confusion over what he should be doing to make things better, and he hints that he is worried that behind everything, it is he who has made all these bad things happen. This emerging compassionate understanding helps firm up a commitment between mother and son to maintain their connectedness and to stick by each other through whatever might transpire in the future.

> **Jacinta/Wendy: Diverted Attention**
> Wendy and her friend, Sally, are driving to a meeting one evening.
> "Wendy, I'm not quite sure how to say this. You know when Elliott spent a couple of days with us last week? You know how he doesn't usually talk much? Well, one night we called him to dinner but he didn't come. James then walked up to his room and politely asked him to turn the computer off. Well, he suddenly just started yelling at James, saying he was an idiot and control freak."
> "That's not like him."
> "Yeah, exactly. I asked him what's wrong and he ran out of the room crying, not saying anything. Look, I know you and Jacinta are having a hard time, but Elliott's going through a lot too, and somehow he's being left out."
> "Oh, Sal, I think you're right. We've been so tied up with Jacinta's problems we've sort of left him to look after himself. He's too young to make sense of all this."

Change and Power

As discussed earlier, top-down imposed change has limited effectiveness primarily because of difficulties associated with uncertain ownership. Imposed change is embedded in other people's solutions and is driven by their concerns—concerns that may not coincide with the needs of the people affected. Top-down imposed change has a tendency to emphasize more the power of

Danny/Jack: Going It Alone

One evening Danny comes marching in with a black look across his face. Jack sits down and waits for him to erupt.

"They're all bastards, all of them. As if I haven't got enough to worry about. They all want to make it that much harder."

"Bad day at work?"

"The boss is at me about coming in late, Julie is talking about restricting my visits to the kids, the lawyers are bugging me to start sorting things out..."

"You know what could help you sort things out?"

"Oh don't you start. A few drinks are all I have left to enjoy anymore."

"Danny, we've been over this. I don't want to spoil your fun, but as you admitted before, there is a real connection between these troubles you're having and your drinking."

"I know, sorry," he mutters. "I didn't mean to dump on you, and I am still trying to look at this differently."

Danny/Jack: Court Orders

In a quiet moment, Jack asks Danny, "Do you remember last year when you were drunk and stoned most of the time, and Julie and I tried to get the courts to send you to treatment?"

"Yeah, all I remember was how angry I was with you two. I thought, how dare you get the courts involved? It didn't make me think for a moment about the reasons you filed the orders. All I thought about was how to stop you."

"But we were desperate and thought it would only be a matter of time before you seriously hurt yourself or somebody else."

"And I didn't care. Even if the courts had supported the order, I would have ignored anyone who tried to get to me."

the instigator, which can result in reinforcing the sense of helplessness of the people affected in terms of both their ability to deal with problems and their position within the social system. Alternatively, when plans for change emerge among those affected, ownership of the initiative is not an issue, and even a small modicum of success is likely to lead to ongoing commitment. In the example in the inset box, Danny's ongoing addictive relationship to alcohol and cannabis has obstructed him from forming any real commitment to change despite threats of losing his job, his marriage, access to his children, and ownership of his home. He has in the past perceived the invitation to change as having been imposed on him, and accordingly he has had no serious interest in complying. It is not until, in a moment of critical reflection, he realizes that change might have some advantages that he begins to look at it as a prospect and begins to "own" where this might lead.[14]

One of the problems here is that in a fragmented social system, the resources to contemplate, plan, and implement a change are severely constrained. The person in the addictive relationship is often too preoccupied with avoiding and responding to crises to embrace alternative perspectives. As illustrated in the inset box, as Danny's addictive relationship intensified, his partner, Julie, and his father, Jack, were experiencing increasing helplessness. As one crisis followed another they could not see how their own influence alone could challenge Danny's commitment. Accordingly they were increasingly tempted to resort to heavy-handed top-down strategies. They figured that perhaps an intervention supported by court orders might be sufficient to jolt Danny into reconsidering his position. Their attempt did not achieve their goal, but it did achieve something else. What often matters in such circumstances is not whether the strategy achieved its desired effect, but more that collective action paves the way for increased social connectedness. Even for strategies that involve imposed change, they require people to combine their energies, and, while Danny balked at being forced into treatment, the attempt still brought Jack and Julie together in a way that could set them up for future joint initiatives. While it is possible that their disappointment with the outcome could lead into further fragmentation as a result of feelings of hopelessness or perhaps blame, the decision to move together has opened up for them both the possibility of decisions and of action.

Counterreactions

Particle change focuses on what is possible within the body and mind of the individual. Social change focuses on the system of interconnected relationships and assumes that changes at one point, particularly changes in power and strength, will lead to reactions in other parts of a system. As in the natural world, changing one part of the ecology will trigger reactions that have consequences for other parts of the ecology, so in the social world changes at one point will ripple across a system and lead to changes at other points. This interconnectedness contributes to the adaptability and strength of a system, but it can also contribute to its capacity to resist change. In a system with highly rigid and asymmetrical relationships, as in addictive systems, dominance itself can be deployed to quash any activity that hints at alternative arrangements. For example, when reconnections occur between intimates that then lead to some form of collective action, even if it only involves a gentle questioning, the possibility of new arrangements can be expected to provoke counterreactions from the person in the addictive relationship. The prospect of having other sources of strength in the system is problematic because it could create a beach-head for intimates to mount a more serious challenge. As illustrated in the inset box at the bottom, Jacinta is highly sensitized to any hint of challenging sources of strength and as soon as that strength emerges, counterreactions are required to split and fragment the identified source (Sally) and neutralize its potential.

Counterreactions to emerging sources of strength that might threaten an addictive relationship can take a variety of forms. They may involve previously used strategies such as the use of violence and

---

Wendy/Jacinta: Punishment

Wendy's friend, Sally, is talking to her over coffee one morning. "About 2 months ago, I asked Jacinta about her gambling."

"You were brave. I'd given up on that."

"To my surprise she said she thought it wasn't that bad; she just enjoys a flutter now and then."

"Yeah, right."

"I told her how upset we were about the disruption it was causing in her life. How it was affecting you and Elliott, and how she needed to change."

"Umm, I bet she walked out."

"Sort of… she just listened quietly then left without saying anything. What she really felt came later. I don't know if you have noticed, but when I'm at your place she no longer talks to me; she takes no interest in my life, excludes me from conversations, and chats pointedly with James. I feel hurt because we have known each other a long time, but she treats me as if I don't even exist."

Bert/Joan: Opening Discussion

Joan is talking over the phone to her sister, Mary, after Mary had tried speaking to Bert about his drinking.

"Thanks, Mary, for having a go."

"I don't really know if I did any good."

"Well, actually, in a way you did, but not quite how you intended."

"He seemed to be listening to some of what I said."

"Maybe… well, no. I think he just didn't want you to think he was listening. When he got home he ripped into me, accusing me of talking behind his back and threatening me if I ever talked to you about him again."

"Oh, Joan, I'm sorry."

"No, it's okay. I can't expect more. It's how he always behaves. Later he was into his grog again and then he started yelling and throwing things."

"I'm so sorry. I'll never do it again. I had no idea."

other controlling tactics. These could include major incidents of abuse—levels of abuse that intimates may take a lifetime to come to terms with. As illustrated in the inset box, Joan is confiding more regularly with her sister Mary and Mary is now feeling confident enough to speak openly with Bert about his drinking and its effects on the family. During the conversation Bert is polite and appears to be listening, but afterward he severely punishes Joan with hours of verbal abuse and threats of violence. He claims she had no right to talk to people outside the home and forbids her to talk with Mary or anyone else about his drinking. When Mary hears of Bert's reaction from Joan, she feels enormously remorseful about what she has done; she never intended to endanger her sister. So together they resolve that it is too unsafe to talk with him again and that they would need to be secretive about their contact with each other. Bert's counterreaction serves the double purpose of blocking Joan and Mary's current collective action and of reducing the likelihood that their relationship will strengthen and lead to further action or threats to his addictive relationship.

Controlling counterreactions can also take more subtle forms. In response to perceived challenges, the person in the addictive relationship might initiate complex mind games that exploit vulnerabilities in intimates with regard to their self-esteem, insecurities, and need for affection. For example, a man reacting to his wife's challenge might begin to openly flirt with women because he knows she has previously felt some sexual insecurity. Alternatively, the person in the addictive relationship might seek to move intimates away from the source of threat. The main aim here is to interrupt proximity and thereby undermine the potential for closeness. For example, in the inset box, Danny feels threatened when he finds out that his 12-year-old daughter has been talking to their neighbor about his drinking. The involvement of the neighbors adds another layer of what he sees as posing a threat to his addictive relationship. He recognizes he cannot do much about the neighbors, but he can manage their involvement by making contact more difficult for his daughter. His planned counterreaction involves exaggerating the impact of the neighbor's involvement and linking it to the status of his relationship to Julie. Other similar counterreactions might involve: selling the house and moving the family to another town where no one knows them, changing jobs in response to pressure from work colleagues, and forcing intimates to mix with other people by forming new interests. In these ways emergent sources of social strength are thereby neutralized, and those involved learn

---

Danny/Jack: What's Eating You?

During one of his visits, Danny is sullen and moody. Julie asks him, "What's eating you?"

"Did you know that Adrienne has been speaking to the Burtons next door about what's going on with us."

"I know she's upset about us separating."

"I ran into Ruth Burton in the supermarket and she kept plugging me about how we are getting on and about my drinking. It's none of her friggin' business."

"Well, Adrienne is upset and she needs to talk to someone."

"Look, we don't need them involved. I want you to stop Adrienne going over to their place. It's not helpful."

"I'm not doing that. She gets on so well with them."

"If you won't, I'm going to point out to her that talking to them is going to make it much tougher for us and will make it less likely that we'll patch things up."

the hard way about the consequences of trying to develop these connections.

Another common counterreaction involves the conditional withdrawal of involvement with intimates. In response to a perceived threat, the person in the addictive relationship could spend longer time intoxicated, be absent from home for longer periods, and participate less in family activities and conversations. For example, in Danny's situation he could devote more of his time to extended periods of intoxication, leading to a range of unpleasant incidents that cause embarrassment, chaos, and hurt for intimates and a crisis in confidence in terms of any collective response. This is a high-risk strategy, particularly when the strength among intimates is well developed. Intimates could use these absences as opportunities to strengthen their connectedness and plan collective action. While Danny is regularly drunk, it gives his family the time, and a reason, to plan an approach. However, when intimate connections are weak, these conditional absences can serve to effectively isolate and discipline intimates who are contemplating change.

Guidelines for Effective Collective Action

Within the addictive system, the strongest opportunity for change is at the phase of intimate reconnection. Any improvements in social connection achieved here will influence how the intimate cycle will proceed in the future. However, while laying the foundations for a move into reintegration, the strengthening of intimate connections and subsequent action does not necessarily lead to changes in the addictive relationship. What will tend to happen is that the intimate cycle rotates faster leading, to more frequent collective action and crises but with reducing impacts on intimates as long as they continue to build their connectedness. This encourages the person in the addictive relationship to experiment with replacement and reversion, but *Several* it may take several years before a genuine opportunity for reintegration *attempts at* emerges. Based on earlier discussions, the following discussion provides *collective* three suggestions for each of five periods leading up to, during, and after *action is* collective action: (1) expectations, (2) preparation, (3) collective action, (4) *usually* handling crisis, and (5) responding to aftereffects. *required before reintegration emerges*

Expectations

What can people connected into an addictive social system expect when, moving forward, they attempt to develop connections for the purpose of collective action?

1. *Do not expect success in the short term.* Well-formed addictive relationships have attained a level of utmost priority for the people in them, and it typically takes multiple crises for them to form an adequate commitment to change. Similarly, their first attempts at breaking away from the addictive substance/process, while initially successful, tend to result in reversion mainly because the task of reforming relationships involves considerably more time and energy than anticipated. Furthermore, the reconnections between intimates that are formed can often be washed away quickly in the counterreaction using a variety of fragmentation strategies.

2. *Individual challenges are least effective.* The intimate who mounts a challenge alone is unlikely to have sufficient strength to threaten the addictive relationship. Additionally, these solo attempts are easily identified and counteracted, and the intimate is likely to be progressively isolated within the system. To make matters worse, the lack of success leads to intense feelings of helplessness with a high likelihood of buying into particle responsibility messages such as: "It's all my fault" and "Maybe I'm being unfair."

3. *Expect counterreactions.* Any attempts to form or reform focal points of connectedness in the addictive social system have the potential to threaten the addictive relationship, particularly when they become obvious through collective action. It is therefore predictable that attempts by intimates to strengthen relationships will yield responses that involve the use of intimacy management strategies. Intimates planning collective action need to look carefully at how their alliances are going to respond to counterreactions and to aim as much as possible to build relationships that can endure attempts at fragmentation.

Preparation

The more prepared and the stronger the links between people involved, the less likely that subsequent counterreactions and crises will fragment these links. Consequently, to maximize the impact and to enable future action, effective collective action requires careful preparation and planning.

Preparation helps reinforce collective strength & prepare for counterreactions

1. *Allow time before taking collective action.* The strength of intimate reconnections are critical to ensuring that initiatives—whether successful or not—do not result in further fragmentation. While reconnecting, intimates require considerable time to talk through with others involved similarities and differences in their experiences. It is not unusual for some family members to require long periods of reflection and discussion before they are ready to engage with others in the system. Furthermore, the initial connections are not always strong enough to withstand an immediate crisis. While discussion about what course of action to take might start early in the reconnection, it is still prudent to

allow the various connecting strands of intimacy to consolidate before exposing them to challenge.

2. *Connect as many layers as possible*: Typically, the first attempts at reconnection and collective action occur between close intimates, and as their relationship strengthens they can connect not only with other intimates but also with other concerned people in their neighborhood and community. This is where addiction practitioners can play a critical role. In their meetings with family members, practitioners can help modify expectations to avoid fragmenting failures and to assist in linking them with others such as employers, physicians, schoolteachers, ministers, and respected extended family members. For example, the practitioner could facilitate a meeting with the person in an addictive relationship where not only family but also community members have a say regarding how the addictive system is impacting on them. Such a meeting would involve connections across three layers: intimates, neighborhood, and community. These options are explored further in Chapter 13.

3. *Keep "one's powder dry"*: A group of intimates bound by multiple strands is more difficult to fragment than a couple of people linked by one strand. The stronger the sense of unity and accord, the less likely fragmenting counterreactions will be effective. Accordingly, the length of time devoted to reconnecting with intimates and other associates before attempting collective action can make a difference in terms of the strength achieved. While the use of lies and deception risk replicating and reinforcing current intimacy management strategies, connecting intimates could still avoid active inclusion of the person in the addictive relationship in the process. The process could remain open, and the person can be told that discussions are occurring and that he or she can join in at anytime. Avoiding active assertions of the reconnection reduces the likelihood of early counterreactions and allows time for the strength of the collective to build.

Take time to ensure collective links have attained adequate strength

Collective Action

When as many parties that seem likely to get involve are firmly connected and when the group as a whole feels adequately prepared, the scene is set to experiment with collective action.

1. *Get ready for crises*: Preparation for fragmenting counterreactions is important even in situations that are relatively stable. It could be that the stability is a product of the lack of perceived threat to the addictive relationship, and once a serious challenge is mounted the counterreactions are likely to be just as severe as in less stable situations. Those contemplating collective action need to prepare for counterreactions by identifying their likely form and planning how best to respond to each scenario.

2. *Avoid overstretching collective resolve*: Care needs to be taken to ensure that the plan of action is fully owned by all those who participate. If one person drives the action further than where others in the group are willing to go, it has the potential for splitting the strength of the group and providing opportunities for counterreactions to fragment the emerging alliances. For example, one family member might want to state to the person that they can only remain in the home if they stop using drugs. Other members may not be ready for such an ultimatum. If the group moves ahead on this action and it becomes obvious that not all involved agree, defiance of their stance provides a basis for the person in the addictive relationship to fragment the group and to highlight the group's powerlessness.

Avoid ambitious strategies that risk spliting the collective

3. *Plan a sequence of step-up responses*: Collective action could occur as one part of several cycles of crises, reappraisals, and reconnections, or alternatively, a sequence of collective actions could be planned for just one rotation. This opportunity requires a relatively well-formed level of collective strength. For example, the sequence might start with a period where all concerned avoid supporting or protecting the person from the consequences of their intoxication, followed by an invitation to attend a series of family meetings, followed by involvement of outside community and addiction practitioners, followed by family involvement with service interventions.

Handling Crisis

The predictable attempts to protect the addictive relationship through fragmenting counterreactions will generate crises of varying proportions.

1. *Recognize strategies aimed at fragmentation*: Counterreactions will target perceived sources of threat, and the people involved are likely to feel pressured to distance themselves from the collective action and return to quiet compliance. To reduce the opportunities of fragmentation, it helps to begin identifying and naming these strategies through discussion and review.

2. *Keep in constant contact*: Organized collective action will be new in the system and has the potential to provoke unprecedented levels of perceived threat. This can be new territory where the reactions of the person in the addictive relationship are difficult to predict. In moving into an action phase, those involved need to have procedures that ensure they keep talking among themselves and planning together how to respond as events unfold. Such communication also reduces the opportunity for splitting the collective. Communication procedures could include pre-planned meetings, daily phone or email contact, and ways of getting

together during crises (such as violence, suicide attempts, and police involvements).

3. *Avoid "painting oneself into a corner"*: Strong ultimatums are tempting strategies to include in collective action: "Get treatment or I'm leaving you" "Do something or we will report you to the police." They suffer from three major limitations: first, the person in the addictive relationship may choose nominally to comply, which can lead to immobilizing confusion over whether the compliance is genuine or not; second, the person in the addictive relationship may feel helplessly trapped and responds to the situation with exaggerated and extreme counterreactions; and third, the ultimatum needs to be a response that every member of the group is committed to following through on, otherwise the group's future actions will not be taken seriously. Actions are more viable when collective responses are proportional and follow as a logical consequence of impacts from commitment to the addictive relationship.

Responding to Aftereffects

Each attempt at collective action, particularly an early attempt, is unlikely to fully succeed in promoting reintegration. What matters more in the long run is the ability of those involved to strengthen their connections and to engage more layers in preparation for future attempts.

Make sure building connections continues even when strategies fail

1. *Avoid blame and shame*: Following a collective action and its resulting counterreactions and crisis, those involved can often experience disappointment at how little has changed. It is tempting then to attribute responsibility and perhaps blame others in the group. This temptation needs to be anticipated and avoided as much as possible because such blame could provide the seed for future fragmentation. The lack of change needs to be seen as part of the process, and if nothing else, it has helped the group gauge the strength of the addictive relationship.

2. *Prepare for further reconnection*: For each collective action it is likely that counterreactions are at least partially successful at fragmenting the group. Those involved may feel chastised, frightened, confused, and possibly easily persuaded to view the collective action as foolish and futile. Furthermore, the counterreactions may expose potential rifts in the group. For example, a half-hearted attempt at collective action may split intimates into those who support the initiative and those who are more skeptical. These differences are easily exploited. Consequently, those who were involved will need time to reconnect, analyze what went on, and talk through their differences, before they are prepared to consider how they would undertake future collective action.

3. *Review the possibility for reintegration*: Although at first, embracing a reintegration is a low probability, it is a low probability at first, there is always a

chance that the person in the addictive relationship will choose this crisis as the moment to make a serious attempt at change. This is a critical moment. A genuine willingness to engage in reintegration opens up a new range of risks and opportunities for intimates. Those involved in the collective action would then need time to consider whether and how they would like to be involved in the reintegration process. Because of past disappointments some may choose to keep their distance from the process, others may choose to connect slowly, giving themselves space to feel comfortable with how it unfolds, and others may be open to full participation straight away. Again, to avoid opportunities for fragmentation, the group will need space to discuss and accept the different positions taken by others involved.

Chapter 10

Reintegration

Now I am out of element
And far from anything my own,
My sources drained of all content,
The pieces of my spirit strewn

All random, wasted, and dispersed,
The particles of being lie;
My special heaven is reversed,
I move beneath an evil sky.

This flat land has become a pit
Wherein I am beset by harm,
The heart must rally to my wit
And rout the spectre of alarm.

Theodore Roethke, "Against Disaster"[1]

As outlined in Chapter 4, reintegration is the slow process of reestablishing intimacies in social system previously dominated by an addictive relationship. For the person leaving this all-consuming involvement, reintegration involves journeying from a singular asymmetrical intimacy to a social world of multiple symmetrical relationships. It is a long and difficult voyage that will require many steps both forward and backward before balanced and multiple connections can be achieved. For intimates, there are two paths of reintegration depending on whether or not they choose to remain associated with the addictive system. For those who choose to stay, reintegration focuses primarily on steadily intensifying the relationship with their affected loved one as he or she moves progressively out of the addictive relationship. For those who choose to leave, the pathway can also engage them in a long voyage focusing on establishing a new array of connections. While separation is an important process in itself, the following discussion will focus on intimate reintegration for those who choose to remain in the integrating social system.

What is Reintegration?

The social character of reintegration means that it is relationships that matter, and with relationships the onus or responsibility for change relies on the involvement or two or more parties, mostly more than two because the layers of neighborhood, community, and society also play a role.

171

P.J. Adams, Fragmented Intimacy: Addiction in a Social World
© Springer 2008

Recovery Versus Reintegration

Metaphors help describe and explain the world around us.[2] Metaphors exploit the similarities between objects (or complexes of objects) to describe or explain abstract concepts in concrete terms and with familiar concepts. The language employed by social scientists makes frequent use of metaphors.[3] Psychologists employ simple and concrete metaphors as a means of describing more complicated cognitive and experiential processes.[4] For example, spatial metaphors are phrases such as "personal space," "mental distance," and "depth of processing"; container metaphors are "memory capacity," "perceptual defense," and "inner experience." A common metaphor in mental health involves describing the aftereffects of psychosocial distress or trauma in terms of processes associated with physical disease and injury. People or "patients" affected are seen as having an inner malfunction, an "illness" or "inner wound," for which they require "treatment" or "therapy" by trained treatment professionals who over time lead them in a process of "recovery." This disease metaphor is useful in coordinating professional efforts and in managing patient expectations, but when adopted in a literal or fixed fashion, it can stand as an obstacle to benefiting from alternative ways of looking at such issues. As argued in Chapter 2, by focusing primarily on the individual, the predominant acceptance of disease and other particle-oriented metaphors risk obscuring approaches that view mental concerns in terms of social relationships.

Relational metaphors lead to a more complex and dynamic interpretation of addictive relationships. Instead of limiting explanations to the qualities of individual particles, they widen the focus onto the nature of relationships between such particles. For example, in everyday speech, military metaphors are often used to describe aspects of a marriage with references to events such as ongoing "conflict," verbal "attack," obeying "orders," and so forth. Other common sources of relational metaphors include references to parent–child dynamics (as when referring to a "patronizing" friend or "dependency" relationships), and employer–employee dynamics (as in "going on strike" and holding a family "meeting"). Relational metaphors also play a vital role in developing explanations in the social sciences; for instance, in sociology the metaphor of a "structure" is commonly used in phrases such as "government structures" and "class structures"; health sciences frequently make use of the concept of "system" in reference to objects such as "the health system" and "body systems"; and psychology addresses the complexity of interconnection in the natural world with reference to terms such as social "ecology" and neural "networks."

Reintegration is a relational metaphor for re-connecting intimacies

The relational metaphor of *integration* emphasizes the opportunities of social connection at several levels. At one level it highlights the interactional possibilities between two objects or two people; what one person does is integrated with what another person does. For example, the coauthors of a book need to integrate their ideas and writing styles. In a similar fashion the reforming of symmetrical intimacies on a one-to-one basis with others in the addictive system comprises a key part of a reintegration process. At another level it highlights the potential for individuals to integrate within a system. For example, a new student requires a period of integration into a school environment, just as the person in the addictive relationship needs time to reintegrate into the family system. At yet another level it highlights the possibilities of integration between two systems. This can be observed when a large company merges with a smaller one, or when countries are reformed as happened when East Germany and West Germany were reunited. Similarly, the complex of relationships surrounding each person in an addictive system and their relationships with people and systems in outside layers all require reintegrating in ways that support the complex of relationships across the system at the cost of the strength of the addictive relationship.

The slight variation of the metaphor from "integration" to "reintegration" changes the emphasis from establishing new relationships to suggesting that connections that were once lost are now being restored. For most people in addictive relationships old intimacies are still at hand and capable of restoration. For some with longer and more intense relationships to an addictive substance/process, old connections may have been damaged beyond repair or require too great an effort to undertake early in a reintegration. For example, the use of controlling tactics may have created too much fear for family members to consider any type of reengagement. Nonetheless, since reintegration needs to happen between individuals, between groups of people, and within the broader social context, the notion of reintegration remains a more accurate description.

Purpose of Reintegration

Reintegration is a process of socialization—or more accurately resocialization—involving those who have found their lives fragmented through attachments to an addictive system. It aims to move people out of a world dominated by a single asymmetrical relationship to a world rich in multiple and symmetrical interconnections. It is an immense undertaking because it involves not only dismantling the power of the addictive relationship but also *Reintegration* rebuilding the very basis on which personal strength and personal identity are *aims to* formed. By the nature and magnitude of these tasks it therefore requires the *restore* people participating in the reintegration to sustain considerable effort over *relationships* long periods of time—a significant challenge particularly when it is likely to *fragmented* involve extended periods of setback and disappointment. *by addictive*

Reintegration is organized around two main goals: building multiple *processes* relationships and ensuring that they are symmetrical. The first goal seeks to enable the emergence of multiple and multilayered social connections. A person in an addictive relationship typically maintains a broad range of connections to family, friends, and work, but these relationships tend not to function as relationships with meaning and value in their own right; as the addictive relationship intensifies, these other relationships function more as second-order relationships that service and protect the one dominant relationship. The task in reintegration is to reestablish these relationships as having importance and value in their own right. Similarly, for intimates many of their relationships have deteriorated through fragmentation into connections that serve other purposes; for example, they help protect, avoid, and camouflage the reality of family life. Reintegration also opens a pathway to multiple relationships with value for them their own right.

The second goal of reintegration is to ensure that the emerging relationships are symmetrical—meaning that they are balanced and as much as possible free from *power over* control and other intimacy management strategies. As explored in previous chapters, the singular axis structure of the addictive social system is held together by a complex array of intimacy management strategies, which then lead to imbalances and asymmetries in the connecting strands of intimacy. For example, as illustrated in the inset box, Wendy reports experiencing a level of closeness that is not reciprocated by her partner. Jacinta is more preoccupied with her addictive relationship to gambling. Wendy wants to believe the behaviors Jacinta used to feign closeness and commitment, in order for the relationship to continue as it has in the past. Beyond these deceptions Wendy is beginning to recognize that a return to symmetrical relationships will require both her and Jacinta to let go of this control and progressively to open themselves to the full emotional potential of symmetrical intimacy. For people already feeling vulnerable and exposed by threats to the addictive relationship, the prospect of adding further layers of vulnerability is highly unattractive. The reintegration process requires a long and careful progression, advancing slowly step by step.

> **Jacinta/Wendy: I Still Felt Close**
> Wendy is speaking with her friend, Sally.
> "You know, Sally, even when Jacinta's gambling got bad, for a long time I still had strong feelings for her."
> "That was surprising when she was treating you so badly."
> "Yeah, in hindsight. But at the time I believed, or wanted to believe all her stories. I knew things were going bad for her, so I wanted to be loyal and caring..."
> "... so you just allowed yourself to be persuaded."
> "Yeah, and besides the problems, she seemed real close. But in hindsight I think she put it all on."

Six Phases of Reintegration

Earlier chapters have plotted the double cycles of fragmentation for people in addictive relationships and surrounding intimates, and reintegration was identified as an option in both cycles. In contrast to understandings of recovery, reintegration is seen here as a social process; the focus is not on one individual but on multiples of people across several social layers. This means the gaze now needs to shift away from personal perspectives to looking at how the social connections interact as a whole within the addictive system. To assist in this, Figure 10.1, has unraveled the double cycles and divided the process of reintegration into six phases. The first three phases—

collective action, crisis, and reappraisal—have been transferred across from the double cycles. They represent the lead up to reintegration and were discussed in more detail in earlier chapters. Similarly the possibility of reversion back to the addictive social structure is represented as a progressively fading option at the bottom of the

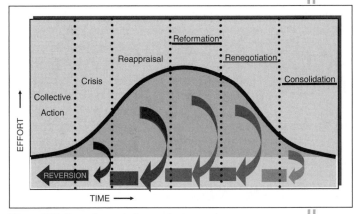

Figure 10.1 Reversion and phases of reintegration

diagram. The three new phases—reformation, renegotiation, and consolidation—are underlined because they represent the central components of reintegration.

All six of these phases take time. For some families several of the phases may take years. For others they may take only a few months. However, for most families immersed in a well-formed addictive system, moving through the various phases of reforming these fragmented relationships is likely to entail a process that takes 5 to 10 years. Furthermore, in contrast to the episodic involvement with addiction services, the process requires some level of support throughout its lengthy progression. This need for ongoing support is the focus of the next three chapters. The following discussion describes the six phases of reintegration and illustrates them with the circumstances in Jacinta and Wendy's addictive system.

Phase 1: Collective Action

As described in the previous chapter, collective action is critical to setting the scene for reintegration. Without pressure the person in the addictive relationship remains captured by the power of that relationship. The incentive for change usually has to come from elsewhere and probably as a result of collective action involving intimates or others with neighborhood or community connections.

Another reason for identifying collective action is that intimates are often the first to openly recognize and discuss the asymmetries or social imbalances introduced by the addictive relationship. This may happen long before—perhaps years before—people in the addictive relationships begin seriously contemplating their impact. For example, Wendy has been discussing with Sally her dissatisfactions with Jacinta's gambling. Through these discussions Wendy

Jacinta/Wendy: A Friendly Meeting

Wendy, Sally, and James meet with Jacinta to discuss the effects of her gambling. Sally starts by stating, "You know all of us here care for you very deeply and want only the best for your future."

"Yes, you really matter to us, Jacinta," says James.

"But we are worried that your gambling is hurting Wendy and Elliott, who we also care about, and we feel you will eventually lose both of them."

Jacinta is listening quietly and casting the occasional disapproving look in Wendy's direction. Wendy adds tearfully, "I can't go on like this. I live in constant fear now of losing the house; I don't know what you are up to in the evenings and there is such tension whenever we do spend time together. I can't go on like this; I can't deal with this and work full-time and care for Elliott."

Jacinta, head bowed staring at the table, responds slowly, "Is this an ultimatum, is this what you are saying?"

"No, no. It's just what's true for me, I can't go on like this much longer."

"And why do you need these two involved?"

"I need them because I've talked to you about this before and you haven't taken me seriously."

"Okay, okay. I get it. Now leave me alone and I'll think about it."

decides that continuing in the relationship as it stands is unacceptable. She and Sally begin considering what actions they might take together. They invite Sally's partner James into the discussions and conclude together that they need some way of emphasizing to Jacinta the seriousness of Wendy's position. The inset box presents the conversation of their first attempt at collective action, and while it is unlikely to be enough for Jacinta to seriously consider change, it does signal the intent of this group to challenge the status quo and demonstrates to them that different things can be attempted when they join forces. Similarly, in future attempts they will probably find that their efforts are insufficient to unsettle Jacinta's attachment to the addictive substance/process. They might need to cycle several times through crisis, reappraisal and reconnection before they gather sufficient momentum in their collective action to engage her in contemplating change.

Collective action can occur across several of the layers, and sometimes the main impetus may come from outside the circle of intimates or the family. It might require the combined strength of court action, medical recommendations, and efforts by employers before sufficient impetus is generated to prompt consideration of change. For example, the arrival of bailiffs at Wendy and Jacinta's home may provide the opportunity for the friendship collective to deliver a more powerful message. However, more often it comes as a result of multilayered collective action involving members of the immediate family, neighborhood, and community. For example, in subsequent collective actions, Wendy and her friends might engage Jacinta's current employer, her general practitioner, and concerned neighbors. They all repeat a similar message, that continuing in the addictive relationship to gambling is unsustainable, and eventually with the repetition of the message Jacinta is forced to consider it.

Phase 2: Crisis

Crisis is brought about through a combination of collective action and subsequent counterreactions by the person in the addictive relationship. These responses initiate a period of uncertainty and confusion that affect everyone involved. Crises vary in size and duration depending on the potency of the strategies employed in collective action and counterreactions. The extent of the crisis also makes it clear how important the addictive relationship has become. The person in a well-formed addictive relationship is capable of upping the ante until those mounting the challenge back down. For example, as illustrated in the inset box, Wendy's challenge, backed up by her friend, prompted an exaggerated counterreaction in which Jacinta threatened Wendy with her ultimate fear of losing both her and her son. Other possible counteractions could include violent outbursts, emotional abuse, legal threats, threats of leaving, and sometimes suicide attempts. To maximize the potential benefit of crises, those involved need to recognize that few crises lead automatically to reintegration. A crisis creates a momentary window of opportunity for change, but in addictive systems where so much is invested in the addictive relationship, an interest in change does not come easily. To avoid energy-sapping disappointments, those involved can benefit from seeing the crisis as part of a cycling process in which while one attempt fails to prompt change, next time around, and with stronger collective planning, the person in the addictive relationship could respond differently.

> ### Jacinta/Wendy: The Aftermath
> "Wendy, what happened yesterday after we left?"
>
> "Oh, Sally, I'm so confused. I've been up half the night. Jacinta just kept going on and on, asking me why I involved you two. She is adamant that I had no right and that it was our private business."
>
> "Did she discuss what we were getting at?"
>
> "No, she didn't mention it. She was more interested in why you were there. She says that you never really liked her and that you're always poisoning my head with negative views of her."
>
> "That's not true. I go back even further with her, I..."
>
> "She said I must cut off all contact with you, otherwise she will leave with Elliott and prevent me from having any contact with him. I'm really scared now. You know how much I love Elliott."
>
> "So are we going to stop meeting?"
>
> "No, no. I need this contact. Maybe we'll just keep it quiet for awhile."

Phase 3: Reappraisal

Chapter 4 identified reappraisal as a post-crisis period that both parties—the person in the addictive relationship and surrounding intimates—opt either to return to or continue with previous arrangements (reversion), or to change them (reintegration or separation). For the person in the addictive relationship reappraisal is a critical period because the outcome ultimately determines whether or not the addictive system will continue. Other people cannot make this decision and as far as the addictive system is concerned, they are forced to wait until circumstances and opportunities transpire to prompt a rethink. For example, as illustrated in the

> ### Jacinta/Wendy: A Dilemma
> Late one night, after hearing what she thought was sobbing, Sally opens her front door to find Jacinta sitting on the steps.
>
> "Oh, Sally, I don't know where else to turn."
>
> "Jacinta, come in, you must be freezing."
>
> "Last night, after the bailiffs took away our furniture again, I saw Elliott sitting with red eyes on the empty floor. He was just sitting there, staring at where the TV used to be. He looked at me all confused. I could see the pain in his eyes... I could see in his eyes a future where he would grow up hating me for all the turmoil I created." Sally sits down next to her.
>
> "We've all talked to you about this many times."
>
> "But this time," pointing to her chest, "it hit me deep inside. I now see I can't continue gambling and be a good mother. I know that changing is going to be hard... so hard. I don't think I have the strength."

inset box above, following repeated collective actions involving Wendy, their friends, neighbors, and others, Jacinta has found it increasingly more difficult to divert and ignore their concerns. But it was not until she was confronted with the loss of something she treasured above all else—her relationship with her son—that she was finally ready to embrace the prospect of change. While her next moves might not lead to a sustained reintegration—her reappraisal could result in her reasserting her current commitment to gambling—the decision does mark a critical moment and one that opens future reappraisals to similar considerations.

Phase 4: Reformation

Reformation is the core phase of a reintegration process. What happens here will determine the strength and success of what follows. For this reason the next section is devoted entirely to a fuller description of reformation. To introduce it briefly, the aim of reformation is to work progressively away from the asymmetrical world of an addictive social system and to rediscover the world of multiple, symmetrical relationships. Reformation is a social process and as such involves both the person leaving the addictive relationship and other intimates. In the early stages, transitional replacement provides temporary stability to enable the slow process of reforming social connections to get underway.

As illustrated in the inset box, when Jacinta first stops gambling she buries herself in her job and working at home. The involvement holds the system together and prevents it from spinning back into fragmentation and crisis, while those involved can devote their attention to building connections. This can also be observed in the transitional reliance on particular hobbies (hiking, meditation) or on regular sessions with an addiction counselor. With a counselor the sessions can provide a stable base on which the person leaving an addictive relationship can gradually reestablish connections to intimates, friends, and meaningful occupational activities. As connections are reformed, the compulsion to stay connected to a singular axis can be relinquished and slowly the broad array of multiple symmetrical relationships spread and reform.

Jacinta/Wendy: Working Hard

One evening Wendy says, "I'm really pleased you've managed to stop gambling these last couple of weeks, but since you've stopped, I'm worried about how much time you spend working."

"We need the money, and things have to get done."

"Yes, but there are limits. You've increased your hours at the supermarket, and when you come home, you keep slaving away right into the night. You're also at it all weekend. We're not really spending time together and you have no time for anything else, including getting together with friends."

"At least it keeps me from thinking about gambling."

"But you need more than this, we need you more than this. What would happen if things went wrong at work? What would you do?"

"I guess if anything went horribly wrong I'd probably go back to gambling."

Phase 5: Renegotiation

Attention and energy in the early years of reintegration focuses on the task of reforming intimacies and ensuring that connections with the addictive substance/process are slowly diminishing. As these changes stabilize, the focus of attention then switches to looking into the future and to wondering more about the quality of relationships in this reformed world. The reentry of the person from the addictive relationship into the world of multiple and symmetrical relationships has profound effects on relationships for everyone involved. Furthermore, for some, the types of relationships that are emerging may not be what they expected or what they want. This leads them to begin questioning the direction of the reintegration. As illustrated in the inset box above, not everyone involved will feel comfortable with the way relationships are reforming.

> **Jacinta/Wendy: I Knew What to Expect**
> Wendy is growing increasingly uncomfortable with always focusing on Jacinta's issues. "At least when you were out gambling I knew what you were up to."
> "No, you didn't."
> "What I mean is I knew what to expect, and I knew it was you who was troubled."
> "So you think it's better then than now?"
> "No, not that. What you are doing is great. I admire it. It's more to do with how we are as a couple."
> "What do you mean?"
> "It's almost like you are more superior to me now. I'm the one who isn't honest enough. I'm the one who manipulates. I'm the one who keeps secrets, I'm … I'm just not sure about us anymore, or whether I'm ready for this type of relationship."

For some intimates the pace of reconnection is too fast and, based on past disappointments, they are unsure of whether they can trust the changes enough to expose themselves to closer intimacy. Reversion could occur at any stage, and the closer they are the more vulnerable they become. For others, attention may have focused so much on leaving the addictive relationship that other relationships have been neglected. For instance, a couple may have placed issues in their marriage on hold until the reformation is established. When this appears to have stabilized, they may then feel ready to address marital issues. Others may feel that as intimacy management strategies diminish and as honest communication improves, this is the time to address fundamental relationship issues. This is the time that parents begin talking through issues of harm and neglect of children, couples examine issues of conflict and communication, and the family members start exploring what they want from their relationships in the future.

Phase 6: Consolidation

Once the course of commitments have been set—the child does or does not want to reconcile with the parent, partners do or do not wish to continue their commitment to each other, friends are or are not willing to remain close—reintegration enters the lengthy phase of consolidation. This phase is important in ensuring that the reformed system is truly robust and is capable of withstanding the emotionally volatile effects associated with experiences such as boredom, loneliness, and bereavement. Since this phase is likely to take many years, it is easy for periods with reduced social connectedness to creep in and thereby set up the conditions for a reversion. For example, instead of ensuring a balance of connections in different domains, a person might have opted to invest more and more energy into one single relationship; perhaps with a new lover or with work (see the inset box before the previous box above). With high reliance on these singular connections, any major troubles could threaten the balance within the system as a whole. For this reason, consolidation requires procedures that ensure that the goals of reintegration are reinforced and that all those involved maintain a constant level of vigilance regarding the quality and diversity of connectedness. These procedures can involve regular meetings with a mentor to help review progress, attending group meetings for support, or taking time out by oneself to consider the strength and weaknesses of the overall progress with this reintegration.

Reforming Intimacies

Multilayered interconnections prevent recapture by the single axis addictive system

The multiple and multilayered connections that are established during reintegration are critical to preventing recapture by a single dominant asymmetrical relationship. For example, a person whose reintegration focuses only around work relationships runs the risk of replicating the single axis structure of the previous addictive relationship and thereby sets the scene for a reversion. The restoration of intimacies is the defining phase in reintegration and consequently warrants closer examination.

Entering Reintegration

For reintegration to occur, there must be points at which the person leaving an addictive relationship can reconnect. It therefore requires the willing engagement of others immediately surrounding the addictive relationship. Without these points of contact the person is likely to remain stuck in replacement mode with the only other option being reversion. But the timing of attempts at reintegration can be an issue. For instance, the person in the addictive relationship might be prepared for reintegration, but intimates are reluctant to participate because of past experiences of disappointment and humiliation. As illustrated in the inset box above, these timing issues can initially put intimates in a difficult position. If they jump straight into reforming intimacies, they risk unprotected exposure to the effects of a reversion. If they remain aloof, the opportunity for reconnection may pass. Do they go along with it or do they play it safe? Their ambivalence might mean that in the initial stages the person intent on leaving an addictive relationship is forced to remain in a replacement holding pattern until the intimates feel trusting and confident enough to participate.

Intimates may also have difficulty with the power dynamics associated with the timing of the reintegration. For example, an adolescent son had yearned for many years for his father to change, but the fact that it was his father who decided when the reintegration would begin has left him feeling that yet again it is his father who calls the shots. As described in the dialogue in the inset box above, Wendy's participation requires her to adjust her life again around Jacinta's decision to change. Jacinta's choice reinforces the helplessness Wendy has been feeling all along. Part of her questions submitting yet again to Jacinta's agenda. In such circumstances it may be a matter of allowing intimates like Wendy enough time to accept the changes and for the Jacinta to provide sufficient acknowledgment of how difficult it must be for her.

> **Jacinta/Wendy: Control of Timing**
>
> Wendy is discussing with Jacinta some of the difficulties she is having adjusting to her change.
>
> "I've waited and waited for you to look at changing, and now you make the decision when it suits you."
>
> "Okay, I understand. But I'm here now and it's not too late."
>
> "You can just wait. That's what I feel. I had to wait, so you should too. Besides I'm not sure if I'm ready."
>
> "Oh, come on. This is what you always wanted."
>
> "Look, you've controlled so much in my life over the last few years. You've come and gone as you liked, you've spent all our money, you've always told me what to do…"
>
> "Okay, but you must agree I have changed, I don't do that anymore."
>
> "Yes, this is why I'm telling you. I'm not your dog to come and go on command. I really needed you 3 years ago and you weren't there. I don't think it's fair that you automatically expect me to support you now."

For those in particularly intense and long-lasting addictive relationships, the main historical intimacies may no longer be available. For example, the person's partner and children may have given up contact long ago and may have no interest in resuming any kind of connection. Alternatively, in some situations the main intimacies are affected by past negative experiences, such as sexual and emotional abuse, making them too difficult a place to pursue in the early stages of reformation. In these situations, reintegration needs to focus more on forming new relationships rather than reforming old ones. Considering the time it takes for most people to form stable intimacies, this pathway will necessarily be slow and involve gradual increases in peripheral closeness until the opportunities for deeper involvements emerge. As described in Chapter 4, this is likely to start with meeting people through new interests or by frequenting local venues. Slowly acquaintances become associates, associates become friends, and from there the opportunities for new intimacies begin to reveal themselves.

Transitional Replacement

Chapter 4 identified the dangers of reversion when one addictive substance/process is simply replaced with another—alcohol with cannabis, compulsive sex with gambling, or heroin with tranquilizers. It

Jacinta/Wendy: Swapping

Jacinta is reflecting on her gambling.

"Wendy, I never told you this, but during the year before I stopped gambling, I was actually worried about it and I did try to change."

"You never told me that," Wendy replies, looking surprised.

"I didn't want to give you the satisfaction of knowing. I thought if I simply stopped gambling, everything would be okay. So, for a whole month I stopped playing the machines."

"But you still went out at night. I don't remember *that* changing."

"Well, yeah. That was the problem. I went to the bars, mixed with the same people, but instead of gambling, I drank heavily."

"Oh, I do remember worrying that you might get breathalyzed coming home."

"But it grew harder and harder to watch everyone else enjoying the slot machines. I still stuck to it and I proved how strong I could be. Then, one day, I thought, 'I don't really enjoy drinking like this, and I'm not really achieving anything, so, what the hell, why not get back on the machines.' Well, quick as a flash I was back gambling as much as I ever was."

also identified how in the initial phases of a reintegration, the reforming of social connections takes considerable time and that most people require some form of transitional replacement (replacement for the purpose of change) in order to hold the system together as this readjustment takes place. Typically, people attempting to leave addictive relationships will experiment initially with partial attempts at change. Their early efforts often involve making changes on their own and implemented in their own particular ways. They also tend to focus on changing only one small part of the addictive system rather than seeing that it is the whole system that will require attention. At this stage they perhaps view addictive substances/processes as merely one dimension of their lives, and as such, see changing the addictive relationship as a self-administered surgical operation where the unwanted relationship is removed without needing to interfere with the system as a whole. In the inset box above, Jacinta describes an early attempt to stop gambling without trying to change anything else within the system. She initially succeeds in her goal but then finds that there is little in place to prevent her from reverting back to previous arrangements. While these experiments in compartmentalized change are often not sustained, they are an important part of the process in helping those involved recognize the scale of effort that will be required for a full reintegration.

Since the strength of attachment in an addictive relationship has had a long history of dominance, it may be difficult to find an alternative that can compete with the reliability, availability, flexibility, and convenience of an addictive substance/process. For example, the ever-present availability of alcohol and its automatic effects on the mind and the body maintain a sizable advantage over the slow-moving nature of social relationships. To provide adequate strength, transitional replacement might need to be made up of combinations of connections. For example, for early replacement twelve-step programs advocate accessing the combined strength of regular group meetings, spiritual connectedness, membership of a fellowship, and as well as the guidance of a mentor ("kindred spirit"). This combination caters to the varying ways that needs are met by addictive substances/processes and to changes in needs as the reintegration proceeds.

Reductions in Intimacy Management

While the addictive relationship was in its ascendancy, relationships with intimates functioned more as a means to an end, rather than intimacy being an end in itself. The repertoire of intimacy management strategies can include the use of violence and other controlling tactics, such as the frequent use of deception, strategic intoxication, other forms of absence, and the manipulation that leads to fragmentation. People who have relied heavily on these strategies are unlikely to shift quickly and will have difficulties accepting the reductions in control. For them letting go of control is likely to feel a little like walking naked in a forest, with little protection from the negative emotional potency of open intimacies. For this reason, the use of some intimacy management strategies is likely to continue in the early stages of a reintegration, reinforcing for intimates their fears that the reformation is not genuine and that they should keep their distance. For example, a man who has controlled his family through shouting and disparagement may have difficulty refraining from doing so when he is stressed or threatened, which has the effect of undermining the trust intimates feel in the reintegration process. However, with the help of other mentors, as he slowly learns to identify these strategies and makes less use of them, he finds other intimates willing to engage more closely. Examples of alternative control messages are listed in the inset box above.

> **No Control Self-Talk**
> - "I don't want to live close to people who are frightened of me."
> - "I can let people be the way they choose to be."
> - "Hearing other people's negative feelings is not going to harm me."
> - "I don't have to take responsibility for other people's anger."
> - "I can be strong and they can be strong."

As the intimacy management strategies become less frequent, surrounding intimates will feel less constrained and will begin communicating their inner world more directly. This may happen in ways the person leaving the addictive relationship never expected. It functions similar to the way sediment might accumulate in a disused pipe; when the pipe is cleared, what first comes out is all the waste materials that have accumulated over time. When fear is no longer an obstacle, the intimate's first communications may consist of all the accumulated hurt and pain experienced during years of living in an addictive environment. This is not encouraging to hear, particularly when a person is seeking reassurance and support. The person would be strongly tempted to silence such talk using previous controlling tactics. Nonetheless, progress can continue as long as the person is supported in recognizing that hearing past grievances is a necessary part of the process, and that this is just a zone that one needs to move through before open and symmetrical intimacies are possible.

Cascading Reformations

Chapter 4 described reintegration in terms of a cascade of reconnections that progressively shift connectedness away from the unitary axis structure of an addictive system to a system where there are multiple symmetrical linkages.

The pace of a reintegration involves a fine balance between moving too fast and thereby risking replication of asymmetrical intimacies, or moving too slow, which then allows the power of the addictive relationship to remain strong and ready to reassert itself whenever the process falters. Either of these directions can lead to reversion back into the structure of an addictive system. Transitional replacement of the addictive substance/process with other objects (such as the support of friends, family, or spiritual attachments) helps to hold things together on a temporary basis. The real work involves the gradual reestablishment of a multilayered network of connections. This could start with the easy, ready-to-hand, and promising connections already available within the context. As these connections are reestablished, the people involved will need to keep gently encouraging each other to continue and to make sure a range of symmetrical relationships are forming.

The reformation of individual social connections will, by the very nature of the process, take time because the participants in the connection need to feel they can trust the process. If someone feels things are moving too fast they are liable to either withdraw their involvement or try to control the situation. For example in the inset box below, Wendy indicates she is having difficulty adjusting to the speed and intensity at which their physical intimacy has been reformed. Mistakes in timing and communication are understandably common, and participants may need regular discussions to review problems and look at ways to avoid reversions. For example, a person may attempt a total break from the addictive relationship without any form of replacement with the result that during the next period of difficulty he or she is forced to revert back to reliance on the addictive substance/process. Alternatively, another person may rush into intense new intimacies (such as new romances), but in so doing risks either replicating the single axis-structure of addictive systems or has difficulty managing the intensity of feeling without resorting to controlling tactics.

The four connecting strands of intimacy (closeness, compassion, commitment, and accord) play a critical role in the cascading reformation of multiple, symmetrical intimacies. In the early stages, efforts need to focus on improving closeness and particularly with assisting intimates to feel physically, emotionally, and psychologically safe with the person leaving the addictive relationship. Later, the focus shifts to improvements in receptivity and compassion, but for all parties this typically poses enormous challenges. Similar to the sudden transition from a dimly lit room to brilliant sunlight, too sudden an exposure to the emotions of other people can be overwhelming and could prompt consideration of reverting back to controlling tactics. The next shift involves a reorientation from commitment to the addictive relationship to commitment to a range of other

> **Jacinta/Wendy: Don't Rush**
>
> During a dinner out to celebrate 6 months without gambling, Jacinta say, "Wendy, when we're in bed together, I have this strange feeling that you don't really want to be close to me."
>
> "I do really... but things have changed so quickly. A couple of months ago we hardly spent any time in bed awake together. Now it's every night. I'm finding it a bit intense."
>
> "But I'm feeling so strongly towards you again. I want, no, I need to show it."
>
> "I'm sorry. I am pleased and I do want to be close, but it has been such a sudden change."
>
> "Don't you trust that I've changed?"
>
> "No... well partly that. But more that I need some time to get used to the change."

intimate connections. This too is no easy process. Old commitments to alliances with drug using and drinking buddies, and to well-ingrained patterns of behavior, are not easy to let go of, and a commitment to these emerging intimacies may seem alien and unrewarding. A sense of accord and unity with other intimates is usually the last strand to emerge, and it provides further incentive for the reintegration process. However, since it tends to emerge at later stages, it does not play a major role in the early and middle stages of reformation.

Enabling Closeness and Compassion

In the early stages of a reformation, strategies aimed at improving closeness and compassion play a significant role in building the capacity for intimacy. The connecting strands of commitment and accord emerge later in the process and they are more an outcome of improvements in the other two strands. *Closeness* Improvements in closeness and compassion both rely on an improved ability *compassion* in the area of communicating emotions. Since the emotional needs differ for *play a* people with different roles in the reintegrating social system, the needs of the *particularly* person leaving the addictive relationship, the needs of other intimates, and the *important* needs of broader social involvements are discussed separately. *role in* *reintegration*

The Person Leaving an Addictive Relationship

A surprising amount has been published on the psychological processes and practices associated with reintegration, particularly during reformation.[5] These publications have mostly taken the form of books based on the writer's own experience of reintegration (recovery) and marketed as self-help guides. The books make many recommendations but tend to share a common view that improved emotional competence is critical to undertaking a reintegration. This task applies particularly to relearning how to respond to one's own feelings and the feelings of other intimates. They also identify that this relearning requires those involved to take on a number of key attitudinal stances and attitudes that reduce the likelihood of returning to emotion controlling and other intimacy management strategies. These stances also play a vital role in reducing the generalized emotions of fear, resentment, and shame discussed in Chapter 6. The following subsections discuss some of the main recommended attitudinal stances aimed at improving the capacity to enter into multiple and symmetrical intimacies.

Openness

A stance of openness to emotions is difficult in the early stages. It involves embracing all feelings, negative and positive, without resorting to familiar strategies used in the past to control them, such as intoxication, violence, or strategic absences. For most people, this stance is achieved through successive graded exposures to feelings, blocking them whenever they seem overpowering, but working steadily through to less avoidance. Writing and talking about them as much as possible can also help to improve clarity and judgment on their appropriateness.

Nonattachment

The stance of non-attachment does not mean avoiding emotions; on the contrary it means embracing them but in a way that does not involve controlling them. The stance involves seeing emotions as a natural part of belonging to a social world; they do no harm and contribute strongly to the meaning of a connection. Feelings can come and go like images on a mirror. They require no containment or capture.

Humility

The shift from a stance of pride to a stance of humility plays a critical role in reducing the control of both feelings and relationships. It runs totally against the grain according to how intimacies were managed in the past, so maintaining humility is a constant struggle in a reintegration process. For example, a dangerous entry point for pride can occur when the person claims responsibility for successes in a reformation. This can often lead to premature exposure to the addictive substance/process with a high risk of reversion.

Honesty

The stance of honesty involves communication freed up from intimacy management strategies such as lying, evasion, and other forms of deception. For example, it was in the past commonplace to speak about addictive relationships in ways that minimize or justify their impacts (see inset box). Communication now seeks full and frank disclosures of the negative effects of the addictive relationship and to pursue recognition of the person's role in enabling it to continue.

Minimizing and Justifying
- "My drug use was never that bad."
- "I'm not alcoholic because I never drink in the morning."
- "It was just my drinking that caused problems."
- "I remained loyal to my family and never abused them."
- "You'd gamble too if you'd gone through what I've had to endure."

Critical Responsibility

The term *critical* is included here because not all perceptions of responsibility are accurate and people may need to carefully examine their part in events before their responsibility in them becomes clear. Once responsibility is clearly identified, the challenge then is one of owning the effects. For example, a person might claim diminished responsibility for shameful acts (such as abuse and disloyalty) on the basis that they were helplessly trapped in an addictive relationship. This perception is inconsistent with attempting a reintegration. While it helps reduce levels of shame, it also acts both as a means of controlling feelings and as a strategy for minimizing the strong effects that addictive behavior has had on intimates.

Forgiveness

The flip side of critical responsibility is the capacity to let go of feelings associated with grievances and perceived violations. This is a difficult socio-emotional process that normally involves repeated attempts at talking the events over with other people, acknowledging their impacts, and establishing rituals that aid the process of acceptance to emerge and to be communicated to others. For example, during reintegration resentments from childhood toward a parent's abuse and neglect may surface strongly as the person opens up more to feelings. The reformation process requires these feelings to be embraced and it may take considerable talking and symbolic gestures before these resentments reduce in potency.

Communication for Intimates

During reintegration, intimates are faced with the task of reconnecting both with the person leaving an addictive relationship and with other intimates whose relationships have been fragmented by intimacy management strategies. The isolation and fear that have been experienced within the addictive system have led to feelings being suppressed similar to the way a wet blanket extinguishes a flaring fire. Following the removal of the blanket it takes time for feelings to reignite and for intimates to perceive their situations as safe. Several of the attitudinal stances listed above would also play a role for the reintegration process of intimates, particularly openness and forgiveness. The self-help literature guiding intimates is less prolific than resources for personal recovery,[6] but recommendations include some of the following:

Emotions have often been suppressed like a wet blanket over a fire

Keeping Safe

A stance of vigilance and attention to safety issues is recommended, particularly in the early stages of reforming intimate connections. The single axis social structure left by an addictive relationship is still in place, and reversion remains a solid prospect. Accordingly, a prudent approach would avoid rushing too quickly into intimacy and risking negative exposures. Instead, opportunities for closeness are handled slowly bit by bit.

Graded Exposure

A careful way to proceed is to grade emotional exposures to the person leaving an addictive relationship according to the level of control the person feels over the level of exposure. If it proceeds too fast and feels unsafe, intimates retreat back into the isolation that had provided them protection previously. Since rapid exposures can contribute to reversions, subsequent reappraisals also provide an opportunity to assess whether reforming connections are occurring too rapidly and whether they should be sequenced more slowly.

Reciprocity

A stance of reciprocity can provide a guide to the rate of entry into intimacy. Progress in attempts at drawing closer to others within the family system is matched by the recipient with perhaps slightly additional effort to keep the process rolling. For example, an adolescent begins to talk to her mother about feelings regarding the chaos the mother's addictive relationship had inflicted on the home. The mother returns this overture by increasing her availability perhaps by devoting more time to common activities or communicating more about her inner life.

Critical Responsibility

Intimates are likely to take more responsibility for negative events than they deserve. This is a product of the isolation and intimacy management strategies they have experienced over long periods of time. For example, a husband might feel that it was his inadequacies that had contributed to difficulties in the marriage. As he reconnects with his wife in an increasingly forthright and direct manner, he will require time to think and talk through the extent to which he contributed to problems and how much was due to his wife's commitment to an addictive substance/process.

Acceptance

Reintegration requires intimates to embrace acceptance of a wide range of difficult issues. The process of acceptance resembles forgiveness and grieving, in that it takes time and a number of rituals of expression before its key objectives feel settled in a person's mind. For example, a man who had grown up in an addictive system may require several years of involvement in thinking, talking, and writing about the deprivations of his childhood before he feels ready to discuss them openly with his parents.

Communication for Others

The wider social world of neighborhood, community, and society can all play important roles in aiding a family system in reintegrating from addictive relationships. There are fewer publications on these roles than on the roles of family members, but based on the discussions in this book, the following attitudinal stances are recommended.

Communities play a role in setting the scene for reintegration

Nonjudgmental

Negative judgments regarding addictive relationships (such as "all addicts are weak and undeserving") increase the isolation affected families experience within their communities. In some ways this is remarkable because the addictive relationships are common enough for large portions of society to be affected. Activities that involve either challenging discriminatory views or promoting open discussion on addictive relationships would contribute to more reintegration-friendly environments.

Understanding

Connected with being nonjudgmental is the need for increased societal understanding of the nature of addictive relationships and what it takes to reintegrate. Government agencies and other major organizations (non-governmental organizations, welfare and treatment organizations, universities) could foster activities that improve understanding such as public education campaigns, improved (less particle oriented) media depictions of addictive relationships, and open debate on key issues.

Receptiveness

To assist in reducing the isolation experienced in an addictive system, the willingness of outsiders to engage with people previously in addictive relationships in talking about their reintegration process can make a big difference to how connected people feel in a broader context. This could be encouraged through the sharing of stories of reintegration through television and newspaper articles, publication of narratives in book collections, and open acknowledgment and celebration of those who take on a reintegration.

Domains of Connectedness

An integrated social system differs from an addictive one in that it requires connections that are multiple and symmetrical. By *multiple* is meant connection across several different territories or domains. While reforming relationships with intimates occupies the core part of reintegration, reconnection in other domains can also play a pivotal role. Within each domain lie multiple opportunities for connection. By *symmetrical* is meant connections that are no longer managed or controlled; the object of connection moves from functioning as a utility in the addictive family system to attaining the status of an object in its own right. Alongside the domain of intimacy already discussed above, there are four other domains of connectedness: occupational, physical, communal, and inner connectedness. (These are also discussed in Chapter 13 in outlining the domains of inquiry in conducting a social assessment.)

Occupational Connectedness

The nature of a person's daily activities and involvements with others plays a key role in the person's well-being. As an addictive relationship intensifies, occupational connectedness typically deteriorates. Relationships with employers are compromised through the effects of intoxication or through work-related controlling tactics such as deceit and social manipulation. As illustrated in the inset box, Cathy's access to heroin is the primary purpose of her efforts at getting money. As her body increased its tolerance to heroin, her need for more money led her into petty pilfering and stealing at work. This in turn led to her eventual dismissal from her job, forcing her to widen her involvement with the handing and selling of drugs. For many like Cathy, this pattern of uncertain work involvements and poor work relationships can develop into a routine: find work, get into difficulties, lose the job, then move onto the next one. Alternatively, others in addictive relationships keep their

---

Cathy/Dion: Earning Money

Dion and Cathy are speaking over lunch.

"Mom, how come you never seem to have a job."

"I do get jobs, sometimes."

"No, they never seem to last very long."

"It didn't start out that way. Before I started using I had a job as a shop assistant. Then when I did start, at first I had enough in my salary for drugs. But later there just wasn't enough money to keep up."

"You needed a better job."

"At 18 that wasn't likely. So I started stealing goods from the store and selling them. I was eventually caught and that's when I started getting involved in with your dad."

"But you could have kept trying?"

"I did try to hold jobs, but they were never enough, and more and more I had to spend the time on other things that would bring in more money."

jobs but display deteriorating work relationships and performance; they experience a level of isolation that suits their need for camouflage all the while keeping their job performance just above the level that would result in being fired. A natural outcome of work transience is long periods of unemployment, a reliance on state benefits, and involvement in crime—all of which adds further to their isolation and noninvolvement with others.

Reintegration engages a person in establishing a symmetrical relationship with occupational attachments. Both the person and the occupational setting should benefit equally from the connections. Work is no longer simply a means of financing consumption of an addictive substance/process or a way to camouflage the reality of addictive relationships. These goals no longer count. What really matters is the extent to which work connects with other activities and other people in ways that are meaningful and rewarding. As the reintegration proceeds, these new expectations prompt a reevaluation of the longer term purposes in an occupation or career, and in many cases interest will shift away from the occupation as a means of making money and shift towards the creative or altruistic dimensions of the work. The new purposes often foster interests in new careers and associated training, a stronger commitment to work colleagues, and in return enjoyment of work less as a means to an end but as an activity in its own right.

Physical Connectedness

The place of people in society is determined in part by their health, their activities, their social identity, and their social involvement.[7] People in addictive relationships neglect their health (see inset box), because of their focus on the addictive relationship. Good health is no longer a priority. As the addictive relationship intensifies, their health deteriorates because of poor fitness, poor nutrition, frequent injuries, and high stress.

Reintegration includes reformation of a relationship to the body. This involves committing attention and time to activities that reestablish a symmetrical and balanced relationship with the body. Activities that help achieve this balance include regular exercise and physical activity, meditation and relaxation, positive sexual experiences, improved diet and nutrition, and pastimes that reduce stress and tension.[8] While these may initially appear forced and contrived, over time they generate a strengthening sense of accord with the body and add another connecting fiber to the world as a whole. Another dimension of physical reintegration involves reconnecting with the locality and place. Previously the

> ### Danny/Jack: Letting Things Go
> One weekend, while watching TV, Jack says, "Danny, I'm worried about how often you've been getting sick lately. You're not looking after yourself."
> "I know, I know. I've really let things go. In the past I would have worried a lot about putting on so much weight and always looking a wreck."
> "You don't get out much anymore."
> "I used to enjoy hiking and playing sports. But there doesn't seem to be any point anymore. It's not that I don't care; I get down about it sometimes. But when it comes to doing anything I just feel it has no meaning; my life's pointless anyway. I'll just take it as it comes."

emphasis on place in addictive systems had been on its usefulness for protective and other survival purposes. During reintegration this changes to becoming a meaningful involvement in its own right. For example, time is invested in connecting with the surrounding natural environment, in responding to the look and feel of the place, and in recalling past involvements.

Communal Connectedness

> **Bert/Joan: Awkward Involvements**
>
> Joan is chatting with her sister, Mary, over the phone.
>
> "Joan, just because Bert no longer gets involved or goes out anymore doesn't mean you've got to do the same."
>
> "There was a time I had lots of interests: tennis, basketball coaching, quilting, school committees. I'd go out to films, meet up with friends, go on garden walks."
>
> "Well, why not now?"
>
> "I suppose I've gradually lost contact with all my friends and don't feel interested in any of these things anymore. They seem silly and indulgent compared to what else is going on."
>
> "Oh, come on. You need these things."
>
> "Really, Mary, you don't understand. I feel so ashamed of how we are living and Bert makes it damn awkward for me to have contact with anyone outside the home."

Communal connectedness refers to links with a broader circle of people—friends, neighbors, work colleagues, agency workers, and others in the neighborhood and local community. For those leaving high-intensity addictive relationships, where there has been strong attrition of other social connections, this domain provides a key starting point in the process of reintegration. This loss of connectedness also occurs for others in the addictive system (see inset box). As described with the other domains, cascading involvements here might begin with new hobbies, then move on to linking in with community activities and spending time with neighbors, then involve regular participation and commitment to local organizations (clubs, sports, and crafts). While these nonintimate relationships may appear contrived and trivial at first, over time they generate stronger attachments that provide a base for later intimacies. An additional aspect to communal connectedness is its potential to strengthen and accelerate emerging bonds within a circle of intimates. Involvements outside the home can create a focal point for shared involvement with others in the family. For example, a father joins a local soccer club and brings his son with him. Their mutual involvement with other members brings them closer to talking openly with each other.

Inner Connectedness

In the preceding chapter reference was made to the power within as a major source of strength and support for initiating a process of change. This reservoir of inner strength can also be viewed as a domain of connectedness, but not with someone or something outside, but with something within (or more vaguely as awareness of a connection within). Twelve-step approaches identify spiritual connectedness as critically important in providing the backbone to a reintegration process, and many authors have backed this up by claiming a spiritual awakening was a crucial point in their own journey out of an addictive relationship.[9] For some, this connection will come in the form of specific religious or mystical experiences during which people feel they are merging with a greater whole (see inset box[10]). For others it will be experienced more as a spiritual dimension of their life, a constant presence that imbues everything else. For others it is more a vague sense of being guided or looked after by something or some greater purpose. Activities that enable this awareness to involve include creating space for reflection and finding time alone for prayer, meditation, and going for walks. As with the domain of social connectedness, the power of this awareness can be overwhelming, and the person may be tempted to block these moments with mind-controlling strategies such as distractions and obsessional thoughts; however, as openness to the inner world of thoughts and feelings improves, so also openness to spiritual awareness becomes more likely.

> ### Jacinta/Wendy: Becoming One
> Wendy is talking with her friend, Sally, about an experience she couldn't understand.
> "The other day I was walking by myself along the river, you know that long track surrounded by trees, when I had this strange feeling that I can't make sense of."
> "You'd been smoking that stuff again."
> "No, it wasn't like that. I'd been by myself for about an hour, my head drifting mindlessly across different topics, when all of a sudden... now you might think me crazy... when all of a sudden I felt as if I had had merged into the trees. I felt as though I had become one with everything."
> "Well, I suppose those feelings happens from time to time."
> "No, this involved a very strong and meaningful sense of oneness. It was vibrant, exhilarating; it seemed to me that something or someone fundamental was communicating with me. I don't know what sense to make of it; all I know is that it made me feel strong and somehow connected with a greater whole."

This concludes the three chapters on families and communities, which have laid the basis for looking at how a social understanding of addictive relationships leads to intervention possibilities.

Part IV
Applications

Chapter 11

Family Resources

Everything else in my life improved.... I no longer had to do things I hated, like steal money or borrow money with no intention of paying it back, or skip work because I was too sick, or end up in bed with some horrible man that I wouldn't have gone near if I hadn't been out of my skull. I never woke up racked with shame and guilt about the way I'd behaved the night before. I had my dignity back....

Mine was no longer an existence where I had to lie constantly. Drugs had put a wall between me and everyone else. A wall that wasn't just chemical, but made of secrecy, mistrust and dishonesty.

(Marian Keyes, "Rachel's Holiday")

The previous three parts of the book have stepped out from under the mantle of particle orientations and explored what it might mean to interpret addictions in a social frame. Part IV explores how this work might be applied to assist people in their struggles with addictive relationships and their attempts at reintegration. This chapter provides an overview of the approaches and resources that an individual or family can make use of in challenging an addictive relationship (namely the relationship between a person and an addictive substance/process). The chapter is divided into three sections, starting with what is currently available and moving toward what is desirable for the future. The first section examines the social components that already exist in various self-help approaches to reintegration. The second section summarizes family and other social interventions that have been developed by researchers in conjunction with addiction services. The third section makes use of the content developed in earlier chapters to outline how people in an addictive social system can monitor their own response through the phases of reappraisal, reconnection, and collective action. The family situation with Jack, Danny and Julie, and their two children, Adrienne and Luke, will be used to illustrate the different opportunities.

Social Resources from Inner Power

When individuals and families take on a challenge as daunting (and as long lasting) as reintegration from addictive relationships, they need to look carefully at what is going to sustain their efforts both through the difficult initial phases

P.J. Adams, Fragmented Intimacy: Addiction in a Social World
© Springer 2008

and in the years to come. Several self-help approaches are oriented around the strength offered by inner connectedness in mounting a reintegration.

Twelve Steps

By far the most important and most influential resource for people in addictive relationships and their families has been the twelve-step movement, which originated in the midwestern United States in the 1930s. The movement has spawned several variants for people in a wide range of different types of addictive relationship. The main variants include Alcoholics Anonymous (AA), Narcotics Anonymous (NA), Gamblers Anonymous (GA), Sex and Love Addicts Anonymous (SLAA).[2] The approach has also been applied, controversially and with less uptake, to other mental well-being issues through programs such as Codependency Anonymous (CoDA), Overeater's Anonymous (OA) and the mental health recovery program called GROW.[3] The movement has also been adapted for family members living next to loved ones who have entered into addictive relationships. These include Al-Anon for alcohol, Alateen for adolescents, Nar-Anon for other drugs, and Adult Children of Alcoholics (ACoA). From a community development point of view, with minimal organization and funding, the twelve-step movement has achieved an impressive spread throughout the world, now claiming over two million active members and over 100,000 groups meeting weekly.[4] This growth over 80 years is an impressive achievement.

People in the twelve-step movement attend regular meetings in which they are welcomed to declare their addiction (addictive relationship), talk about their experience of recovery (reintegration), and support others with their progress. The meetings provide a focal point for "working the program" by discussing their ongoing progress in continuing to incorporate guidance from the twelve steps as an alternative pathway to pursuing an addictive relationship. As listed in the inset box, the first three steps focus on recognizing how the addictive relationship has led to unmanageable deteriorations in a person's quality of life and on the need to identify and connect with a source of inner power

---

AA and Al-Anon's Twelve Steps

1. We admitted we were powerless over alcohol—that our lives had become unmanageable.
2. We came to believe that a Power greater than ourselves could restore us to sanity.
3. We made a decision to turn our will and our lives over to the care of God *as we understood Him*.
4. We made a searching and fearless moral inventory of ourselves.
5. We admitted to God, to ourselves, and to another human being the exact nature of our wrongs.
6. We were entirely ready to have God remove all these defects of character.
7. We humbly asked Him to remove our shortcomings.
8. We made a list of all persons we had harmed, and became willing to make amends to them all.
9. We made direct amends to such people wherever possible, except when to do so would injure them or others.
10. We continued to take personal inventory, and when we were wrong, promptly admitted it.
11. We sought through prayer and meditation to improve our conscious contact with God *as we understood Him* praying only for knowledge of His will for us and the power to carry that out.
12. Having had a spiritual awakening as the result of these steps, we tried to carry this message to alcoholics and to practice these principles in all our affairs.

that could act as a bridge to change. A person reaches what they understand as "rock bottom"—a critical moment, a pivotal crisis—in which it becomes clear that continuing in the addictive relationship will lead to ruin. The next four steps (four to seven) focus on the identification of harms occurring in the addictive system. Most importantly this involves acknowledging the use of intimacy management strategies and the effect of these on loved ones. The next two steps (eight and nine) refer most explicitly to social dimensions and focus on the processes of acceptance and forgiveness as they apply to reforming connectedness with intimates. The final three steps (ten to twelve) focus on consolidating the spiritual and emotional dimensions of the program into everyday life.

People who attend twelve-step groups are inducted into what Mariana Valverde refers to as "a fully-fledged, lifelong social identity".[5] The groups provide a network of involvements that makes up a micro-society, thereby resembling more a cultural event than a form of therapy. Entrants are introduced to new ways of relating that for most participants include new values and new patterns of socializing. Participants often socialize outside meetings in their own circles; they adopt common catch phrases ("a day at a time"; "let bygones be bygone"); they make use of a common vocabulary to describe different aspects of their change process ("recovery," "dry drunks," "white knuckling"), and they plug into a system of mentorship by connecting with a chosen "sponsor", a person who acts as a guide and whose reintegration they admire. Furthermore, members all share in a common understanding that commitment to an addictive relationship is best understood as a progressive and enduring "disease" that has infected all aspects of their lives. For most entrants, these elements involve a radical reorientation of how they use their time and the way they relate to others. It opens up opportunities for reforming both communal and inner connectedness and lays a pathway to reforming intimacies. As depicted in the inset box, during Danny's brief involvement with AA, he had difficulty applying the twelve steps but was still able to access the social potential offered in the meetings.

The twelve-step movement's adoption of a disease model and its focus on changes within the individual suggest that the approach is firmly placed in a particle paradigm. It is the individual that suffers this lifelong disease, and it is through a process of individual recovery that the disease can be managed. Nonetheless, categorizing the approach as particle-oriented overlooks important aspects of how the movement operates. It is better seen as a hybrid that straddles both particle and social understandings of addiction. Its particle orientation is evident in its emphasis on the pivotal role of the individual, but its social dimensions can be seen in its emphasis

> **Danny/Jack: Social power in AA**
> While separated from his wife, Julie, Danny is living with his father, Jack, and one night over dinner he comments, "Dad, when I was going to those AA meetings…"
> "I was sorry you didn't carry on."
> "… I didn't really get into all this talk of disease and God. That wasn't me. But I tell you what I did find helpful and that was talking at meetings."
> "That's because you're with other people in the same boat."
> "Yeah, to some extent. But I found just being around other people who were getting their lives together made me want to do the same. When I talked and when they listened I had a sense that I wasn't alone and that change was possible."

on practices that reestablish intimacies. In the first place, the addictive relation-ship is not seen as a medical condition that requires the expertise of others to cure. It is conceived much as it is depicted in this book, as a powerful relation-ship that only the person in it has the ability to change. Professionals have a secondary role and are useful only insofar as they are able to support people in discovering their own inner power. In the second place, spirituality is empha-sized as an important source of strength and power, and as such is approached as a relationship—an inner relationship—that contributes as part of a nexus of other relationships. For example, talk often focuses on the person's relation-ship to a higher power and how this connection impacts on relationships at home, at work, and with friends. In the third place, the use of this inner power is primarily focused on relationships; it aims to mobilize inner connectedness as a means of achieving other forms of connectedness. For example, the key attitudinal stances of honesty, humility, and forgiveness are aimed at providing a base for reforming noncontrolling symmetrical intimacies.

The twelve-step approach incorporates strong social processes

While much of the understanding underpinning the twelve-step move-ment can be seen in social terms, some of its practices are inconsistent with a social orientation and thereby run the risk of enabling fragmentation. For example, while family members are welcomed at meetings, the person in the addictive relationship and family members tend to attend separate meetings. This practice is understandable in the early phases, when individual attendance at meetings serves a replacement function,[6] but in the longer term it could act to reduce the closeness and commitment between family members. Another limiting aspect in social terms is the emphasis on anonymity. Anonymity can be seen as a response to the widespread negative attitudes and stigma associ-ated with addictive relationships; by being anonymous the scrutiny of others becomes less of an obstacle to attendance. But anonymity also reinforces this stigma by reducing the visibility of addictive systems and indirectly endorsing the need for secrecy. A related limitation is the movement's active avoidance of relationships and affiliations with political movements, churches, health services, media, and other organizations. Through the guidelines laid out in their "twelve traditions," the movement steps away from involvements that divert it from its core commitment to recovery (reintegration). Nonetheless, this also involves a distancing of its relationship to other social layers around the addictive system, such as neighborhoods and community networks, and effectively prevents liaisons developing with other resources for reintegration through services and social agencies.

Emotional Detachment

Al-Anon has adapted the twelve-step program into a guide for intimates on their path through addictive environments and on to reintegration. Instead of focusing on the person in the addictive relationship, attention shifts to the relationship between the intimate and the addictive relationship. The twelve steps then substitute "alcohol" (or other addictive substances/processes) with the relationship their loved ones have with these objects. Accordingly, the key to reintegration for intimates involves the gradual relinquishing of investment in and control of this relationship. Intimates are urged to let go of responsibility for the behavior and consequences associated with their loved one's addictive relationship and to avoid the destructive spiral of trying to control that which is uncontrollable. As presented in the inset box, it is extremely difficult to detach from the downward trajectory of a loved one. Consequently maintaining this stance requires access to the spiritual and emotional resources activated in the twelve steps. These practices—calling on a higher power, recognizing and amending harm, forgiving and reforming honest relationships—are then incorporated into a process aimed at reducing the power of their loved one's addictive relationship in their lives.

In the absence of other alternatives, the Al-Anon pathway of emotional detachment has dominated the common wisdom of how intimates should respond to addictive relation-

> **Danny/Jack: Julie's Dilemma**
> While visiting Julie and the children Jack asks, "Since you left Danny, you still seem very concerned about him."
> "That's the problem, and really why he had to leave. I felt so much for him… perhaps too much."
> "How does that work?"
> "Well, when I was with him I couldn't bear the pain and humiliation of his drinking and drug use any more. He was the closest person to me in the world. Living with him everyday I couldn't stand by and watch him fall."
> "I know what you mean. It was like that with my wife, Rose, God bless her. I had to watch her slowly deteriorate. It pulled me apart."
> "I couldn't bear sitting, waiting, and worrying about him getting caught and going to prison. It scared me constantly when I thought of the damage to his organs and it kept dragging me down whenever he entered these black moods that seemed to go on for days."
> "Yeah, he's still doing that and I don't know what to do."
> "I felt I had to do something. So first off I tried hiding his alcohol, taking over the money so he couldn't afford it and challenging him whenever he went out. It didn't do much good and only made me feel increasingly upset and powerless. Him leaving seemed the only way I was going to stop us both being dragged under."

ships. From discussions in magazines and self-help guides, to advice provided by general practitioners, to recommendations given by addiction counselors, the common message echoes how intimates need to stop "enabling" or supporting the addictive relationship by refocusing their energy onto issues regarding their own well-being and development. Behind this position lies the belief that if allowed to run its own course, the addictive relationship will eventually collapse of its own accord and that attempts by intimates to influence and manipulate events will only add to fragmentation and reinforce feelings of powerlessness and hopelessness. For example, when Julie attempted to restrict Danny's access to alcohol by hiding bottles or blocking access to bank accounts, Danny was then able to use his consequent anger and frustration to justify further consumption. When Julie challenged him going out at night, he was similarly able to use the ensuing argument as just cause for an angry exit. She found that the effort she put into trying to control his addictive relationship was futile and served only to weaken her position. She began to recognize this energy could be better invested by leaving Danny to pursue his own trajectory and focusing on improving her own and her children's circumstances.

In contrast to this common wisdom regarding emotional detachment and self-care, some intimates may experience these expectations as unhelpful in their struggle to remain connected with an addictive family system. Intimates pursue enabling behaviors because of enduring historically driven emotional attachments to the person in the addictive relationship. These attachments can be very intense, perhaps too intense for loved ones to really embrace a process of detachment. As depicted in the inset box, failure at letting go responsibility for the addictive relationship may only result in further feelings of inadequacy. Julie found maintaining a path of detachment virtually impossible when she was living with Danny. Trying to do so only made her feel worse, and separation appeared the only way ahead. Though not experienced by Julie, another difficulty with emotional detachment concerns the common use of violence and other intimacy management strategies. Emotional detachment, if detected, could provide the pretext for abusing or punishing intimates for their attempts at maintaining some degree of distance. For example, a woman who fails to back up or lie for her husband in a court hearing may encounter severe abuse when they return home. Similarly parents who turn down their child's requests for money may find their homes burgled, adding another level of fear to their involvement.

> **Danny/Jack: Detachment**
>
> Jack says, "Julie, I found I could still stay living with Rose and look after myself. Why did you need to split up?"
>
> "As you implied earlier, we're not totally separated. Danny is still visiting a lot and we still care about each other."
>
> "Yes, but why separate?"
>
> "Look, I did try hard for a long time to follow what you said and detach myself from what he was doing. I let him do his own thing, and left him to clean up his own messes, deal with his own money and legal problems and... lots of things. I concentrated on improving my life with the children. But this was the man I love. I couldn't just sit by and let him collapse. I wasn't that tough. As his situation deteriorated I felt myself being pulled apart, bit by bit."
>
> "But things collapsing; this was what he needed."
>
> "I know, I know. I did try, seriously. But it was too hard. I started feeling I was failing at this, on top of everything else."

Codependency and Disease

The codependency movement partially originated from twelve-step approaches, but it draws on a wider base that includes ideas from modern self-help psychologies, psychotherapy, and feminism.[7] The notion of "codependency" takes the Al-Anon concept of "enabling" one step further and argues that a person can form an emotional dependence to other people in ways that mimics an addictive relationship. This is reflected in the way adults who have been brought up in addictive home environments experience a broad range of difficulties with their later intimacies. These difficulties include exaggerated avoidance of conflict, difficulties in trusting people, and compulsions to please. The codependent, it is argued, may go as far as re-creating their familiar childhood environment by forming the distorted and asymmetrical relationships in their adult world, relationships that could include strong attachments to people in addictive relationships, tolerance for poorly reciprocated closeness, and commitment or even acceptance of intimacy controlling strategies. Furthermore, as a legacy from the twelve-step movement, the person who becomes codependent is seen as affected by a disease—a disease that has its own trajectory and can lead onto similar levels of isolation and fragmentation. Accordingly, a self-help process of change typically involves measures that seek to activate inner strengths to empower the person against the multitudinous threats of entrenched relationship asymmetries.

The codependency movement through its many popular publications has acquired a wide following,[8] but one primarily based on individual personal growth rather than building up social networks. In contrast to the twelve-step movement, the emphasis is on psychological processes within an individual and therefore it leans more toward a particle interpretation of addictive relationships. Adherents miss much of the social understandings inherent in AA or Al-Anon, which along with use of the power within still maintain an ongoing focus on socially oriented sources of strength (such as intimate or communal connectedness).[9]

Codependency approaches miss out on the social processes of twelve step approaches

The emphasis on the individual is further reinforced by linking negative attachments under the rubric of an emotional disease. Destructive attachments are viewed as part of an ongoing relational disease that is difficult to quantify but assumed to persist as an abiding presence. Such a view also risks converting normal and customary relationships into some form of pathology. Particularly for women, unhealthy relationships may be a product of a wide range of social processes, such as role expectations and romance norms, that have more to do with social structures that maintain traditional dominance by men rather than an inner inadequacy or dysfunction in a woman. For example, a woman who feels dominated by her partner, by striving to change how she behaves may find herself having very little impact on her partner's commitment to dominance. In a way this individual focus on her pathology conveniently draws attention away from the social structural issues. It risks devaluing both the negative and positive power of social connectedness.

Social Resources Offered by Services

What can people in addictive social systems expect their society to provide to aid the process of reintegration? Several reviews of research interventions have commented on how some of the most effective approaches include social dimensions.[10] For example in a recent review, three of the top eight most effective service approaches involved a clear focus on family functioning.[11] Yet the majority of these approaches still confine their use of social processes to operating as an adjunct to particle-oriented approaches, and they have yet to explore the potential of a purely social orientation.

Perhaps a constraining factor is the extent to which intervention services have been organized according to particle orientations, which in turn limits their capacity to incorporate social approaches. This section looks at three varieties of service approaches: those that focus primarily on changes for the person in the addictive relationship; those that aim at changes for both the person in the addictive relationship and others in the person's life; and those that aim at changes primarily for the person's intimates. The role of the health professional in utilizing social dimensions is explored in more detail in Chapter 13.

For People in Addictive Relationships

By far the majority of addiction services, especially in Western Europe, North America, and Oceania, are driven by approaches that concentrate on reforming individuals. These approaches focus on thinking (e.g., cognitive behavior therapy), on decision making (e.g., motivational enhancement), on resolving emotional issues (e.g., client-centered counseling and psychotherapy), and on the twelve-step movement. While most services acknowledge the importance of families, few include the family in assessment or intervention, and when family members do attend, the services still have an individualistic focus on change. Few of these services have as yet explored the full potential of social processes in their own right. However, recently some approaches have attempted to include social processes as a core part of their methods. Three of which will be explored below are therapeutic micro-communities (TMC), A Relational Intervention Sequence for Engagement (ARISE), and Community Reinforcement and Family Training (CRAFT).

Few addiction services currently adopt a social or family orientation

Therapeutic Micro-Communities (TMC)

The therapeutic micro-community movement[12] emerged in the 1960s in New York and London as a way to assist people with mental health issues to reintegrate back into normal life. It arose partially as a response to the pathologizing and alienating effects psychiatric diagnosis and treatments were having on people at that time. The idea of small micro-communities as a means of resocializing alienated people was adopted as an approach to addictive relationships and evolved into live-in rehabilitation programs of durations varying from several months to several years. Whereas TMCs are now less commonly used with mental health issues, they have persisted as a common approach to reintegration from addictive relationships. Many such programs aim to provide a postcrisis replacement opportunity that creates a safe space for reappraising the possibility of mounting a reintegration.

For other participants, particularly those already committed to reintegration, the TMC provides a bridging exposure to acquiring the resources they need to connect with others in their lives. In this relatively controlled environment people in addictive relationships are invited into a process of resocialization where they can safely acquire the skills they need for reestablishing intimacies. The controlled environment enables them to experiment with the attitudinal stances of forgiveness and humility, to begin learning to communicate honestly without controlling tactics, and to clarify their emotional world so they can begin expressing feelings without concealment and impression management.

From a social perspective, the key challenge for TMCs concerns the transition from the program environment back into everyday life. While making significant progress in forming relationships in a controlled environment, this is often not so easy in real life where old patterns of behavior are difficult to modify. As depicted in the inset, Danny made considerable changes during his time in the rehab program, particularly in the way he connected and communicated with others. But once he left, he found these changes contrasted starkly with the lack of change in the relationships that make up his everyday life. In a study I was involved in, a group of thirteen people were interviewed at length some months after they had been discharged from a 3-month residential treatment program.[13] The interviewees conveyed how difficult it was to leave one environment in which they had made considerable progress and return into their circle of intimates where much remained unchanged. They had altered their whole approach to communication and participation in relationships, but others in their lives continued in the same old routines. It was almost as if their success in changing had set them up for a reversion because it highlighted how rigid and fixed the relationships were in their everyday lives.

Rehabilitation programs have recognized the difficulties in transition from micro-communities back into their communities of origin, and many are incorporating strategies such as family weeks, family groups, and family transition counseling. Nonetheless, by removing a person from their social context, TMCs are on the whole more likely to adopt particle-oriented psychological approaches to addiction with only peripheral attention to social perspectives.

> **Danny/Jack: Leaving Rehab**
>
> Following encouragement from Jack and Julie, Danny enters a one-month rehabilitation program. Two months after his discharge, he reverts to his addictive relationship and is trying to explain what had happened to Jack.
>
> "Well, Dad, in rehab I became a different person. For the first time I started communicating what I felt directly to people without bullshitting or covering up."
>
> "That must have been a new experience."
>
> "Yep, it sure was. I was talking straight, and, hey, nothing happened; nobody attacked me and my brain didn't explode. I also stopped trying to control or manipulate people around me; the others made sure of that."
>
> "I noticed how different you were when you came out."
>
> "But when I returned home, I found no one in my life had really changed; sorry, Dad. I said to everybody, 'I don't do that anymore' and 'I'm a different person,' and they just said 'Sure, sure' and they kept on playing their same old games. Why haven't they changed? Why don't they engage like I do? I felt so incredibly frustrated that I'd changed and they hadn't. What's worse, they didn't even see the benefits of my communicating differently. Then it all became too hard and I just had to get back into old routines."

A Relational Intervention Sequence for Engagement (ARISE)

This program developed originally from experience using the Johnson intervention,[14] which involved addiction practitioners coaching groups of people associated with an addictive relationships—intimates and others such as employees and physicians—in techniques of caring confrontation as a means of exerting sufficient influence on the person in the addictive relationship to engage him or her in therapy. These techniques, as with other uses of confrontation, tended to result in a low level of engagement and a high risk of reversion soon after.[15] Interestingly, in a sizable number of applications, despite involving intimates in planning for a confrontational meeting, these meetings did not always need to take place[16]; the process of planning generated its own momentum and the meeting became unnecessary.

Garrett and colleagues looked at the critical ingredients to the Johnson approach and concluded that its effectiveness was more an outcome of social networking than of the confrontational methods.[17] Accordingly, they devised a series of strategies to mobilize social networks around an addictive relationship to engage the person in the relationship in a program of change. These strategies included ways of connecting with other people, working out when best to raise issues, and training in assertiveness to clarify impacts and expectations. By engaging intimates and other associates, ARISE focuses on the collective action phase of the intimate cycle. It illustrates the power that intimate reconnection and can exert on the addictive family system. However, while the approach incorporates social connectedness, it still primarily aims to lead the person in the addictive relationship into a particle-oriented approach to change. The focus is on engaging just the person, not the system of intimates. Their version of collective action does not explore how the whole system of connections could be incorporated into the social process of reintegration.

Some approaches use collective action to engage individuals in particle approaches to change

Community Reinforcement and Family Training (CRAFT)

This program was developed at the University of New Mexico as an extension to the Community Reinforcement Approach (CRA) to addictions.[18] The CRA aims to reorganize the environment for a person in the addictive relationship in a way that tips the balance of incentives away from the addictive substance/process and toward engagement in change.[19] This is achieved through the application of a range of strategies that seek to restore deteriorated connections. These strategies include job skill training, social and recreational counseling, relationship therapy, and training in relapse prevention.[20] Several of these strategies require the support of intimates and others associated with the addictive relationship, particularly in relationship counseling and engagement in new activities and interests. Experience with CRA methods and a series of carefully conducted research studies helped highlight how involvement of intimates was a vital ingredient in its effectiveness,[21] and, in response, elements from family therapy were added as "family training" to form CRAFT.

This program consists of a package of strategies specifically aimed at supporting intimates (and other associates) in realizing their potential in engaging the person in the addictive relationship in a process of change. The main set of procedures (listed in the inset box[22]) develops the role of intimates as catalysts for engaging the person in the addictive relationship in contemplating change. In this way the procedures focus particularly on the reconnection phase of the intimate cycle and, similar to ARISE, aim to engage the person in the addictive relationship in treatment. Applications of the approach have been carefully evaluated and are showing some promising results.[23] However, while CRAFT is on the verge of recognizing the potential a social paradigm, as clearly stated in the inset box, efforts so far center on engaging the drinker or drug user (as a particle) in having treatment; the intimates (called "caring significant others" or CSOs) make up a support team, not a primary focus, so again the social opportunity is neglected.[24]

> **Community Reinforcement and Family Training (CRAFT) Procedures**
> 1. Developing a trusting therapeutic relationship
> 2. Preparing the caring significant other (CSO) [intimate] to recognize and safely respond to any potential for domestic violence, particularly when the behavioral changes are being introduced at home
> 3. Completing two functional analyses: the first to identify the substance user's triggers for using alcohol or drugs and consequences, and the second to profile the user's triggers for nonusing, prosocial behavior and its consequences
> 4. Working to improve communication with the substance user [person in the addictive relationship]
> 5. Showing CSO [intimate] how to effectively use positive reinforcement and negative consequences such that they discourage a loved one's harmful using behavior
> 6. Teaching the CSO [intimate] methods for decreasing stress in general, and emphasizing the importance of having sufficient "rewards" in his or her own life
> 7. Instructing the CSO [intimate] in the most effective ways to suggest treatment to the substance user, and helping to identify the most appropriate times
> 8. Laying the groundwork for having treatment available immediately for the user in the event that the decision is made to begin therapy, and discussing the need for the CSO [intimate] to support the drinker or drug user during treatment (Meyers and Miller, 2001)

Relationships in Addictive Social Systems

A range of service responses focus on the joint involvement of the person in the addictive relationship and other intimates in undertaking change. The following discussion briefly examines three interrelated approaches: family therapy, family life history, and multiple family groups.

Family Therapy

The application of family therapy and other systems-based approaches to addictive social systems have a relatively long history. Families have been subjected to the full gamut of techniques developed in the family therapy movement from the early structural and conjoint therapy approaches, to the more recent cybernetic and narrative approaches.[25] For example, Stanton and his colleagues,[26] using a structural-strategic family therapy model, have devised a range of ways of engaging family members in exploring the effects of varying the way they connect with each other. Working in a similar vein, Marc Galanter combines psychodynamic and cognitive behavioral approaches to developing a supportive network to promote and maintain a change process.[27] A more recent variant involves the use of narrative based therapies,[28] in which understanding and options for change are sifted out from the way people construct and create stories about their relationships.

These and many other family therapy approaches have regularly contributed to the design of a broad range of service interventions, but unlike work with troubled adolescents, such approaches have not flourished as interventions with addictive relationships.[29] Possible explanations for this are multileveled. At one level the extra effort required to meet with families involves far more costs than meeting with individuals. Properly conducted meetings typically require the involvement of at least two well-trained therapists, often meeting after business hours to ensure that as many members as possible can attend, and meeting for longer than individual sessions. At another level, the emphasis in these approaches on practitioners having high levels of training and skill creates the impression that conducting meetings with families is beyond the competence of most addiction practitioners, and accordingly they back away from such work. At a more theoretical level, while family

Family therapy risks obscuring social potential by turning the family into a particle

therapists view the addictive social system in terms of relationships rather than of individuals, several aspects of their practice replicate particle orientations by in effect converting the family into a self-contained particle; the family becomes a thing to work on. This particularization of the family is reinforced with strategies such as the use of mirrors and therapist conferencing, where the family experts analyze family dynamics and administer recommendations aimed at unblocking dysfunctional and enmeshed relationship processes.

Family Life History

Steinglass and his colleague, working from a systems orientation, developed their family life history model based on the idea that the type of addictive system they call "alcoholic families" are best thought of as behavioral systems in which aspects of the addictive relationship have become "central organizing principles around which family life is structured."[30] Chapter 6 explored this interpretation more fully, but to summarize it briefly, the family is seen as an interconnected homeostatic system in which changes at one point lead to effects at another point, which in turn has effects on another, and so on. Accordingly, the presence of an addictive relationship disturbs patterns of normal family development effectively moving the focus from long-term growth to short-term stability. This shift in how a family regulates itself leads to development distortions[31] both for the system itself and for the people who inhabit it. The aim of therapy is to work with the family as a whole (or as complete as possible) to identify these family regulatory behaviors and to work at reshaping them in ways that assist families to move developmentally into the next phase. As with other family approaches, despite the many insights and sophistication of their approach, it has not been widely adopted for the reasons mentioned earlier.

Multiple Family Groups

Multiple family groups have been widely used in residential and community outpatient settings to engage families in the process of change.[32] Often the groups are provided as an adjunct to particle-oriented interventions (such as TMCs or individual counseling). Families are invited to a series of large meetings attended by both the person in the addictive relationship and other intimates. As people get to know each other, they begin to listen to accounts of experiences from other families and discover that much of what other family members talk about parallels their own circumstances. From these *Multiple* accounts they gain access to a wealth of understanding and hear the different *family groups* ways people attempt to deal with similar problems and their positive and *focus on the* negative outcomes. While these groups are often embedded in services with *strengths &* a focus on individuals rather than social networks, the methods used come *expertise* closer to a social approach than family therapy. The emphasis is clearly on *within* expertise emerging from the group rather than the practitioner and decisions *families* about what to do are derived from multiple (and possibly conflicting) perspective. An example of a community-based system of multiple family groups is explored in detail in the next chapter.

For Intimates

Few service interventions have directly and specifically targeted the social potential of intimates in addictive social systems. Since the next chapter is devoted to looking closely at three examples, the following discussion briefly considers two other interrelated approaches: coping skills, and the Stress-Strain-Coping-Support (SSCS) approach.

Coping Skills

Based on their own and other people's research findings, Cronkite and associates[33] have developed a theory of family adaptation to addictive relationships to alcohol. Their early work and research by others point out that reintegration requires a combination of low-stress environments and effective coping skills for intimates before the necessary cohesion is generated for change to persist.[34] However, with the regular cycles of sobriety and intoxication and the longer term cycles of crisis, replacement, and reversion creating chaos and uncertainty, the required ingredients for change never gain a foothold. Cronkite and associates recommend that services for intimates "should be oriented toward strengthening the natural recovery process and improving the life contexts of patients and their ability to manage these contexts."[35] This emphasis on improving the life skills of family members has led to a variety of approaches such as applications of behavior therapy to supporting married couples[36] and psycho-educational strategies.[37]

Stress-Strain-Coping-Support Approach

Continuing the focus on stress, Copello and his associates, through their involvements with the U.K. Alcohol, Drugs, and Family Research Group, developed the Stress-Strain-Coping-Support (SSCS) approach specifically targeting family members (intimates).[38] Their approach concentrates efforts on five steps (see inset box) that aim to empower intimates whose lives have become fragmented within an addictive system. Early evaluation of their approach is indicating that it helps intimates become less stressed, more able to cope, and more willing to participate in collective action.[39] This approach has been developed further into Social Behavior and Network Therapy (SBNT), which involves people in the addictive social system in eight sessions aimed at engaging them in positive social network supports for change.[40] Results for trials of this method have yet to be published. Both these approaches and the coping skills approaches show promising signs in the way they focus specifically on the needs of intimates, but their methods remain primarily individualistic, falling just short of exploring the potential of a social orientation.

> **Stress-Strain-Coping-Support (SSCS) Procedures**
> 1. Giving the family member [intimate] the opportunity to talk about the problem
> 2. Providing relevant information
> 3. Exploring how the family member [intimate] responds to the relative's substance misuse
> 4. Exploring and enhancing social support
> 5. Discussing the possibilities of onward referral for further specialist help (Copello et al., 2005, p. 376)

Social Resources in the Family

A recurring theme is that the family—or the circle of intimates—is the strongest site for promoting reintegration from an addictive relationship. Inner psychological resources and individualized help from services and other community agencies can make a contribution, but since all people live immersed in a social world, social resources offer the most powerful and available source of strength to facilitate change. In the long course of a reintegration, addiction services can provide assistance only intermittently and only in a small part of the reintegration process. With each of the six major phases of reintegration likely to take years (see Chapter 10), the whole process could take a decade or even two. Services can provide help in only part of this process, and these occur generally during the crisis-oriented phases. Support for reintegration needs to emerge from a stronger and more enduring presence, such as the nexus of immediate intimate relationships.

As discussed earlier, addiction services are also impeded by an overriding interpretation of clients as particles, which emphasizes processes within the person, and they devote scant attention to unleashing the potential within social networks. With an eye on how intimates might respond to addictive relationships, the following discussion takes the ideas developed in earlier chapters and translates them into a set of guidelines that family members might use in deciding how to respond. The guidelines begin from the point shortly after a period of crisis and divides recommendations into the three important phases of reappraisal, reconnection, and collective action.

Reappraisal

The period of reappraisal, which immediately follows a sequence of events involving enforced fragmentation and crisis, provides an opportunity for family members to rethink how to respond in an addictive system. Through their recycling experience of multiple crises they gradually form an appreciation of the dominating power of addictive processes. Unfortunately, a full appreciation of this power takes time to acquire, and in the meantime the addictive relationship has managed to firmly anchor itself as the primary axis within the family system. Accordingly, intimates need to prepare themselves for a struggle that may take considerable time and effort before any hope of reintegration is possible. The following recommendations during reappraisal are divided into mindset messages, preparation measures, and action strategies.

Reappraisal involves reviewing past strategies & preparing for new ones

Mindset Messages

- *The addiction is too powerful to tackle on my own*: Connections with others in the family are my strongest resource.
- *Outsiders can support initiatives but are unlikely to change the situations*: services have a limited role, contrary to impressions that they cannot fix addictive social systems, so it is important to avoid passing responsibility over to them and to view them more as contributing in a support role.
- *Change is possible but it is likely to take a long times*: in the fragmented world of an addicted social system the addictive relationship can appear overwhelmingly powerful. The power needs to be understood, but there are

immediate things that can be done to work toward the long-term opportunities for change.

Preparation Measures

- *Discuss the last crisis with others already on board about*: Identify the intimacy management strategies in use during counterreactions.
- *Learn as much as possible about addictive relationships*: Read the relevant literature, watch videos, look for information on the Internet, attend classes or groups, and talk to others who have also experienced addictive social systems.[41]
- *Take care of oneself*: Addictive relationships affect everyone exposed to them and for intimates they typically lead to reductions in personal confidence and optimism. Avoid activities that might increase negativity such as additional stress, overworking, poor nutrition, and other forms of self-neglect.

Action Strategies

- *Consider whether to stay or leave*: Separation from the family system is an option for many and should be included as part of the reappraisal. Observe how other people react and interact; try to work out which relationships within the family matter most and whether they could possibly be interested in change. Try to strengthen the quality of these relationships.
- *Determine where in the system lie the best opportunities for further reconnection*: Ideally focus on the family, but if this looks unlikely, look to wider connections with friends, colleagues, and neighbors.
- *Identify realistic and achievable goals*: Several crisis cycles may occur before the full strength of the addictive relationship is appreciated. Each rotation helps clarify what is achievable and how the larger tasks can be sequenced into a series of small achievable steps.

Reconnection

Reconnection aims to counter the fragmenting effects of intimacy management strategies

Effective use of intimacy management strategies leads intimates to feel cut off and separated from others in the family. For isolated individuals, options are limited; the task of reforming relationships is critical in building the infrastructure for challenging the single axis social structure.

Mindset Messages

- *Communicating and connecting with intimates is important*: To some extent the addictive relationship can be left to run its own course and the focus can shift onto opportunities for connection with other family members.

- *Others may be at different levels of readiness:* In fragmented and disempowered circumstances it takes time for others to recognize where opportunities lie and to find the strength to approach them. Those who first recognize the need to reconnect may need to wait as others achieve the same recognition.
- *Reconnection often requires many attempts:* At first, opening channels of communication are likely to be blocked because this is the normal pattern associated with fragmentation in addictive systems. The intimacy management and other fragmenting processes have had considerable time to separate people, so it may take time and multiple attempts for progress to be made.

The process of family members reconnecting may take time & multiple attempts

Preparation Measures

- *Write stories about the experiences and events:* Story-telling is a powerful way of gaining insight into and strength for dealing with difficult events.[42] Work the stories through and try to telling them from different angles (e.g., first person, third person, as they happen, in the past).
- *Talk to trusted friends, colleagues, and mentors:* The activity of talking increases one's comfort about disclosing and helps clarify what to say when it comes to talking with intimates. Avoid unnecessary conflict or attempts at change that are unlikely to succeed; the focus here is on reconnecting with intimates, and the addictive relationship can take its own course.
- *Collective action can focus on improvements in intimate connectedness:* Those who are connecting might continue to focus on connecting to other intimates before turning their attention to the addictive relationship.

Action Strategies

- *Organize meetings so that people can feel free to talk:* This may require special arrangements such as meeting on neutral territory, increasing safety by using an intermediary, and gradually introducing topics in casual conversation.
- *Avoid projecting blame and responsibility:* Openly acknowledge that addiction is a major problem and is likely to take more than one attempt. Work with intimates where they are and avoid blame when things proceed slower than one would like.
- *Foster closeness and compassion:* Engage in activities that encourage closeness such as going on outings together and spending time listening to each other's stories.

Collective Action

In preparing for collective action, the reconnecting intimates need to be aware that what they choose to do will prompt negative reactions. If the person in the addictive relationship feels sufficiently threatened, the counterreaction is likely to be strong. This in some ways is good because it signals that the collective response is having the desired effect, but it is also a risky period because without support intimates are likely to experience fearfulness and liable to retreat into isolated spaces. When intimates feel sufficiently connected to try challenging the addictive relationship, they also need to look carefully at how they will support each other.

Mindset Messages

- *There are no quick-fix solutions, and what worked for others may not work for one's own circumstances*: Family relationships, let alone those complicated by addictive processes, are complex, dynamic, and multilayered.
- *Addictive relationships are very strong*: Intimates will probably need to support each other in collective action several times.
- Don't underestimate the potency of intimacy management strategies
- *Think of this as a journey*: Avoid pushing people beyond their comfort zones; in the longer term, it is building the relationship that matters, and there will be other opportunities for collective action.

Preparation Measures

- *Clarify the goals of the next action*: Discuss what you would like to happen next if the person in the addictive relationship expresses a genuine interest in change.
- *Formulate an agreed-on plan of action*: Plan each step of the interchange. Clarify each person's role in the action; make sure those involved know what they are supposed to do and say. This might involve identifying the main spokesperson, the person who monitors safety, and the person who works out how to respond.
- *Talk through responses if things go wrong*: Preplan points at which those involved review what is happening, with particular attention to counterreactions and safety.

Action Strategies

- *Back off if connectedness to others weakens*: It is more important for the longer term to maintain team links with other intimates.
- *Keep in constant contact in responding to counterreactions*: Disciplinary counterreactions are likely to be effective particularly in the first few attempts at collective action. This is normal, and constant discussion and support is essential to maintaining connectedness.
- *Avoid blaming others for unsuccessful action*: Most attempts are likely to be unsuccessful, and blaming people might split up the group.

- *Connect as soon as possible for a joint reappraisal*: This feeds immediately into the reconnection phase of the intimate cycle.

While pursuing these processes, besides family involvement in collective action, the opportunities within addictive relationships can be supported through connections into the wider community (see Chapter 12).

Danny and Jack Enter Reintegration

To recap Danny's story so far, Danny's addictive relationship to alcohol and cannabis has led his wife, Julie, to ask him to leave. He then moved in with his father, Jack, on his nearby farm but found it difficult coping with the time apart from Julie and their two children, Adrienne and Luke. His drinking and cannabis use then increased in frequency, leading to trouble at work both in terms of his reliability and his relationship with his boss. His boss subsequently fires him, forcing him to rely on casual jobs he picks up in the neighborhood. As his alcohol and drug consumption continued to increase, signs of physical dependence on alcohol were beginning to emerge, particularly early morning symptoms of withdrawal such as tremors and needing to have a drink at breakfast. Jack, who had already suffered the pain of his wife Rose's similar deterioration, was now deeply troubled by Danny's situation. In the face of Danny's hostile objections, Jack kept pressuring Danny to recognize he had a problem. To please Jack, Danny eventually attended AA for a brief period, and following more pressure he also attended a 1-month live-in rehabilitation program. Despite these efforts and some brief periods of abstinence, Danny's drinking and cannabis use overall continued to increase. Jack, smarting from the previous disappointments, is now beginning to wonder whether he has any hope of saving Danny from self-destruction.

The need for collective effort emerges when individual efforts are unsuccessful

Reappraisal

One Saturday Danny visits the children, expecting that Julie would allow him to take them fishing that afternoon. Julie can see immediately that he has been drinking heavily; his speech is slurred, his gait is unsteady, and he reeks of whiskey. Julie says that there is no way she is going to let him take the children, as he is not in a fit state. Danny starts shouting angrily at her and threatening to take them anyway. Julie, frightened by his manner, phones the police, who arrive quickly and arrest Danny, taking him to the police station where he is detained in a cell overnight. She phones a lawyer and applies for an interim restraining order that will prevent Danny from visiting her or the children in the home. She then phones Jack to explain the latest crisis and seek his support, and about 20 minutes Jack arrives looking ashen, with a stooped posture. To Julie he appears old and broken. Jack had hoped desperately that Danny's treatment attempts would have made a difference. He was feeling despondent about the prospect of Danny changing and this latest crisis appeared to confirm the hopelessness of the situation. As he walked across the fields to Julie's house, he had been deliberating whether to share his feelings of helplessness with Julie and whether together they might make a difference. She too was wondering where to go next. She had hoped that somehow Danny's time apart would help him come to his senses, but instead he only seems to be getting worse. She and Jack begin the process of reappraising their current circumstances, a portion of which is presented in the inset box.

Reconnection

Jack begins visiting Julie and the children more regularly and talks more openly about his concerns regarding Danny. They speak at length about the troubling events that have happened in the past and they discuss their many attempts at change and their disappointments. The children join in the conversations, and Julie encourages the children to talk about their feelings. She also tries not to react to their critical comments and to avoid providing excuses and justifications for Danny. As the children feel more comfortable in the conversations, they share more and begin talking more with each other. At one point Luke presents a picture he had drawn of the family in which Danny stands separate from the family dressed as a devil and throwing hand-grenades at them. Though initially shocked by the image, Julie asks him to explain what it means to him, and slowly the depth of the children's distress unfolds. As Julie's confidence in communicating increases, she begins disclosing more to other people—first a close friend, then her lawyer, and later the family physician. Jack too is prepared to speak with more people about their difficulties. He reconnects with someone in a long-term AA recovery (reintegration) who had

---

Danny/Jack: Opening Discussion

"Julie, I'm so sorry my son is putting you through all this. It happened to Rose and now to him, and I'm the common factor. There must be something I'm doing wrong."

"It's not your fault, Jack. He's addicted and can't help himself. I've tried so hard not to support his addiction. Throwing him out was my trump card, and even that wasn't enough to shake his attachment. He just won't let go."

"Perhaps he'll never let go."

"Hmm, maybe. But I don't want the children to lose their father; you know where all this is heading. There must be something we can do that will make a difference."

"I dunno. Sometimes it feels to me like there's a little switch inside him that if we could just get to it and flick it, he would change his whole approach to things."

"Yeah, but look; he's been to AA, he's had treatment, he's lost his home and family; that's surely enough to flick a switch... if there is a switch."

"Maybe we're thinking of this in the wrong way. Maybe we need to think less about what's happening inside him and more about what is happening on the outside?"

Danny/Jack: Planning a Meeting

"Julie, you know how both of us have been talking to different people and they've introduced lots of new ideas? Well, I think we should get the key people together to plan some course of action."

"Yeah, Jack, I've been wondering that too. If we try anything, we need to make sure we sing the same song, otherwise he'll just split us up again."

"And we both know what it's like to have no impact."

"Mmm, I'd have plenty to say... so would everyone. What we need is someone to keep us focused, focused on deciding what to do."

"I reckon our family doctor would be a good facilitator. She's very good at listening to different points of view, and she knows what Danny is like. If it's okay with you, I'll ask if she'd convene the meeting. Maybe we can meet in her office?"

"I'm okay with that. I suggest we invite two of my friend's and two of yours. What about the children?"

"Not at this stage. I'll tell them about the meeting and what goes on, but I think they are just learning to trust talking with me. It would be too much of a jump."

helped him previously with his wife. Although it is difficult at first, he explains his situation to a couple of his close friends, who to his surprise speak about similar struggles with members of their own family. As depicted in the inset box, above, Jack and Julie then decide to organize a planning meeting where they can pool their ideas and come up with a collective strategy.

Collective Action

Jack and Julie continue to prepare for their first collective meeting with Danny. They invite two friends of Julie's and one of Jack's to attend the planning meeting in the physician's office. They decide not to include Danny just yet. At first the discussion moves haphazardly across different topics: Danny's misdemeanors, the need to hit "rock bottom," what treatments could work, and anger at Danny's intransigence. Several speak of the need to confront Danny about the personal impact of his addiction. Julie expresses some misgivings about this; based on past experiences she knew Danny was unlikely to simply acquiesce to such a challenge. But maybe collectively they could take a stronger position. They resolve that presenting themselves as being united in no longer tolerating his addictive behavior would be enough of a change to prompt some reaction. They then discuss likely counterreactions: he might threaten to kill himself, or leave altogether, or try to hurt or threaten to hurt one of them. They carefully review each possibility and look into how they might respond in each case.

In coming together people share experiences & review ideas for action

Danny and Julie drive to his first meeting at the physician's office. Julie had warned him that others were attending and that they were going to discuss among other things his drinking. Danny knows the physician well and trusts her professionalism, but based on his experience of discussions with Jack, he does not expect much to come out of the meeting. What happened takes him by surprise. During the meeting he hears his father, his estranged wife, and three of their friends talk openly about the impact of his drinking and drug use on their lives.

They also all declare how much they care for and love him, and how difficult it is to stand by and lose him to his addiction. He had never experienced this level of open and frank discussion. He wants to leave, but it would mean losing face, so he sits there listening quietly, trying hard not to show any reaction. He can see they are all of one mind, and he hears them declare they would no longer tolerate his addictive behavior. He feels angry, frustrated, sad, and humiliated, but he sticks resolutely to his position of nonengagement. After the meeting he leaves by himself, saying nothing. No one hears from him until his phone call to Julie that evening (see inset box, next page). Julie is initially unsettled by his threats of legal action. Since the children mean so much to her, she is understandably tempted to apologize and to back down from the declarations of the meeting, but Jack encourages her to hold fast and at the prearranged meeting of the group the next day, she is able to

---

Danny/Jack: Counterreaction

"Julie phones Jack the morning after the meeting."

"Hi, Jack. Look, Danny phoned me earlier in the evening after we met. He didn't say anything about the meeting but said he had met with a lawyer and was planning to pursue full custody of the children."

"Julie, he can't be serious."

"He wasn't drunk. He spoke coolly and calmly. Sort of in a way that really scared me. He sounded serious and I'm terrified that he will take court action."

"Julie, we discussed this earlier. It's just his reaction to being challenged. You know he has little hope of succeeding. He knows this will really shake you up and get you to back off."

"Yeah, but the children mean everything to me. I couldn't sleep last night worrying what to do."

"Look, I reckon we stand firm. We knew something like this was likely to happen, which is why we planned another meeting this afternoon. Let's all talk it through then."

Danny/Jack: Starting Reintegration

"Dad, when I left that meeting, I was angry with you, Julie, and everyone. Really wild. I felt ganged up on and humiliated. I really didn't care if I lived or died."

"When we realized you'd disappeared, we were very worried, and thought we'd gone too far."

"No, no, I can't see how you could have done it otherwise... When I first left what I wanted to do was put the shits up Julie, but later I could see she wasn't buying it. So next I felt I had to leave, so I just took off. I took a tent, sleeping equipment and some food, and camped out in the mountains."

"We had no idea where you'd gone."

"Yeah, sorry about that. For the first two days it was hell; I had the shakes and hot flushes and I was desperate for a drink. Three days later it got easier but I was then wracked with shame and guilt regarding the suffering I'd inflicted. So I continued to want to give in."

"But you stuck with it?"

"Alone there in the mountains, among the trees and the lakes, something began to change. It seemed to me as though I was facing a giant fork in the road. One road led to drug use and destruction, and the other road led to Julie and the children. Unlike before, I couldn't see any middle way. I had to make a choice."

"Yes, isn't that what we've been saying?"

"Okay, okay, I guess you have, but I never heard it, or I always convinced myself I could play it both ways. Over the next week my struggle focused on whether I had the strength to make the choice. But that is where being alone in the wilderness made a difference. Somehow, as my food ran out, I could feel something deep within telling me I would be okay. I don't know how to describe it, but I just felt it was time to move on. From then my fears subsided, or reduced enough for me to know I was ready to commit to one road."

---

review her fears, accept the threats as unrealistic, and together the team reaffirms its commitment to the planned course of action.

Danny then disappears for 2 weeks. At first they assume he has gone on a binge and will reappear in a few days, but 4 days later they have still heard nothing. After worrying about his absence for a week, Jack decides to call another meeting. Back at the physician's office they speak about their concerns for Danny's welfare, but also agree they can do little and that their course is set. A week later Danny arrives at Jack's house, unshaven, ragged, and dirty, but Jack can tell immediately that something has changed. After cleaning himself up, Danny tells Jack what had happened (see inset box).

Danny continues to live with Jack. As the first weeks of Danny's abstinence turn into months and then into years, father and son communicate more freely; they talk about their earlier experiences, share more of their shame and fear, and regularly review progress in rebuilding their relationship. It is not always easy, and at times their discussions erupt into arguments and abuse, but slowly the controlling tactics and other intimacy management strategies subside and the two find themselves connecting in ways that they had never thought possible in the past. Jack's confidence in supporting Danny grows; he helps him find work as a builder in town, he helps fund his study of carpentry at the local night-school, and they go fishing together. Danny also spends more time with Julie and the children. For the first year the children remained suspicious of his intent, but as they see the durability of his change, they begin to trust in his reliable and attentive presence and slowly the emergent closeness and commitment are reciprocated. Similarly, communication between Danny and Julie improves; however, while they would like to return to living all together, they both agree they should live apart until they are fully confident of the changes.

The choices Jack, Julie, and their friends made in deciding on their course of collective action, while prompting a favorable outcome at this stage, come with no guarantee of success. Collective action in other circumstances may be quite different; it might not be suitable to mount an open challenge either because the collective is still weak or there is a significant risk of the recipients harming themselves or others. It is also quite possible that their current reintegration process will flounder, and the addictive system will quickly reassert itself. Nonetheless, what is important is that a group of people have defied the fragmenting effects of an addictive system and chosen to act collectively. This decision alone has important long-term implications for that system. It signals to all those involved that even if fragmentation occurs again, those affected are still capable of reconnecting and by doing so accessing their potential to validate each other's experience and perhaps move toward mounting another challenge. It also sends a clear signal to the person in the addictive relationship that intimacy management strategies will at best be only partially successful and that powerful collective responses will always remain a possibility. In this way the success of a particular collective action matters less than the fact that a group of affected people have come together to share their thoughts and combine their efforts. With the prospect of ongoing collective action as a central feature of change, the next chapter explores how neighborhoods and communities might engage in providing the types of social environments that foster challenges to addictive relationships.

Chapter 12

Mobilizing Communities

I am not an individual,
I am an integral part of the cosmos.
I share divinity with my ancestors, the land, the seas and the skies.
I am not an individual because
I share a tofi with my family, my village, and my nation.
I belong to my family and my family belongs to me.
I belong to a village and my village belongs to me.
I belong to my nation and my nation belongs to me.
This is the essence of my sense of belonging.

(Tui Atua Tupua Tamasese Efi on the Samoan worldview)[1]

The discussion of the opportunities for collective action in Chapter 9 identified the key role community empowerment and social connectedness can play in engaging the strength of neighborhoods and communities. The quotation above by a leading Samoan academic captures the way in which social connectedness and personal identity are intertwined. This chapter explores how these broader layers of social connectedness can contribute to collective actions that challenge addictive relationships. It focuses on three quite different examples of community approaches that have been used to assist and support the long process of reintegration. The first example examines the use of volunteers as a way for addiction services to link in ongoing community support for reintegration. The second example emerged within Croatian and Italian communities as a widespread and organized network aimed at providing long-term support for families undertaking reintegration. The third example describes the application of indigenous understandings of the central value of relationships to develop a variety of strategies to support changes in Māori communities in Aotearoa–New Zealand. Each example was chosen to highlight the diversity of ways that a community might incorporate social approaches in their response to addictive relationships.

Volunteer Networks

One way that services working specifically with addictive relationships can connect with communities is through the development of volunteer networks. Volunteers, who are members of the community, give of their time freely to support those in addictive social contexts reintegrate into multiple

P.J. Adams, *Fragmented Intimacy: Addiction in a Social World*
© Springer 2008

and symmetrical intimacies. Such volunteer networks have the advantages of being financially inexpensive and of providing widespread access to support over long periods of time for individuals and families in their ongoing struggles with reintegration.

The Role of Volunteers

The volunteer role differs substantially from the role of a professional therapist or counselor in that the volunteer forms a transitional contact point for families pursuing their social reintegration back into communities. From a social perspective, there are many advantages in using volunteers in the long-term process of reintegration:

Volunteers provide a means by which communities can support reintegration

- Volunteers are members of the local community and collectively can provide linkages back into that community.
- The low costs associated with volunteers enable support to continue over long periods of time (several years), coverage that paid professionals will seldom be in a position to offer.
- Volunteers are not experts and, when their roles are maintained, are less likely to superimpose their beliefs onto those affected and are more likely to be seen as companions on a similar level.
- Volunteers bring to the reintegration process a wealth of personal experience, native knowledge, and practical understanding that prove important at various stages in reforming intimacies.
- Through their involvement volunteers themselves learn extensively about addictive relationships and bring that useful knowledge back to their own lives, families, neighborhoods, and communities, and thereby provide a knowledge base for assisting others affected by addictive relationships.

Despite these advantages, there are several risks involved in exposing individuals and families to volunteers during the complex social processes involved in reintegration. Volunteers lack advanced professional training and may find themselves (knowingly or unknowingly) out of their depth. Volunteer networks therefore require structures and procedures to ensure that these risks are minimized. For this the following measures are recommended:

- The role of volunteer needs to be carefully maintained to prevent it from sliding into the expert roles of therapist and counselor.
- Some people may not be suitable for the role of volunteer because of firmly held negative beliefs or an inability to respond to the experience of others; they will need to be directed elsewhere.
- Volunteer activities need to run alongside a program of basic training and ongoing education along with a well-designed system of mentoring and supervision.

- Volunteers need to be linked with professional services in order for them to feel supported and to be able to access expert help when required.

The following is an example of a volunteer network linked to a large addiction service.

Donwood Volunteer Groups

In Toronto, Canada,[2] the Donwood[3] provides a range of addiction services that include a 4-week live-in program, a 2-week day program, and a 3-month (3 hours per week) evening program. In 1986 it began recruiting program graduates to work alongside nurse-counselors in offering ongoing support groups to assist clients in their reintegration process once they finished their programs. The success and demand for these groups soon outstripped the availability of counselors, so in response they established a system of long-term groups run entirely by volunteers. The volunteer system quickly became an important aspect of the service and grew into a strong network of over three hundred volunteers. All those graduating from Donwood programs were expected to attend for a period of 2 years.[4] During this time the weekly groups provided a forum for participants to connect with others in their reintegration journeys and to share with each other support and ideas on how to handle the inevitable relationship challenges that emerged. The volunteer facilitators' primary tasks were to assist in group discussions, to enable sharing without domination by any one individual, and to determine if people require additional advice and support from the counseling staff. The network was managed by three Donwood staff members—a manager and two coordinators—along with ongoing support from clinicians. The network recruited volunteers through advertisements, through graduates from their programs, and through reputation and word of mouth.

Volunteer networks provide a longer term complement to counseling

Over the next 13 years the network evolved and developed its procedures. Each group was facilitated by two types of volunteer: a recovery volunteer and a community volunteer. The recovery volunteers were graduates from the Donwood programs, and they needed to have achieved at least 2 years of sobriety before joining the network. Their input into the groups was based on their personal experience in addictive relationships. The community volunteers provided a normalizing balance to the input provided by the recovery volunteers. They were attracted to becoming volunteers perhaps because they had been exposed to other family members in addictive relationships, or because they were seeking training as a stepping stone to other helping roles, such as counseling or social work, or because they wanted to contribute positively to their communities. On average, volunteers stayed with the network for just over 4 years and stated that their continuing involvement was due to their relationships with other volunteers, the satisfaction in helping people change, and their learning through educational opportunities.

Volunteer Selection and Training

The volunteers were important in ensuring that groups were a positive and safe experience for participants. The groups required facilitation by people who were not going to dismiss the experiences of those attending and who would avoid imposing negative judgments or rigid solutions. For example, the volunteer facilitators who participated needed to be responsive to where participants were coming from and needed to avoid promoting rigid approaches.[5] They needed to enable and support participants in discovering their own strategies based on what they personally judged as applicable from the range of options discussed during each meeting. For these reasons the process of becoming a volunteer involved three main phases: selection, training, and ongoing development.

During selection, potential recruits were asked to attend an information session conducted about three times a year.[6] During the session, they were divided into smaller groups with experienced practitioners who posed questions, such as "Why do people become addicted?" and "What do people need to change?" Candidates that espoused rigid and judgmental views about addictions or who seemed incapable of listening or respecting the views of others were advised to contribute their time elsewhere.

During the training phase, every selected volunteer attended a core training program of six 3-hour sessions that focused on listening skills, group facilitation skills, and basic understandings of addictions. After completing training they were progressively exposed to facilitating roles alongside experienced volunteers, along with regular individual supervision sessions with Donwood counselors and therapists.

From then on, ongoing supervision and education was seen as the backbone of the volunteer network. The basic training was followed by more advanced training on a variety of relevant issues such as how to deal with expressions of anger and responding to more complex issues such as addiction to specific drugs or complications associated with mental health issues. At all stages, the coordination team kept in close contact with the volunteers through newsletters and gatherings, and were able to closely monitor and respond to volunteers who were experiencing difficulties or who were wishing to vary the nature of their contribution.

Ongoing supervision & education is the backbone of volunteer networks

Family Involvement

Initially, families could attend the groups if they wished; this enabled them to participate more closely in relationship reintegration and to explore some of their own issues in reforming intimacies. However, since families had not been involved closely in the service programs, they were often lagging behind on the content of discussions, and program graduates found it difficult to speak openly about relationship issues with the families attending.

The network coordinators then began offering separate groups for families, where they could obtain a better understanding of the reintegration process and have a forum in which to talk over their own issues. Later the coordinators worked toward client and family groups being reunited as they approached the end of their 2 years. According to a social orientation, the separation of client activities from family activities limits the clients' capacity in assisting the reformation of intimacies, but in these circumstances this separation followed from the concentration of energy in Donwood programs on the needs of clients rather than on the families' relationships with the clients. If families had been closely included all through the program, then perhaps having separate groups may not have been required.

Community Involvement

The Donwood volunteer network provided a platform for the surrounding community to engage in supporting the long-term process of reintegration. In this way it at least partially adopted the principles of a social approach. However, it stopped short of fully grounding the network in community connectedness. At the time there seemed to be little need to expand beyond the Donwood; the volunteer network was growing and maturing, it had the backup support of the Donwood clinical staff, and it seemed obvious that the groups were vital to the success of all the programs. But in hindsight, this reliance on the Donwood as an institutional base placed the network on unstable footing in terms of its long-term survival. During the late 1990s the provincial government of Ontario, driven by financial concerns, embarked on a program of consolidating major institutions, including hospitals and institutions in the addiction and the mental health sectors.[7] The resultant formation of the Centre for Addiction and Mental Health (CAMH) embedded the network in a far larger and particle-dominated institutional structure, one grounded in clinical expertise and where the idea of service through a network of nonprofessional volunteers was seen as too risky for both the organization and its clientele. Support for the volunteers was withdrawn and in the course of the next 2 years the network dwindled and disappeared.

Over a period of 13 years, from 1986 to 1999, the Donwood volunteer network had flourished and provided long-term assistance to thousands of people affected by addictions. Staff members still speak enthusiastically of the power of such an approach. Expert visitors and hospital auditors had also been impressed, praising the program and presenting it with awards.[8] Unfortunately, the demise of the network occurred before any written documentation or formal evaluation was compiled. Its rise and fall speaks loudly of two critical factors: the power that can be unleashed when systems of community involvement are carefully established, and the dangers of a social approach that is embedded in governance structures driven by particle paradigm (see Chapter 2).

Social approaches remain at risk when embedded in particle paradigm structures

Croatian/Italian Community Clubs

The Croatian/Italian community clubs (*I Club Degli Alcolisti in Tratamentto* [Clubs for Treated Alcoholics][9]) are multiple family support groups for people involved in addictive systems. Over 2500 of these self-help groups currently meet weekly in Italy and Croatia. They operate at a community level and offer both people in addictive relationships and their families a local system of support for achieving abstinence as a pathway to the long-term goal of attaining quality intimacies. The clubs are the best example I know of that consistently apply a social paradigm to addictive relationships. I first heard about them in 1995 in a brief conversation with two Italian visitors,[10] who spoke highly of the widespread influence the clubs were having in Italy and recommended that I visit Italy to observe them first hand. I subsequently organized three visits to study how the clubs operate.[11] Since few reports on the clubs have been published in English, the following discussion is based on the information collected during those visits, backed up by the single book that is available in English.[12]

Club Origins

The club movement is based on a social ecological approach that closely resembles the social approach described in this book. From 1964 to his death in 1996, the club founder, Vladimir Hüdolin, drove a core commitment to responding to addictive systems on a community basis. In his early years he had spent time in England and was strongly influenced by the therapeutic (micro-) community movement that flourished during the late 1950s and early 1960s. He was particularly influenced by the ideas of Maxwell Jones and Joshua Bierer. Their perspective on services questioned the role of highly trained mental health professionals in guiding the rehabilitation of those in need. The presence of such experts can undermine the confidence of families and communities in seeking and committing themselves to their own resources. When given the opportunity and adequate supports, most people derive their own approaches to a problem, and the process of unraveling these solutions is critical to their ownership and confidence in attempting a program of change.

During the early 1960s Hüdolin was in charge of the alcohol and drug services in Zagreb. He was one of a handful of addiction professionals based there who were servicing a large hinterland with many people in addictive systems. Understandably, Hüdolin was searching for innovative ways to maximize the impact of his service on a large and increasing client group. To do this he took the notion of therapeutic communities and extended it beyond the micro-level of a residential treatment program out into the community as a whole. The social unit he used to achieve this outreach was with what he called "clubs." As he stated:

> Clubs are founded on the concept that alcohol-related problems are considered as different types of behavior, life-styles and difficulties arising from problematical

The club movement embraces a social approach to addictive systems

relationships and interactions between ecological systems in communities and families. Consequently, the treatment must start in the environment in which alcoholics live, as both alcoholics and their families are not like patients cut off from society, but are integral components of it.[13]

After Hüdolin formed the first club in Zagreb in 1964, the clubs spread steadily throughout Croatia, Slovenia, and Bosnia, and then in 1979 crossed over into Trieste, from where they spread throughout Italy.[14]

Clubs and Reintegration

Everyone who attends the club is seen as a member of it. But in order to ensure the operation of the club, every person attending is allocated club roles. The following summarizes the key roles:

The Servant Teacher

The servant teacher's role is central to the functioning of club meetings. The term may seem odd, but it accurately describes the role's central function. Servant teachers are not there to run the group, or facilitate, advise, or provide therapy for the families. Servant teachers are there to serve the families, to enable families to run their club in the fashion that assists their change. Also, the servant teacher provides the initial teaching, which introduces new families to the functioning of the clubs (see inset box). From my observations, the club movement actively sets up systems to prevent servant teachers from assuming therapist or advisor roles in meetings. It is central to the clubs that expertise and advice emerge from among the attendees, and is not imposed on the club from one source. The pitfalls of therapizing are repeatedly emphasized in training, in regional meetings, and in supervision sessions.

Servant teachers are required to attend a 50-hour "sensibilization" program during which they are schooled in the basic principles of the club. No formal qualifications are required to become a servant teacher. Servant teachers are either nominated by their communities or apply to the regional office on the basis of their previous experience and facilitation skills. Some who apply are health professionals: physicians, psychologists, and social workers. Others are concerned community members with strong leadership and facilitative skills and perhaps with direct exposure to addictive systems in their own lives. All take on

---

Servant Teachers: Main Tasks
- Listening and promoting the listening of others
- Supporting the members facilitating the meeting
- Connecting with and introducing new members to the clubs
- Maintaining the psychological safety of all those present
- Providing new members with basic information and advice regarding the nature of alcohol and drug dependency
- Reflecting the central purposes of the club movement within the meeting

the task with the understanding that they will not receive any payment, and despite this, many health professionals seek the role as a means of increasing their practice experience. All nominees are interviewed by regional club representatives, and those selected enter into the training program. The coordinator of the training program monitors their performance and may discuss their suitability when concerns arise.

Administrators, Secretaries, and Recorders

Administrators are appointed by a club for 1 year through an informal process of suggestion and nomination. Their primary role is to oversee practical issues regarding the functioning of the club. They might negotiate the use of the room, arrange meetings with members of the local community (the mayor, local physicians), and they usually represent the club at district meetings.

Secretaries, too, are appointed for 1 year through an informal process of suggestion and nomination. Their primary tasks include maintaining roles, managing financial records, and responding to correspondence. Recorders are responsible for recording what happens in a meeting, particularly the main issues and goals that emerged during discussion. They occupy the role for a week, and write up the content in a book ready for the new recorder at the next meeting.

Italian Club Meeting

Late one Saturday we drive to a small town in Northern Italy. The club's servant teacher is waiting outside to show us the way. We pass through a large courtyard to a small room filled with eighteen people. I am introduced and the group welcomes me. A man in his late fifties with his hair waxed back continues what he was saying:

"I have been sober two weeks now. I feel good, my health's improved and things are going great."

A small man across the other side of the room comments:

"My father was alcoholic and always claimed he was changing, so how can you be so sure of change this time."

"Yes, I understand, I am very good at giving up, I've done it lots in the past, but I always manage to drink again a short time later. My skill at giving up is now famous. It will now be known in New Zealand. But this time it is different. This time I really mean to stay stopped for good."

Some group members mutter approval, others remain quiet.

The Process of Club Meetings

Clubs, as autonomous units, do not operate on a formal or fixed set of rules. Clubs are expected to negotiate their own code; however, the servant teachers are provided with some guidelines on what ground rules tend to support effective group process (see inset box). The rules are not rigid. For instance, when a person attends while intoxicated, the club meeting may discuss this openly with the person and negotiate a response that may or may not involve asking the person to leave.

Typical Club Ground Rules
• Punctuality; lateness is disruptive
• No violence
• No smoking
• No drunkenness
• Family members must come as much as possible
• Speaking in the first person ("I think, I feel")
• Speaking in the here and now
• Acknowledge the right to a view and to disagree
• Allowing people to finish what they are saying
• Confidentiality (what is heard here stays here)

With addictive relationships more visible communities have a way to respond to reversions

Clubs also vary in how they respond to members who continue drinking. They tend to try to keep track of a member who experiences a reversion and sometimes they will nominate two or three members who know the person well to provide "friendly visits" to check on whether the person wants assistance. This increased visibility for members makes it harder for them to slip into a reversion. For example, some club members spoke of how when they began to revert, they chose to drive to outside towns where members of their own community would not see them drinking.

Club Regional Structures

The Italian club movement has evolved a national structure with consumer representation at all levels. Every 15 to 20 clubs form a local association with an executive composed of one or two members from each club. The local associations meet monthly and organize supervision and resolve administration issues (such as the formation of new clubs). Members of all clubs meet every 3 months for 2 to 3 hours to share views and present servant teacher certifications. Each local association sends two representatives to a regional executive. They meet regularly to plan regional resources and select and develop training programs for servant teachers and to manage supervision processes. Two members from each regional association are voted in as representatives on a national board which provides an overseeing function and defines mission, policy, and relations with outside organizations such as the government. Since most aspects of the club movement involve voluntary contributions, the whole operation costs very little. The rooms are either offered for free or rented for a nominal fee that is covered by a small contribution from members. The only costs are payment of the health professionals who train and supervise the servant teachers, costs for postage and stationary, travel costs, costs for the publication of a national magazine, as well as each year costs of organizing the national congress at which over 1200 people attend. Together with the club movement in Croatia and those in other European countries (most notably Denmark, Serbia, Slovakia, the Czech Republic, Poland, Russia, and Spain) the European School of Alcohology and Ecological Psychiatry promotes the clubs both in Europe and internationally. It does this through publications[15] and a 3-day training program conducted in English.

Education and Training

Education and training is seen as central to the operation of clubs because it is critical that participants fully appreciate a social paradigm on addictive relationships. Education is organized at several levels. In most regions, families are encouraged to attend introductory education groups to learn about addictive relationships and the club approach to change. These introductory groups are organized differently in different regions, but they usually involve ten evening sessions conducted by a combination of club members and local addiction service staff. All the newly referred families are encouraged to attend the sessions, which together with their club meetings would mean attending two sessions per week for the first 10 weeks.

For the training of servant teachers, one-week (50-hour) intensive basic training courses are run by alcohol and drug professionals (e.g., psychiatrists or psychologists) and experienced servant teachers. These usually occur on a regional basis once every several months. The programs include an introduction to addictive relationships and its effects on family members and detailed coverage of club philosophy. They aim particularly at changing the way people think about addictive relationships, to shift people away from pathology-oriented (particle) approaches to addictive relationships and to introduce them to a social ecological model. The programs typically include informational sessions on addictive processes, practice at listening and other facilitative skills, details on how to access local resources, and organized visits to clubs. Prospective servant teachers are required to attend these courses, plus ongoing training and supervision before they take on a club.

Opportunities for further training and supervision are organized differently in each region and depend on the expertise available. Some regions will provide sessions on specialized topics, such as responding to heroin abuse or people with addictive and mental health issues.

> **I Feel Unsure**
>
> At a club meeting a woman in her mid-forties turns her chair around slightly to address her husband sitting next to her:
>
> "Don't get me wrong, I admire how you have managed to stay sober for three years, but it has been enormously difficult for me too."
>
> "What do you mean?" he responds.
>
> "Well, to be frank, our relationship seems to be getting worse."
>
> "But stopping drinking was always what you said you wanted me to do."
>
> "Yes, but… well, put it like this. When you were drinking I had the upper hand. You were always mucking up then apologizing, and then what I said mattered. Now you always question and challenge what I say and keep pushing for us to communicate better."
>
> "That's what we're meant to be doing."
>
> "…and its very unsettling. I'm not sure I want an intense relationship with you."
>
> Another group member joins in: "But aren't we all striving for better quality relationships"
>
> "Yes, but I don't know if I want this one. It's all new to me… it's out of hand. And why did he change then? Why didn't he stop drinking ten years ago when our children were young. It's his agenda not mine."

Clubs and Community Connectedness

The club operates as a multifamily community, functioning in and connected with a local community. This is a core principle of the clubs. The meetings provide a forum for family members to listen to other family members and to discuss a variety of responses to common problems. In this way families are empowered to review possibilities, to make judgments, and then to come to their own consensus on how to proceed. This means that much of the conversation focuses on the nature of relationships and the interpersonal dynamics associated with reintegration. For example in the inset box above, a woman reports that in the course of a reintegration she is having difficulty adjusting to changes in roles and responsibilities.

The perception that a club is grounded in a specific locality means it is owned by and identified with that community. Club families are likely to know each other and interact outside of their meetings. Furthermore, the club, as an autonomous unit, reflects the social composition of the local community. Communities with unique combinations of people form clubs that reflect this composition. This identification with locality is a key to the ownership and success of the clubs. A specialized club for specific cultures, such as Chinese, gay and lesbian, and youth clubs, would deviate from this important principle. Clubs are locality based, communities within a community, and not a coalition of similar people.

In regions with a high concentration of clubs (those more than one club per 2000 people), the clubs tend to develop a visible presence. Key community members (such as local council members or local physicians) are invited to attend and get to know the people involved. Since people attending clubs socialize outside meetings, over time it would be difficult to find members of those communities who do not know of distant family members or friends who have some relationship to clubs. This high visibility in the community underpins for each club a level of acceptance that makes them a meaningful part of these communities and helps profile addictive relationships as an important issue for them to address. In contrast with the anonymity traditions of the twelve-step movement, clubs endeavor to relate openly with communities and often community members know which families are attending. This reduces the shame and stigma associated with addictive relationships. Clubs also connect strongly with other services in the area, particularly alcohol and drug services (see inset box, above). For instance, outpatient units include club meetings within their programs and encourage people to attend clubs as one of the goals of counseling.

Clubs in Addiction Services

In San Daniele in Northern Italy, Francesco Piani manages a mental health service for the Udine area and this service includes a residential alcohol and drug program. I was invited to attend group sessions, admission interviews, and to talk with staff about the program. I was struck by extent to which the treatment program reflected club philosophy. Staff insisted at admission that family members attend the interview. The interview carefully reviewed any previous involvement with clubs. Community meetings modeled on the clubs were held regularly in the program, and family members were required to attend. Those without available family members invited other members from their local clubs. Furthermore, a social worker in the service was employed with the primary task of referring participants to local clubs upon discharge. Staff commented that similar integration of clubs with specialist alcohol and drug services was occurring in many places throughout Italy.

Twelve-step programs are also available in both Croatian and Italian communities. Since both approaches recognize the importance of family, and aim to support families in maintaining abstinence, many club attendees also attend twelve-step programs, and the choice comes down more to comfort with either a disease (particle) or a social interpretation of addiction.

The other important linkage for clubs is with local primary health professionals such as general practitioners and community nurses.[16] These health professionals (who are trained both in brief intervention skills and club approaches) actively screen for alcohol, drug, gambling, and other addiction issues and help direct affected families to clubs and other associated resources. Since they continue to see members of these families on an ongoing basis, they are also well positioned to provide ongoing support and ensure that club involvement is maintained.[17]

Social Ecology and Intimacy

Clubs espouse an ecological theory of addictions. As in this book, club affiliates see addictions as intense relationships to an addictive substance/process that occurs at the cost of other relationships. Clubs view involvement of intimates and the community as critical at all points in responding to addictive relationships. This commitment to relationships permeates every aspect of their activities. Participants are repeatedly reminded at meetings that the primary goal of clubs is not sobriety but to achieve "quality of life" and "quality of relationships" both within the family and in the surrounding community. At the meetings I attended, the topic of conversation was predominantly about relationship issues: "If you stop drinking, then where do I stand?" "Why can't you trust me now that I have changed?" "It's always you who decides when to change, and I resent your never changing when I needed it." "Why do you keep protecting me from situations where people are drinking?" (See inset box) These relationship issues are seen as the substance of a reintegration process. They matter because collectively people can support each other in strengthening their reconnections. Shortly before his death, Hüdolin, while speaking to the 1995 club convention, related the importance of social connectedness to the processes of spiritual connectedness:

> **I Have Difficulty Trusting**
>
> In the middle of a meeting a tall man in his early thirties walks in straight from work with fresh plaster and paint splats dotted over his clothing.
>
> "We'll, I've been 951 days sober today." Everyone nods approvingly.
>
> His fiancée arrives ten minutes later, and joins in by saying, "It's only two months to our wedding."
>
> An older man at the end of the table, the fiancée's father, then addresses the tall man by saying, "My daughter means everything to me and over the last three years I feel we've grown close and we both know each other very well. Also, I admire what you have achieved in staying sober." He leans forward slightly. "I care for you and in many ways you are the best future husband for my daughter, but in my heart, deep within, I am still afraid that one day you will go back to drinking and my daughter will suffer."
>
> "I wouldn't let that happen."
>
> "I know, you will do everything to avoid it and I'm not saying don't get married. I just want you to know about my fear and my anxiety about the future."

> The person, together with his or her family, drops alcohol and commences to grow and mature, looking for a better quality of life, a better quality of health culture and general culture. In other words a better anthropological spirituality.... Sobriety does not simply mean abstinence, rather it means a blend of the best human anthropospiritual characteristics, including abstinence.[18]

He saw the club movement as supporting a long-term process of ethical and spiritual growth, linking together the various dimensions of reintegration as depicted in the inset box.[19] In terms used in this book, his concept of "anthropological spirituality"[20] can be thought of as an inner power that is derived from social connectedness.

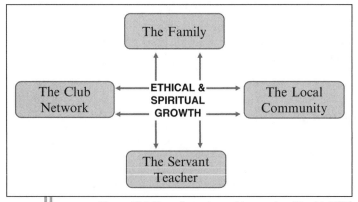

Figure 12.1 Four dimensions of interaction (Cecchi, 2001)

The ecological thinking underlying the approach considers each club as a connecting point in a "net" of interconnections.[21] As depicted in the onset box below, each club provides a node for connecting people in a community, and provides the community with a focal point to tackle the difficulties it faces with addictive relationships. Each of these nodes spreads out as a net across this community and connects with other communities.

While some communities lack clubs, overall this net establishes a supportive presence that enables families and communities to participate in collective action and reintegration. In this way the individuals affected are understood in the context of intimate relationships, family relationships, relationships to the community, and the broader societal, political, and cultural contexts. The health professional connecting with this approach seeks to facilitate individuals, families, and communities in searching out and owning their own responses to the problem at issue. Expertise becomes contested and negotiated according to the contexts in which the problems are being managed.

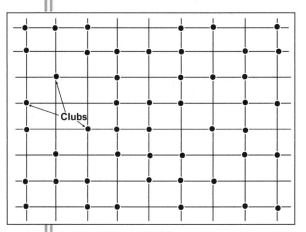

Figure 12.2 The net of interconnectedness

Three interesting concepts have emerged within the clubs as a guide to equipping family members in their attempts at reintegration: solidarity, unity, and love. These three words are often used together and are given considerable weight in club discussions, and while they may have other connotations in Italian, they appear to refer to the core ingredients of intimate reintegration. *Solidarity* refers to the commitment that attendees have to their family, to their club, and to their community. It suggests that while fragmentation processes may tempt people to back away from each other, it is important to maintain commitment to the long-term goals of reconnection. *Unity* refers to the need for people to act together and recognizes that individuals on their own are unlikely to compete with the power of the addictive relationship. *Love* refers to the sense of one-ness and accord people acquire as they share experiences and act together. It encompasses the unifying power that emerges in family relationships and the wider sense of accord with the club movement, the community, and wider society.

What Effect Are Clubs Having?

The club movement, like the twelve-step movement, involves a sprawling number of autonomous entities firmly embedded in different ways within local communities. Their variable composition and social complexity poses multiple challenges to the task of researching and evaluating their impact (not that dissimilar from the challenges faced in assessing the impact of attending twelve-step programs[22]). An obvious indicator of their impact is their success in spreading in sizable numbers within the communities that embrace them. In Croatia, the number of clubs grew steadily through the 1970s and 1980s to about one thousand. They also spread to other parts of the then united Yugoslavia, particularly in Slovenia and in Bosnia-Herzegovina. In 1991, the wars and breakup of Yugoslavia severely reduced the number of clubs.[23] In Italy, the first club started in 1980, and by 2000 there were over 2500 clubs spread all over Italy. This was achieved with minimal government funding and relying virtually entirely on voluntary community and professional support. People from other countries that are exploring the use of clubs (such as Norway, Spain, Brazil, Russia, Bulgaria, and Poland) are having mixed results,[24] but their involvement is relatively recent and they require time to work out how clubs might best fit into their different social environments.

Other countries are exploring how club systems would best suit their circumstances

In 1992 Pierluigi Morisini in Rome and Francesco Piani in Udine initiated an outcome evaluation study (VALCAT—Progetto Nazionale di Valutazione Club Alcolisti in Trattamento) tracking the effectiveness of clubs throughout Italy.[25] Over a 6-year period they collected baseline data on 798 families attending clubs, with the goal of reassessment at 6 months, 18 months, and 3 years. The interview schedules aimed to assess the impact of the clubs across a broad range of social, mental, and health variables. In reporting their results, they found that 73 percent of families benefited consistently well at 18 months and 62 percent of families benefited consistently well at 3 years; 15 percent of families showed improvements that were erratic and inconsistent (due to reversions and other problems) at 18 months and 26 percent at 3 years; 8 percent of families reverted to addictive relationships at 18 months and 5 percent at 3 years. The number lost to follow-up or death for the entire period was only 7 percent at 3 years, indicating that families are closely engaged and retained in clubs.

The results from the VALCAT evaluation are promising and contrast with evaluations of other social approaches (such as family therapy), which have struggled to demonstrate effectiveness. However, research into the effectiveness of clubs at an early phase; this is only one study, it does not contrast the clubs' methods with other approaches, and little is known as to which critical factors contribute most to change. Compared with other social approaches (as discussed in Chapter 11), clubs make considerably more use of neighborhood and community connectedness, and this, I suspect, is the strongest contributor to its apparent effectiveness. Perhaps both the club movement and other social approaches to addictive relationships could benefit from closer collaborations in future research.

An Indigenous Approach

A third community-based approach highlights how in many cultural contexts the power of social connectedness is already a high priority and thus readily available to assist in both resisting and reintegrating from the fragmenting impacts of addictive relationships. In many traditional societies, such as those of Chinese and Indian origin, high value is placed on the power of collective approaches, and family and community connectedness is often mobilized in addressing threats to well-being.[26] For first nation and other indigenous populations, this capacity is particularly important because their communities tend to have been fragmented by the effects of colonization and urbanization, and this fragmentation creates environments in which addictive relationships flourish, thereby contributing to further alienation and deprivation. This section provides a brief overview of how Māori, the indigenous people of Aotearoa–New Zealand, are employing social connectedness to build their resilience to fragmentation from addictive relationships.[27]

> **Proverb:** *Whakatauāki*
> *Ēhara taku toa I te toa takitahi*
> *Engari taku toa he toa takitini*
> My strength is not the strength of one
> But my strength is the strength of many

The Māori Context

Aotearoa–New Zealand is a small nation of approximately four million people situated low in the Pacific and at least a 3-hour jet flight from the coast of its nearest neighbor, Australia. Its geographic isolation is the basis for both what constrains it and makes it unique. Its land mass covers an area of roughly the size of England and Scotland combined, and it consists of two main islands stretching from north to south across subtropical and temperate climates. Mountain ranges run up the middle of both islands and are flanked by foothills, uplands, and fertile lowlands. Its moderate climate together with its regular rainfall supports the growth of a vigorous plant life that, prior to the intrusion of humans, had supported the evolution of a unique flora and fauna.

The first settlement of Aotearoa–New Zealand by Polynesian peoples (Māori) occurred about 1200 years ago. These "people of many islands" had mastered the skills of ocean navigation that enabled them to progressively occupy the larger islands of the south Pacific.[28] Māori ancestors arrived in Aotearoa–New Zealand in a series of emigrations and established small communities in coastal areas. The villages steadily expanded in accordance with the growth of their economies, which relied on either hunting and fishing or mixed gardening. These enterprising people, referred to today generally as Māori but in reality made up of many different tribal groups *(iwi)*, gradually established a complex system of tribal communities *(hapū)* linked by kinship connections and trade throughout the extent of Aotearoa–New Zealand. Their day-to-day routines were strongly organized according to status and obligations within extended family networks *(whānau)*. By the fifteenth century a network of over 6000 *pā* (fortified villages) had formed, which relied heavily on transportation and communication using large canoes and path systems.[29]

With the arrival of Europeans *(Pākehā)* in the late eighteenth century, following a period of contact and initial settlement, increasing numbers of Europeans occupied the land for extraction industries and agriculture. In 1840 the Treaty of Waitangi was signed between Māori and the British Crown. For the British, the Treaty provided a means by which to legitimate their rule and their ongoing appropriation of land, while for Māori, working off a different translation, it protected their sovereignty over vital interests (land, water, and other resources). Subsequently, Maori, as for indigenous people in North America, were swamped by waves of mass European migrations, and as a consequence of land confiscations, wars against the British, and deaths from unfamiliar European diseases, they soon found themselves a poor and disenfranchised minority in their own land.[30] In the first half of the twentieth century, this disenfranchisement was compounded by the imposition of European values and practices through education and progressive urbanization. These processes caused significant distress and contributed to relatively poor health and social well-being.

Colonization & urbanization fragments the strength of indigenous peoples

The second half of the twentieth century was marked by the increasing recognition that many of the difficulties Māori faced as a people were a product of deterioration in their cultural base and that improvements were unlikely to come via European systems. This led to a broad upwelling of Māori identity that included a renaissance of Māori culture *(tikanga)* and cultural practices *(kaupapa)*, demands for Europeans to honor the original Treaty, the return where possible of confiscated land, and reorienting key resources such as education and health around Māori social systems. It is in the midst of this period that distinctively Māori approaches to addictive relationships began to emerge.

With the backdrop of the rise Māori consciousness and cultural owner-ship, I have been of two minds about whether to discuss their social approaches to addiction. I am not of Māori origin; my forebears migrated to Aotearoa–New Zealand from the British Isles in the 1840s. Furthermore, there is a real danger of explaining one part of a Māori worldview and imposing it without recognizing its interconnections with other parts of that world (this is the issue of incommensurability mentioned in Chapter 2). This could lead to misleading and culturally demeaning impressions. However, in the context of what is being proposed in this book, my purpose here is not to provide definitive coverage, but rather to point out how strongly cultural perspectives include social principles. I believe a social orientation shares many commonalities with Māori approaches to health, and on the basis of these commonalities they warrant some exploration.[31] The following discus-sion, therefore, provides a brief glimpse of what is a far more rich and com-plex picture, but a glimpse that reinforces the value of a social orientation.

Connectedness and Whānaungatanga

For Māori generally, the care and maintenance of relationships takes a very high priority. As captured by the commonly used proverb *(whakatauāki)* in the inset box,[32] many other concerns of the world intrude, but ultimately it is rela-tionships with people that really matter. Relationships are not confined to the current circle of intimates. Connectedness is understood in broad terms as encompassing a range of different types of relationships that include the wider extended family, those who are dead, those who are yet to come, the land, and a spiritual realm. As stated by Pam Armstrong: "Maori health and well-being is found in valu-ing traditional belief systems, as a holistic phe-nomenon that values the interconnection between spirituality, nature, ceremonialism and kinship."[33]

> **Proverb:** *Whakatauāki*
> *Hutia te rito o te harakeke*
> *Kei hea te kōmako e kō?*
> *Māu e ui mai*
> *He aha te mea nui o tenei ao?*
> *Māku e ki ātu*
> *He tangata, he tangata, he tangata*
> If you pull out the heart of the flax bush
> Where will the bellbird sing?
> You ask me:
> What is the greatest thing of this world?
> I reply
> People, people, people

The concept of *whānaungatanga* focuses on connectedness to *whānau* (family - pronounced far'noh), but this is seen as involving far more than ties to family. It includes broader links to both the extended family group *(hapū)* and tribal identities *(iwi)*, and through these links out into the social world as a whole.

Whānaungatanga is fundamental to *Maori*. It is the basis of Māori as a people and a society. It is from this basis that Māori are able to interpret their true sense of belong-ing through, identifying, realizing and experiencing, their kin-based associations and interrelationships. *Whānaungatanga* stresses the importance of interrelationships of people and their roles within their communities plus their interconnection to *whenua* or their environment and out into the spiritual realm: *nga atuā*. It is the process from which they develop their collective strength that enables them to transcend their ethnic culture and become part of the universal world of culture.[34]

For Māori, a strong sense of social connectedness permeates all aspects of living; all relationships are treasured for their own intrinsic value and their value is reinforced repeatedly through a variety of common cultural practices. For example, personal introductions include the naming of one's extended family *(whānau)*, one's river *(awa)*, and one's mountain *(maunga)*. Thus river catchments are used as a way of graphically defining the land and the environment of primary relationships to which one belongs. Another strategy that establishes connections involves recounting one's genealogy *(whakapapa)* as a way both of connecting the past, the present, and the future, and of looking for connections with other people.

For Maori social connectedness permeates all aspects of living

In the processes of connecting, two concepts play an important role: *tapu* and *mana*. *Tapu* has no clear equivalent in European cultures. It is at times translated as referring to what is "holy" and "sacred," and therefore linked to practices associated with boundaries and restrictions. However, these understandings refer to surface manifestations; at a deeper level *tapu* refers to the intrinsic being in everything and everyone. It is "being with potentiality for power" and for that reason, respect for *tapu* is an essential ingredient to social connection. *Mana* (roughly translated as "power") refers to sources of power that include and extend beyond social understandings of power:

> *Mana* is essentially power to effect, to order, to achieve. *Mana* has purpose. It is spiritual power that has effect on the physical, it is spiritual power which proceeds from *tapu* as its source. Where there is *tapu* there is *mana*.[35]

The functions of *mana* are closely linked to those of *tapu*:

> If *tapu* represents potential, *mana* represents the development of that potential, therefore the more one develops their potential for being, the greater their *mana*. The word *mana* is used in different contexts and the various translations include: authority, control, influence, prestige, power, psychic force, effectual, binding, authority, having influence or power, vested with effective authority, be effectual, take effect, be avenged. These are all aspects of *mana*.[36]

When people and their relationships are strong, when their intrinsic being is empowered, and the various levels of connectedness are in balance, then they are understood to have *mana* (power to effect), and the well-being of themselves and the people they connect with is enhanced.

Fragmentation and Noa

Since taking care of relationships is given such high priority, any activities that involve the possibility of splitting or fragmentation need to be carefully monitored. The threat that people in relationships lose their social connectedness and become *Noa* is a major concern. Michael Shirres writing about *noa* describes it as being free from the restrictions that circumscribe *tapu*. He writes, "*Noa* is directly opposed, not to *tapu* itself, but to the restrictions which follows on from the recognition of *tapu*. *Noa* basically means 'free from restriction' and can be something positive or negative."[37]

For *noa* in the positive sense, people have their own intrinsic *tapu* that needs to be acknowledged and respected. Many of Māori social rituals aim to ensure this is honored. *Noa* in the negative sense occurs when a person's intrinsic *tapu* is violated. According to Shirres: "This 'trampling' on the *tapu* of another is itself seen as a way of increasing one's own *tapu* while diminishing the intrinsic *tapu* of the other. With the weakening of the intrinsic *tapu* there is the weakening of the power of restrictions.... The other person then becomes *noa*, or 'free from restriction' in a negative way and able to be treated as *otaota*, as 'rubbish.'"[38] This means that the failure to acknowledge *tapu* will lead to diminishing one person compared to another in ways that lead to social fragmentation. Addictive relationships involve an intensification of one central relationship at the cost of other relationships. In this way they inevitably diminish the intrinsic *tapu* not only of the person in the addictive relationship but also of surrounding intimates. The people involved become disconnected from one another, they become *noa* (in the negative sense) and their *tapu* and *mana* become impoverished. For a people already fragmented through cultural dominance, the presence of an addictive relationship compounds the sense of alienation and it does not take much more for addictive social systems to finish the process.

Fragmentation in addictive systems compounds alienation from other sources

Reintegration and Hohourongo

A leading Maori academic, Mason Durie, describes Maori health development proceeding along two pathways: *whānau* development, "the enhancement of critical *whānau* capacities," and *whānau* healing, "the conversion of dysfunctional patterns into less harmful practices."[39] A key point he repeatedly emphasizes is that social reintegration along both paths must also involve cultural restoration (cultural reintegration). The second path, *whānau* healing, is the key process in reintegrating from addictive relationships:

> Healing can occur at more than one level: body tissues heal, individuals heal, both physically and spiritually, and healing also occurs for groups. *Whānau* healing... involves processes of appraisal, confrontation, and deliberation, as well as reconstruction of *whānau* values and standing. Unlike family therapy, which often leads to a concentrated examination of micro-communication and the elaboration of underlying feelings and attitudes, the energy in *whānau* healing flows outwards, away from intensity and raw emotion towards shared ownership of whatever problems are unearthed.[40]

It is in the process of healing that *hohourongo* is understood to occur. *Hohou* means to bind or lash together, and *rongo* means peace, so joined *hohourongo* refers to a binding peace, a process of achieving peaceful reintegration and restoration of *whanau* interconnectedness.[41] *Hohourongo* helps sustain *whānau* in situations of stress and fragmentation, but it also critical to reforming damaged interpersonal links.

In the course of reintegrating from addictive relationships, *hohourongo* can play a crucial role in facilitating reconnections. The cultural dynamics regarding how this is achieved are detailed and complex, but to describe some of the dimensions briefly, social integration and reintegration are achieved through three primary principles: *tika* (roughly "proper process"), *pono* (integrity), and *aroha* (love or compassion). *Tika* is important because it guides the way relationships are formed:

> *Tika* regulates our relationship in all things. Our relationship to other people, our relationship to other created things, and the link with the source of being. If *tika* is observed then *tapu* is addressed. *Tika* applies to the principle, the process, the goal, and the stages.[42]

If the processes used to reform fragmented relationships lack *tika*, then they risk further deterioration. *Tika* is why cultural guidance is so important when attempting to reintegrate. The related concept of *pono* (integrity) refers to the commitment required to enable *tika* to be followed.

> *Pono* is integrity, faithfulness to *tika* and/or *aroha*. It is the virtue that motivates and challenges us. It means knowing what is just, knowing what has to be done to achieve *tika* and then having the personal courage to do what is necessary to ensure *tika* is carried out.[43]

Aroha refers to the binding processes of love, compassion and empathy that bring people together into a sense of common accord.

> *Aroha* is the principle of compassion and is exercised simultaneously with *tika* and *pono* enhances one's (inner being) *tapu* plus the well-being of others. The feeling of well-being gives one a sense of joy, contentment and peace of mind.[44]

Aroha, therefore, is a powerful force in reforming and reconciling deteriorated relationships within addictive social systems.

Love & compassion are powerful forces in reforming & reconciling fragmented relationships

For Māori these three primary principles for establishing relationships, *tika, pono*, and *aroha*, provide a guiding base for achieving *hohourongo* and the types of reconnections that counter the fragmenting power of addictive relationships. There are many other aspects to this process that are beyond the scope of this book. The key reason for discussing them briefly here is to point out that the building blocks for undertaking a reintegration are already well established within this cultural perspective. The challenge for the wider study of addictive systems is to find ways to avoid importing and imposing models and frameworks that might block or divert from the potential of what already exists.

Whānaungatanga in Action

Māori actualize *whānaungatanga* in all aspects of their daily life and ensure that it permeates all corners of their communities. Accordingly, in their response to the fragmentation associated with addictive relationships, *whānaungatanga* is automatically drawn as a resource to counter deteriorations and asymmetries in *whānau* connectedness.[45] However, in many situations this fragmentation is compounded by the effects of colonization and associated poverty and cultural marginalization, leaving many *whānau* in weakened positions regarding their capacity to draw on *whānaungatanga*. To tip the balance, a range of community-based initiatives are attempting to assist families in unlocking their connectedness potential.[46] The following discussion touches briefly on three quite different examples of community approaches that harness the power of *whānaungatanga* in responding to addictive relationships.

The Tātou Network

Tātou (or more fully *"He Ope Awhina Ia Tātou: Whānau* supporting *whānau* affected by alcohol and drug problems") originated in 1998 in Northland (the upper regions of Aotearoa–New Zealand)[47] with the main purpose of strengthening community connectedness around *whānau* affected by addictive relationships. While the instigators of the approach were influenced by what they had heard about clubs in Italy, they sought to develop the network as much as possible within a Māori framework.[48] Initially, five communities were chosen based on their interest in participating. In each community regular *whānau hui* (family meetings) in which all people belonging to addictive social systems were invited to connect to and support each other in collective action.

The *Tātou kaiawhina* (coordinators) worked at linking with families and linking *Tātou* to other services and community initiatives within each location. These were supported with regional networking meetings that focused on training and supporting them in their role. Over time other communities joined the network, and other activities and initiatives were included. Over its 5 years of operation, the *Tātou* network faced many difficulties,[49] particularly in its relationship to particle-oriented addiction and other health services, which maintained expectations that change could only occur through treatment from experts working in treatment settings. As funding support dwindled, *Tātou* activities faded out in several locations, but in those locations where its activities were strongly embedded into Māori community networks, *Tātou* continued, and in some locations mutated and merged with other community initiatives.[50]

Colonized people may also be subject to dominant particle orientations to addiction

Community Action on Youth and Drugs (CAYAD) Projects

The CAYAD projects employ community action principles of empowerment to strengthen the capacity of youth in specific communities to avoid harm from alcohol and drugs.[51] The types of activities vary, depending on the needs and choices of the community, but aim typically to increase community awareness of drug issues, to improve responsiveness in schools and community organizations, and to empower a sense of inclusion and the voice of young people within those locations. While not specifically Māori, many of the projects occurred in Māori communities, and consequently the principles of *whānaungatanga* played a significant role. For example, in one small Northland community, Whangaruru, social and cultural connectedness were fostered in projects such as involving heavy cannabis users in sports and cultural activities (such as long canoe competitions, *waka ama*, or traditional dance, *kapa haka*) and in strengthening *Marae* (Māori community focal point) economic development and youth employment through ventures such as mussel farms. In 1998, six initial sites for CAYAD were implemented in different parts of Aotearoa–New Zealand—four rural and two urban. Evaluation of these found reduced drug problems in schools, reduced crime, improved attitudes toward drugs, and improved coordination between community organizations.[52] This success has led to CAYAD projects being developed in a further eighteen sites.

Kaupapa Māori Addiction Services

Kaupapa Māori addiction services set out to base their interventions on Māori beliefs values and practices and require that their development is governed and managed by Māori organizations.[53] For their purposes cultural reintegration is a prerequisite to durable social reintegration. While in theory, as services, these programs risk functioning separately from their base communities, in practice they work in a closely integrated fashion with Māori community networks. *Whānau* (family networks) are included in activities as much as possible and in ways that differentiate them significantly from the particle approaches of European equivalents. For example, *kaupapa* Māori services in Northland build much of their interventions around *whānau hui* (family meetings) where not only immediate intimates, but concerned extended family members and others in the community are engaged and encouraged to participate. The meetings use cultural protocols to establish an environment of trust, honesty and respect within which the power of connectedness *(whānaungatanga)* can emerge.[54] These services also seek to link as much as possible to subtribal *(hāpu)* structures, thereby facilitating ongoing social and cultural links into the community. For example, in the Hawkes Bay on the East Coast of the North Island, *hāpu kaumaatua* (subtribal elders) play a critical role in guiding the development of services and advising on protocols.

Cultural approaches are embedded in broader social networks & structures

This chapter reported on three mobilizing communities, but I must remind the reader that I am an outsider in all three. As an outsider, I am able to describe in broad terms the nature of these initiatives and their congruence with the assumptions in a social paradigm. What I am unable to do is capture the full meaning and depth of these approaches for the people who live within them. As described here, they provide more a beacon for what might be possible in other contexts. The next chapter takes our understanding of a social paradigm and applies it to another specific context, that of the specialist alcohol and drug service. It focuses on the ways that practitioners might open up social opportunities in their contact with clients.

Chapter 13

Applications to Practice

We propose that one of the most significant barriers to family involvement in routine addiction treatment results from the commonly held notion among service providers that family members are "adjuncts" and are not central to addiction treatment services.... Models of alcohol and drug problems need to place the role of the social environment as central and as important as that played by individual factors.

(*Alex Copello and Jim Orford, 2002*[1])

The initiation of a therapeutic relationship between an addiction practitioner and someone in an addictive relationship often provides the first step in the processes of resocialization and reintegration. But in many circumstances introducing a therapeutic relationship—a relationship with high intimacy potential—adds further fragmentation into the addictive social system. Family members who are bewildered and frustrated by their loved one's deteriorating behavior, and are buoyed up by expectations and hope that these services can fix addictions, are only too willing to hand over their involvement to addiction professionals. The practitioner's presence and the prospect of quick solutions provide them with some reprieve, and they willingly withdraw to allow the practitioner to exercise his or her knowledge and skills. While family members may have little idea of what is happening during a mysterious sequence of counseling sessions, they are reassured by the prospect of change and their confidence is reinforced when after several sessions the behavior of their loved one seems to improve. However, a little later their confidence is rocked when, following a series of sessions or time in a residential rehabilitation program the therapeutic relationship draws to a close and by implication the responsibility is handed back to the family. Their loved one returns, and acts differently for a while, but in time returns to old routines, which leads on eventually to the addictive relationship reasserting itself. Now, facing a full reversion, the intimates are left wondering whether there is any real prospect for change. What hope is there when not even addiction services with all their wisdom and resources are able to make things different? In their despondency they continue to distance themselves from their loved one, and their fragmented world seems more solid and powerful than ever.

This chapter is a departure from the previous chapters, which focused on the potency of social networks to influence the course of an addictive relationship. The site of deterioration and the opportunity for change has been firmly located within the social world, particularly the social processes in intimate relationships; this orientation remains the primary preoccupation of

P.J. Adams, *Fragmented Intimacy: Addiction in a Social World*
© Springer 2008

the book. This chapter, however, temporarily shifts attention away from social networks and asks whether there are realistic opportunities for specialist addiction services to contribute to the social dimensions of a reintegration. In recognition that most addiction practitioners work in systems that focus on individuals rather than relationships, the chapter examines how it is still possible for practitioners to operate using a social orientation.

Barriers to Socially Inclusive Practice

The primary barrier to social inclusion with addictions is the dominance of a particle paradigm in research, teaching, and addiction services. As discussed in Chapter 2, the paradigm itself is not the issue; its many theories and strategies have contributed positively to a broad range of approaches to intervention. The problem lies more with its dominance, which permeates every aspect of addiction services and allows little room for other alternatives. For example, in most community addiction services practitioners meet one-to-one with clients for 55-minutes sessions in small offices that are seldom suitable for meeting more that two clients at a time.[2] The clients are either "addicts" (people in addictive relationships) or "significant others" (intimates), who are treated as individual cases in their own right. The sessions are typically held in clinics that resemble either hospital ward/outpatient environments or offices in general practice venues. The reception environments are typically small and

Service environments & practices provide little encouragement for family inclusion

family unfriendly, with an emphasis on record keeping and clinical efficiency. While the assistance of experts in one-to-one sessions has an important contribution in initiating a change process, it has arguably of less value in the longer process of maintaining change. In many ways, the long-term success of an intervention is determined by the extent to which it is integrated into patterns and supports within a person's life. The individual counseling environment can contribute only in a limited way to this process of reintegration.

To conceptualize the potential role of specialist services, practitioner involvements need to be positioned within all six phases of reintegration that were identified in Chapter 10 (see inset box). Each phase could take months up to possibly a couple of years, and the whole process, with some reversions, could take ten years or more.

The practitioner's first involvement could be with a family member who attends a couple of counseling sessions to learn how best to respond to the person in the addictive relationship. The next involvement might occur during a crisis in which the person in the addictive relationship might attend one or two sessions to help determine how to balance the demands of the addictive relationship with the demands of the family system. After the crisis passes, the person might then agree to attend a series of psychoeducational group sessions (probably without other family members). In response to a subsequent reversion the person might then choose to enter a 1- or 2-month residential rehabilitation

program followed by two
sets of aftercare coun-
seling sessions aimed at
reinforcing the changes
made in the program.
The final involvement
could take the form of
couples or family sessions
in which the couple or
family attempts to read-
just marital relationships
or to renegotiate family
issues such as a history of
violence and abuse.

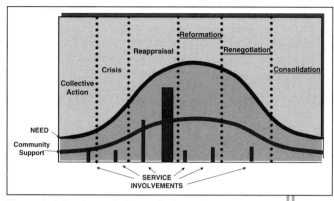

Figure 13.1 Services and phases of reintegration

As represented by the curves in the inset box above, each service involvement
comprises only a small episodic point of contact across the whole process. Of
high significance is the ongoing responses and support provided by community
members, particularly those who comprise the person's immediate circle of intimates. This wider orientation suggests that one of the service practitioner's key
challenges is to find ways of integrating what happens in sessions with what happens in the person's social world. The two levels of involvement need to interact;
otherwise the effort misses out on the social potential of combined collective
action—or worse, the levels could end up working against each other. To sustain
the changes negotiated in counseling sessions, they will need to be linked to the
ways family and friends are responding; what happens outside needs to be reinforced by counseling recommendations, and vice versa. If other parts of the
social system fail to connect, it is difficult to see how social and community
supports can be integrated with the supports provided by services.

Why is the Social World Excluded?

The reasons why services tend to exclude families and other social world
connections are multilayered and complex. The following subsections consider
four contributing factors that play varying roles according to the context.

Practitioner Allegiance to Particle Explanations

Practitioner allegiance to one-to-one particle approaches is surprisingly
consistent and resilient throughout the world,[3] and on closer inspection the
reasons are not difficult to identify. In terms of practitioner training, addiction textbooks adopt thoroughly particle approaches,[4] and the intervention
techniques that are taught focus on individual approaches to assessment and
counseling. Furthermore training programs are mostly situated in either

medical or psychology faculties where academic allegiance to particle orientations is very strong. In terms of ongoing professional development, skills training options focus on individual counseling techniques, and professional conferences and symposia address particle approaches. Added to this, medical and psychology professional associations tend to operate around the understanding of clients as individuals and that their responsibilities are focused primarily at that level and not at the other levels of responsibility as discussed in Chapter 9. Taken together, these influences provide strong legitimacy for individualized approaches and provide very little encouragement for social perspectives.

Funding Strategies Discourage Involvement

Services often consider family inclusion as complicated & expensive

The rise of managed care and third-party payers has reshaped the health systems in many countries. One effect this has had is a move toward identifying unitized volume outputs as the benchmark for performance. This has meant that service funding has been increasingly determined by the number of clients seen, and a successful service is one that can maximize the volume of clients while minimizing the costs to the organization. In such a world the involvement of families is hard to justify. It is too expensive and too operationally complex to devote all the extra time and effort it takes to engage multiples of people; working with individuals is far more efficient. For instance, working with families might entail making several phone calls in order to find a time that suits everyone; the sessions will be longer and require larger offices with family-friendly features; and the practitioners will need training in working with families. In a unitized, volume-funded service, there are few incentives for undertaking these extra demands.

Services Are Expected to "Fix It"

A common expectation is that addiction services "fix" or "treat" addictions. This is an extraordinary expectation, and one that is very hard to substantiate.[5] The majority of people in addictive relationships remain addicted despite the best efforts of counseling services, and in the long term it is the addictive social systems, particularly intimates within the family, that bear the burden of care. Nonetheless, the public understandably continues to expect addiction services to have the answers and the cures for addictions. If people injure their legs, they go to the hospital and they are fixed; when people contract cancer, it may not always be cured, but the public can expect the best possible care. With addictions, specialists can intervene effectively, and the families can expect that services will administer the best available procedures. Families wonder why they need to be involved. Thus the importance and potency of social processes are overlooked.

Stigmatization

Addictive relationships are stigmatizing for all involved. They carry with them a sense of failure, guilt, and judgment. To become involved as a family member could be perceived as entering this morass or as a declaration of guilt. For example, a woman struggling with her partner's addictive relationship to alcohol has enough to contend with in maintaining her survival, but the idea that she might in some way be contributing to the problem would merely reinforce a growing sense of failure. Attending addiction services can be seen as admitting that in some way she is at least partly responsible for the addictive relationship.

Social Engagement

Practitioners should seek stronger social inclusion so as to prevent further social fragmentation of intimate relationships in the addictive system. Also, by working alongside other intimates, the practitioner validates the process of reintegration. This section discusses ways in which practitioners in particle-oriented services can incorporate a social perspective into their practice. The first subsection focuses on engaging environments, and the next two outline options in assessment and ways of working.

Team Culture

The openness of a practitioner team to embracing alternative forms of practice varies according to the culture and ethos that has emerged between team members over time. Practitioners wishing to take on a social approach may need first to look carefully at their team environment. Practitioners who seek to include families but are working in teams wedded uncritically to a particle paradigm are likely to experience problems with their colleagues. Their attempts at social inclusion are likely at best to be seen as somewhat strange or at worst obstructed because they are seen as unnecessary or inefficient.[6] They are certainly unlikely to shift the team's devotion to an individual focus. A more practical approach is either to work with families on one's own or to join up with others who are open to social perspectives. However, this practical response means that whatever is developed remains specific to the individuals involved, and as soon as they move on, hard-won family initiatives tend to dwindle and disappear.

Team culture may need to change before embracing social approaches

The main challenge for social approaches is that, for them to become a durable part of a service, they need commitment from a team as a whole. Treatment as normally delivered is a complex social event involving a number of paid employees interacting with one another and interacting with clients (who are embedded in another complex social event referred to here as the addictive system). These social involvements typically include interacting with receptionists, assessment counselors, and treatment counselors; attending meetings involving other family members; and having group contact with other clients and sometimes follow-up contacts and sessions. In residential programs, the social dimensions are even stronger and typically include more intense 24-hour interactions. Within this multilayered social environment of an addiction service, team philosophy and team culture play an important role. Before implementing a social approach, a service would need to look carefully at its team culture and determine whether work needs to be done in understanding and thinking about how they might incorporate a social approach. In most circumstances a considerable amount of training, observation, and mentoring may be required before a team forms a collective appreciation of its goals, and this appreciation is essential to ensure a positive and supportive response to the methods.

Maximizing the First Contact

The first time a family member makes contact with an addiction service is a critical moment in the social development of an addictive system. It marks the point at which a person in that system has moved beyond the circle of intimates and has sought contact with an independent resource that has the potential to threaten the addictive relationship. It is therefore a moment of trepidation for that person, who has learned from past experience that threats to the addictive relationship most likely lead to strong counterreactions. Often this first contact is by phone (other possibilities are by mail, email, or by an unarranged visit). In many services the contact is handled by receptionists, although in some services this contact is backed up by duty counselors or a triage team. Since at their first contact many family members may not know what to expect, what is said on that occasion can set the scene for much of what follows.

> **Cathy/Dion: First Contact**
>
> "Hello, my name is Cathy, and I'd like to make an appointment to talk to someone in your service."
>
> "Yes, certainly, we have a duty officer who could see you today."
>
> "Yes. Today would be fine."
>
> "One thing we ask is that you bring other people in your life to the first meeting. It is very important that they are involved."
>
> "That's… that's going to be a bit harder to arrange."
>
> "Our service is committed to involving other people because it is more likely to lead to lasting changes."
>
> "Oh, OK. I guess I could ask my son to come along as well. Would that be okay?"
>
> "Great, we'll set the time for…"

Consequently, it is critical in the first phone contact that the expectation of social inclusion be established. The way the initial phone contact is handled (whether by a volunteer, a receptionist, or a counselor) establishes the tone and expectations for future involvement. If the person is handled as an isolated individual—as a particle—this reinforces general public expectations of individualized care—as would be expected when going to an optometrist or a chiropractor. If setting the appointment is perceived as similar to going to a doctor or dentist, then one person attending alone is the likely outcome. If it is perceived more like a meeting such as attending a school interview, then coming with others is more probable. In the example in the inset box above, Cathy was initially seeking to attend by herself, but the service worker makes it clear that the service's usual practice is to involve others too, and with this prompt Cathy is easily persuaded to bring Dion to the first session.

The main problem with seeing individuals alone in the first session is that it tacitly states that it is the individual rather than the relationship that is important. Practice strategies based on seeing addictions as social events need to be actively pursued because by default most services revert to particle approaches. *Establishing* Furthermore, the moment the person establishes a relationship with someone *an individual* in a service, on the phone or in person, this sends a strong message to others *relationship* in the addictive system that the service delivery is focused on that one person, *at first* and that family involvement is unnecessary. The family members see a relation- *contact* ship forming that excludes them; whether they see this as desirable or not, it *signals* means that in any subsequent attempts to include them they will feel like awk- *exclusion of* ward outsiders and may express strong reluctance to getting involved. *others*

Several strategies can help promote greater involvement. One strategy involves developing a service policy that declares that clients would only be seen if they attend with other people in their lives. In other words, individuals would not be seen unless they found others to come with them. Such a policy could be included on signs, in advertisements, on service brochures, and on Web sites. For example, I observed services connected to Croatian/Italian clubs state to new clients that they could not proceed with assessment and intervention planning until they came together with others in their lives. For those in stronger addictive relationships where connection to others had been lost, the practitioners invited clients to attend their first session with someone in a local club, with the expectation that club members would facilitate involvement with the relevant clubs and thereby linking them back into community. Admittedly, the requirement for others to attend is a strong policy and one that would require strong commitment by a full team. A weaker alternative could involve stating the desirability of family attendance, but leaving it to the client to decide whether to bring somebody else. The downside to this approach is that since arranging for other people to attend involves more effort, the majority of clients are likely to opt to come alone, therapy setting the precedent for ongoing individual contact.

Responding to Safety Issues

Another issue that needs to be carefully considered in taking on a social approach is whether wider involvements might place people in situations that put them physically, psychologically, or socially at risk. These risks include the possibility of prompting further physical, sexual or emotional abuse, the possibility of suicide and other self-harm, and the possibility of hostile retributions after sessions. The worrying potential of many of these risks is shared by approaches based in both particle and social paradigms, and the standard protocols for risk assessment should automatically come into play.[7] Nonetheless, there are some dimensions of risk that may be unfamiliar to practitioners who normally operate within a particle orientation. In particular, family sessions can themselves create opportunities for controlling tactics and counterreactions such as subtle disparagement, intimidation, and misrepresentations. They can provide further occasions for dominant members to claim ownership of or appropriate the experience of other members, and use the event as a means of controlling their thinking and feelings.[8] Accordingly, practitioners need to maintain vigilance regarding the way language is being used in sessions and to monitor the effects conversations are having on those attending. For example, during the phone conversation in the inset box above, Joan is asked to bring Bert to the first session. At this stage she is unprepared to state that she is being beaten regularly by Bert and she knows he will punish her severely for seeking outside help. The counselor, sensitive to this possibility, notices her hesitancy and responds by suggesting that he might be brought later. This enables further exploration of potential safety issues during the first session.

Bert/Joan: Safety

Joan has finally reached a point where she is seeking help from an addiction service. During her initial phone call the service's duty counselor states:

"Our service seeks as much as possible to include other family members. Would it be possible for your husband to also attend?"

"Ah... I could ask him... I really wouldn't know how he'd react..."

"Are you fearful of how he might react?"

"Um... I guess I am. He does have strong views, and he won't like this sort of thing."

"Sounds like at this stage it would be better to not include him. Are there other people you would like to attend?"

"I hadn't thought about that, but now you mention it, I am really worried about my two children."

"We would be really pleased to include them in the meeting."

"Yes, yes. It would be good for them to come, but I'll check it with them first."

Despite efforts to avoid joint sessions with people actively abusing intimates, such family members who are actively violent to others in that system are still likely to end up entering a service. During the course of an initial session a variety of strategies can be employed to protect those attending from tactics aimed at controlling or appropriating other's experience. A routine strategy could involve carefully checking the reality of each person who attends and ensuring that he or she is relating his or her experience in his or her own words and without indications of fearfulness or reprocessing by others present. In situations where one person appears evasive and hesitant, then the practitioner could check what is going on by conferring briefly with each person alone, arranging separate sessions, or speaking confidentially by phone to the hesitant person after the session. It is possible that the person is being punished for what he or she said or might say during sessions, or that the family member feels rushed beyond where he or she is comfortable in going in terms of collective action. Whatever the effects, the practitioner needs to proceed cautiously and with awareness that what happens and is discussed in sessions does not always match what is going on in the home.

Preparing the Environment

For many families, common particle understandings of addictions and past experiences of health service environments already prompt a reluctance to be involved. Consequently family members will be strongly sensitized to aspects in the environment that imply their presence is unnecessary. For this reason family inclusive service environments need to be designed in ways that convey a strong welcome to families.

Family inclusive service environments convey a strong welcome to families

Venue Design

Most addiction services are denied the luxury of designing their own venue and tend to have moved into buildings that were originally designed for other purposes, such as hospital clinics, offices, or homes. If services do have the opportunity to influence the design, then they have the opportunity to plan for a large reception and waiting area, with separated spaces where families can sit and wait comfortably with each other, and session rooms with ample space to accommodate large families. Rooms adjacent to the reception area could include a playroom for children, and feeding and changing rooms for babies. Easy access by public transportation and parking areas for those who drive are also important considerations. For services that are adapting older buildings, larger waiting and playing areas can also be created with innovative changes to existing reception and adjacent room spaces.

Room Layout

Ideally, meeting rooms should be large enough to accommodate five or more people, have chairs that allow flexible seating arrangements, and have spaces where children could play or draw. Including child-size table and chairs, toys, and drawing paper will increase the comfort and involvement of children. Since the offices in many service settings are too small for these types of meetings, group rooms or meeting rooms can be adapted to provide an appropriate space, but this will require some planning around issues regarding room arrangements and room bookings.

Timing

Arranging meetings with couples or families is more complex than arranging individual sessions. Working people may find it difficult to take time off during the day. This becomes even more complicated with the inclusion of broader networks of people, such as employers, work colleagues, physicians, and other involved parties. Staff members in socially inclusive services would need to be highly flexible in their working hours, so that meetings could be held outside normal office hours, either in the evenings or on weekends. Also, in working with groups, determining each person's context and negotiating collective action take longer than the standard 1-hour session.

Social Assessment

Social assessment is a vital part of working with addictive relationships. However, service settings with predominantly a particle paradigm orientation relegate social concerns to supplementary roles. Relationships are brought into the picture only when it looks like they will interfere with particle treatment methods (such as compliance with medication or retention in counseling). Despite this secondary interest, social assessment could operate alongside other particle-based assessments as a form of assessment in its own right and it could contribute to intervention planning in a cooperative manner (in the manner of the double helix as described in the next chapter). Social assessment has its own goals and data collection methods. If handled as an independent process, its conclusions are likely to shed a different—but often complementary—light on how services might proceed. The following discussion describes how practitioners can provide a social assessment.

Social assessment provides different but complementary information to particle assessment

Assessment Goals

A social assessment focuses primarily on the way in which the person in the addictive relationship connects into the addictive social system. The assessment pivots around three primary questions:

- What is the extent of fragmentation experienced by intimates?
- What is the strength of the addictive relationship?
- What are the capacities within the addictive social system for a reintegration?

The first question seeks to ascertain the resources in the addictive social system for collective action. The second question has a bearing on the pace at which collective action and a reintegration are planned. The third question determines which relationships becomes the focus for the reintegration.

Participation of Intimates

Ideally social assessment involves participation of both the person in the addictive relationship and the person's intimates. Involvement of the intimates is critical to understanding the structure and processes in the addictive social system, and to planning and implementing a reintegration. If at all possible, all parties should be present at all assessment sessions and everyone's views and judgment should be sought. In reality and despite best efforts, having all parties present is not always possible either because the addictive relationship is so advanced that the intimates are no longer connected or because the person in the addictive relationship or other intimates are unwilling to attend.

In situations where the person in the addictive relationship is not present, the strength of the addictive relationship can only be indirectly assessed, and attention is focused more on levels of experienced fragmentation and opportunities for collective action. When the intimates are not present, the strengths in the addictive social system can only be guessed at, and obtaining information for planning of a reintegration may require other strategies, such as phone conversations or contacts through nonintimates such as key extended family members, physicians, or employers. One approach that might increase the likelihood for all parties to attend is to arrange meetings in outside neutral and less clinical settings such as in the home or in local settings such as a community center.

Dimensions of Strength

As discussed throughout this book, the severity and strength of an addictive relationship can be assessed by examining the degree of symmetry and the degree of multiplicity of the addicted person's other relationships. The more asymmetrical these relationships, particularly with intimates, the more entrenched the intimacy management strategies. The stronger the unitary focus around the addictive substance/process, the stronger the commitment and the more likely for other connections to have deteriorated and fragmented. Accordingly, questions aimed at assessing asymmetry and unitary focus can give some idea of how large a task it is going to be to mount a reintegration.

Asymmetry & lack of multiplicity are indicators for the strength of an addictive relationship

The inset box provides a checklist of the types of queries that elicit information regarding the extent of asymmetry in relationships. Responses to each of the questions can be provided by both the person in the addictive relationship and by other intimates. As explored in Chapters 5 and 6, the focus here is on ascertaining the strength of the strands of intimacy (closeness, compassion, commitment, and accord). For example, strong asymmetry

---

Asymmetry Checklist
- Does the person express compassion toward other intimates? (yes = low asymmetry)
- Does the person spend meaningful time with other intimates? (yes = low)
- Is the commitment to each relationship matched by both parties? (yes = low)
- Are there events occurring that signal low commitment to intimate relationships (e.g., unfaithfulness, betrayal, unreliability)? (yes = high)
- Is the accord expressed by intimates reciprocated by the person in the addictive relationship? (yes = low)
- Is violence (physical, sexual, or emotional) occurring toward intimates? (yes = high)

would be indicated when parents express strong devotion to and accord with their daughter who is in an addictive relationship to morphine, but the daughter communicates little regard for her parents.

The questions in the next inset box provide guidance to checking the extent to which the addictive relationship has come to dominate the social system. It assumes that the fewer significant other relationships occurring in the system, the more likely the addictive relationship has become the central axis around which other relationships play secondary roles. Correspondingly, the more significant relationships the person has with people or activities unrelated to the addictive relationship, the weaker its strength. Furthermore, the more strength and variety of other involvements, the greater the opportunities to mount a reintegration. For example, people heavily involved in sports activities that have nothing to do with their addictive relationships have an alternative base for connectedness, and this may later play a critical role in their reintegration.

> **Unitary Focus Checklist**
> - Do friends, family, and other associates play important roles in protecting the addictive relationship? (yes = high focus)
> - Are there key people still connected but unrelated to the addictive relationship? (yes = low)
> - Is much available time devoted to acquiring and consuming the addictive substance/process? (yes = high)
> - Are there activities not associated with the addictive substance/process? (yes = low)

Topic Domain Reviews

A topic domain review seeks information to help assess the capacities within the addictive social system to mount a reintegration. Chapter 10 introduced five domains of connectedness with which to reform multiple and symmetrical relationships. Examples of cue questions that could be asked in each topic domain are listed in the inset box below. The following discussion summarizes the content that might be sought in each domain.

Intimate Connectedness

Questions here seek to determine where on the various layers of social connectedness the points of intimate connectedness are still occurring. The first layer of potential intimacy occurs in the immediate family. Which family members remain connected? What is the quality of these relationships? How might they be involved? The second layer concerns relationships with very close friends and colleagues. How important are they to the person? What roles do they play within the social system? The third layer relates to intimacy links into the broader neighborhood and community. Key people with mentoring and supporting roles may have connections but are not members of the immediate family or close friends. For example, a young man might identify an uncle or a professional such as a teacher or a coach as playing an important role in his life.

Occupational Connectedness

People's occupational involvements play a critical role in constructing their social identity and in determining the manner of their involvement with their social environment. *Occupation* refers not only to paid employment but also to activities outside employment such as home management, hobbies and interests, daily routines (such as modes of eating and traveling, entertainment choices), and major events (such as celebrations and cultural ceremonies). The details help piece together a picture of how time is used and the key points of connectedness that occur throughout the day.

Topic Domain Cue Questions

Intimate connectedness:
- *Which people do you feel closest to in your life?*
- *How are these relationships going?*
- *Who do you think you can talk to about your experiences?*

Occupational connectedness:
- *What activities are you involved in most days?*
- *How meaningful to you are these activities?*
- *What sort of relationship do you have with your employer?*

Physical connectedness:
- *When do you feel in touch or out of touch with your body?*
- *What is happening when you feel stressed out?*
- *What are you doing to keep fit and healthy?*

Communal connectedness:
- *Which circles of friends, colleagues, and neighbors do you connect with most days?*
- *How many of these are unrelated to the addictive relationship?*
- *Which health and community professionals do you see?*

Inner connectedness:
- *Are there inner spaces that help you in times of trouble?*
- *What keeps you going when things get rough?*
- *Do you have moments of linking to a power greater than yourself?*

Physical Connectedness

Physical connectedness is associated with the physicality of the body and the space it occupies. The social meaning of the body and its position in space is an area that is attracting attention in the social sciences[9] and is increasingly seen as an important factor contributing to a person's stance on life in general. When people dislike their body and treat it as an obstacle or something to be controlled, this can limit their options for social integration. For example, people who neglect their body by not attending to health care, gaining excessive weight, and living stressful lives are likely to experience overwhelmingly negative interactions with their body that discourage them from other involvements such as exercise and socializing. Furthermore, physical connectedness can often play an important role in other opportunities. For example, joining a squash club to improve fitness may lead to getting to know other players, linking a person with other activities, and gradually building up opportunities for friendships that may evolve into intimate friendships.

Communal Connectedness

Communal connectedness refers to the broader, nonintimate, links to other layers of family, friends, neighbors, work colleagues, and community.

This form of connectedness provides the substance from which a person's global sense of communal identity is constructed. Although not as intense as the smaller circle of intimates, collectively it has strong significance because contacts are more variable and they occur more often. Inquiry here focuses on the frequency, quantity, and extended episodes of exposure people have to these relationships. How often do they socialize in broader circles? Do they socialize with people unrelated to their addictive substance/process? What understanding do these broader circles have of addictive relationships? Communal connectedness is important in planning the first stages of reintegration, particularly for people in strongly fragmented social systems where intimacies are problematic or nonexistent.

Communal connected-ness often provides the initial resource for reintegration

Inner Connectedness

The domain of inner emotional and spiritual connectedness for most people contributes positively to their sense of involvement in the world and can play a pivotal role in the first few years of a reintegration. However, talk of spiritual connectedness may not suit everyone, and the language conventions used to express it varies significantly according to spiritual and cultural perspectives.[10] A safer form of inquiry would adopt a more neutral starting point by focusing not on the source but on the effects of this domain of connectedness: effects such as inner strength, fortitude in difficult times, and coping strategies. Accordingly, the types of questions asked might include: Are there inner psychological spaces to which a person goes when things go bad? What inner resources have helped in keeping a person afloat in the past? Has the person had moments where he or she sensed some inner source of strength? Twelve-step programs identify inner connectedness as providing the backbone to a reintegration (recovery) process.

Assessment Process

The process of conducting a social assessment needs to incorporate interviewing techniques that enable flexibility, while at the same time remaining focused on the three primary questions driving the assessment. The diagram in the inset box provides a guide for how to sequence the parts of a social assessment while at the same time remaining flexible and responsive to the issues as they arise. The approach assumes the practitioner has well-developed interviewing skills and is competent in avoiding an interrogatory style. The recommended sequence begins with openers onto one domain and then moves flexibly through each domain at a surface level, transitioning from time to time to explore relevant domains in more depth.

Openers

In a social assessment the interviewer (represented as an eye in the diagram) begins the session with a nonthreatening preface ("Thank you for coming today") and then perhaps circles around addressing each person present in the room, making a connection and asking about nonthreatening topics in their lives (sports, school, jobs). This initial round establishes the speaking rights of all those present and establishes whether they are in agreement or were forced into attending. For those who feel coerced to come, their unwillingness needs to be acknowledged before moving on.

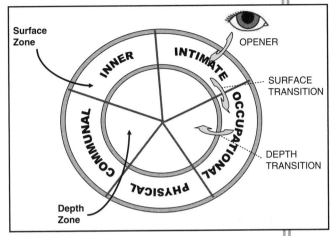

Figure 13.2 Interview question domains

Surface Zone

The next phase of the social assessment determines the surface zone for each of the five topic sectors, forming a general picture of social connections and gauging where those present have the energy to speak more fully. Early in the session those attending may only feel comfortable talking in the communal domain about their involvement with the neighborhood or their school. As they feel more comfortable, they become more willing to discuss other topic domains such as occupational and physical involvements. It may take longer for them to warm up to discussion of intimate and inner connectedness.

Surface Transitions

Surface transitions enable the interview to progress across the surface zone, thereby gaining an overview of the person's current social circumstances. The first major topic transition in an interview is critical. Those attending may have engaged in discussion on these first issues because they seem most pressing and accordingly they may not initially wish to move away from them. The sequenced use of standard interviewing skills can help make the transitions appear smooth and natural. For example, an effective sequence for the first major transition could begin with the use of a validation ("What you are saying is important and we need to talk about it more...")

followed by an explanation ("...but for me to understand what is going on I need to ask you something about how you are getting on at home") finishing by asking permission ("Is it okay with all of you if we talk about the family relationships?"). The validation reduces the chance that clients will perceive the transition as dismissing what is currently being discussed; the explanation provides a reason for the transition, and asking permission, though rhetorical and unlikely to prompt a response, conveys receptiveness to clients influencing the direction of the interview.

Depth Zone

Depth transitions are important in ascertaining levels of asymmetry and unitary focus in the addictive system. The interviewer may decide to concentrate on one topic sector either because it holds most relevance to the current situation or because those present appear to have the most energy for discussing it. For some interviews, where there is a high level of rapport, a depth transition could occur early on. Where the assessment relationship takes longer to establish, the interviewer could make several surface transitions, moving across several sectors, looking carefully at which depth transition would be most productive and where the client appears to have most energy, but only exploring them at depth when clients appear ready to do so.

Depth Transitions

Passive listening skills facilitate depth transitions

Depth transitions move into material that is more intimate and emotionally charged than surface content. In the beginning, the interviewer is unlikely to know where these critical issues will emerge. They may involve events that happened long ago; they may involve feelings regarding resentment, neglect, abandonment, and injustice; or they may relate to a major crisis that is currently occurring (such as separation or abuse). Some family members may be unaware of the events or the feelings associated with them. To open these discussions, the practitioner relies heavily on the guidance and energy of the family members. The skill set required focuses mainly on passive listening skills such as reflection, paraphrasing, validation, and the use of silence, while at the same time managing the boundaries and turn-taking within the session so each person attending has an opportunity to safely express a perspective on the issues.

Genograms

Genograms are an effective way to explore both the strength of the addictive relationships and capacities within the addictive social system. A genogram maps out a person's connections to different intimates along with wider connections to friends and family (see the end of Chapter 1). They are a valuable way of exploring several of the topic sectors at once, but they are particularly helpful in fleshing out the current configuration of intimacies. They work best if they are displayed so that all present can see them and contribute to their construction. This can be done by drawing the genogram on a large sheet of paper or on a blackboard or by mapping them out with objects in the room.

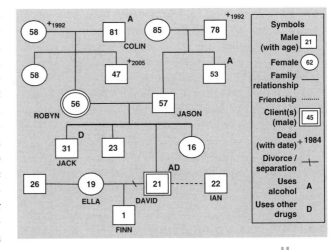

Figure 13.3 Example of a client genogram

The inset box is an example of a genogram. As can be seen it provides an easily accessed and visual way of recording a large amount of relational information. In this system David is in an addictive relationship to alcohol and other drugs. He attends the session with his mother, Robyn, during which they constructed this genogram together. David had separated 9 months earlier from Ella, who is now in a new relationship and caring for their son. His drug use had deteriorated since the separation, and he is now rooming with his friend Ian. It has been a difficult time for his mother. Her younger brother had recently died in a car accident and previous struggles with her eldest son Jack's problems with amphetamine use and her memories of growing up with her father's addictive relationship to alcohol led her into worrying desperately that her son was going to have similar problems. In addition to the information displayed here, other relevant layers (such as key friends and key activities) can be added. The identification of addictive relationships elsewhere in the system is important not only in understanding origins but also in helping to locate potential spots of expertise within the system that might be engaged in assisting with change. All this information can be recorded quickly and the genogram can function as a schema for all future efforts.

Reintegration Plans

The outcome of the social assessment is a reintegration plan. Such a plan determines the strengths and capacities within the social system and sets up a framework for achievable steps in a process of social reintegration. The primary input here for an addiction practitioner is in helping participants achieve a realistic balance between accounting for the strength of the addictive relationship and taking on identified opportunities for change. The focus for planning is driven by two key considerations: First, the "case" or "client" at issue does not refer to the person in the addictive relationship or other associated (particular) people; the "case" at all times refers to the addictive system (whether multiples of people are involved or not). Second, the goals in the plan are not imposed from the judgment of the practitioner; goals throughout are negotiated outcomes that emerge from the input of all those who participate (including the practitioner).

A reintegration plan aims to break the process into clear and manageable steps. This requires drawing a timeline. The plan could be broken down into as many steps as people feel is necessary, but the plan should at a minimum involve descriptions of the agreed-on current concerns, and short- and long-term objectives.

In a reintegration plan the "case" is not the individual but the addictive system

Current Concerns

Members of the addictive system, in most cases family members, need to form a consensus about the key concerns that are affecting them within each topic domain. These concerns are identified primarily on the basis of their ability to block or impede the various forms of connectedness. The initial discussions may focus on individual needs, but as these are identified, the practitioner can help guide family members to talk these through in terms of how they affect the family system as a whole.

Short-Term Objectives

Short-term objectives target improvements in connectedness that are either readily accessible or critical for future reintegration opportunities. For example, the first attempted reconnection may focus more on links between family members and not on those with the person in the addictive relationship. Improvements in broader family connectedness may be required before a safe and well-managed grouping is capable of competing with the addictive relationship. Care needs to be taken to ensure that the short-term objectives are clear and specific enough to gauge whether they are being achieved, and they should be sequenced in achievable steps where probable success encourages further progressions.

Long-Term Objectives

While the pathway to reintegration is long and likely to involve numerous setbacks, the process still needs to be shaped by where people believe it will take them in the end. The setting of long-term objectives enables opportunities for those involved to reach some consensus on where they understand their efforts will ultimately lead.

Two Case Examples

The development of goals in an integration plan will be illustrated with two of the family systems that end up coming to a service, namely Cathy/Dion and Bert/Joan.

Cathy/Dion

Dion wants to travel overseas with his partner, Lisa, but he is worried about leaving his stepsister Shannon in Cathy's care while she continues to pursue her disorderly lifestyle associated with her addictive relationship to heroin. Cathy too is increasingly dissatisfied with her lifestyle. Heroin probably killed her partner, Robert, and several of her other friends had suffered serious overdoses and blood infections. She has grown tired of the endless cycle of scoring, trouble, and criminal involvements, and is thinking of ways she might disconnect from her drug networks. Importantly, for the first time she is seriously considering switching to methadone not just as a means of responding to a crisis or filling in when drugs are scarce but as a means of giving her space to establish a new life. She has made contact with a local drug treatment service that has arranged for her and Dion to attend sessions for a full drug assessment. As part of this assessment, the practitioner conducts a

Reintegration Goals for Cathy/Dion

Sectors	Current	Short Term	Long Term
Intimate	Low levels of closeness between all family members	Cathy and the children to share discussion and activities on a more regular basis.	They increase their closeness and commitment as the addictive relationship weakens
Occupational	Cathy has no qualifications and only ever worked casually	The family supports Cathy in studying cooking at the local polytechnic.	Cathy enters a new career as a restaurant chef.
Physical	Cathy sees herself as poorly groomed, unfit, and unattractive.	Cathy and Dion take an interest in their grooming and undertake regular exercise	Cathy takes up a regular sporting activity
Communal	Both Cathy and Dion have few outside friends and interests	Cathy joins a local book club and helps Dion plan his travels.	They establish a circle of friends maintained by regular dinners and outings
Inner	Cathy has lost any sense of emotional or spiritual connectedness	Cathy puts aside time for reading self-help and spiritual books	The family supports Cathy in instituting regular time out to attend to her inner needs

social assessment that identified the stepped goals as summarized in the inset box above.

During the subsequent months Cathy stabilizes her intake of methadone and finds herself slowly disengaging from her drug networks. This provides her with more time to focus on reconnecting with her children and planning her future. While she struggles at times, with Dion and Lisa's encouragement she enrolls in school and gets a part-time job working in a restaurant. Over the course of the next 3 years, as her connectedness to her family and her neighborhood strengthen, she begins to consider a stepped withdrawal from her methadone use.

Bert/Joan

Bert's addictive relationship to alcohol had continued without reprieve. He was resorting more and more to violence and other controlling strategies to manage his family, particularly Joan. She presented more frequently to her family doctor with injuries inflicted by Bert, and following a more serious beating than previously, which involved broken ribs, her doctor convinced her to seek specialist help. She made contact with her local alcohol and other drug service and attended two sessions with her two teenage children, Donald and Fiona. The inset box summarizes the reintegration goals agreed on during the sessions.

During the sessions with her children, to her surprise Joan discovers that Donald and Fiona were already comfortable discussing Bert's drinking; she is the one who needed to catch up. As they shared more in sessions, she begins to feel less overwhelmed and starts to consider her own needs for a change. She experiences some difficulties

Reintegration Goals Joan, Donald and Fiona			
Sectors	Current	Short Term	Long Term
Intimate	Bert's abuse has left little room for closeness and compassion within the home	Joan and the children talk through their experiences and feelings about the abuse	Joan and the children decide whether they are going to continue to live with Bert
Occupational	The family has very little savings and Joan is struggling in her work as a teacher	Joan assesses their financial position, starts her own savings account and works at reducing stress at work	Joan works towards financial control and self-sufficiency separate from Bert.
Physical	Joan feels flattened and overwhelmed by what is happening and is neglecting her health	Joan plans time for herself, takes up golf again, and attends a women's support group	Joan is physically and mentally strong enough to participate in collective action
Communal	Joan and her children feel isolated and disconnected	They all begin pursuing interests and hobbies outside the home	The family build friendships in their local community
Inner	Joan feels her life has little purpose or direction	Joan spends more time with an old friend talking through where she is heading	Joan feels more strongly grounded in herself and more prepared for collective action

dealing with the negative feelings the children expresses toward her, but she slowly begins to understand it from their perspective. As she pursues her reintegration goals she finds her connections with her children and friends improving, but she does not feel confident about a collective action with Bert. As her involvements multiply, Bert's drinking and abuse get worse. She begins discussing with the children and with friends whether it is realistic to challenge Bert's addictive relationship, but because of her fear and his unrelenting drunkenness she concludes that mounting a meaningful challenge would be impractical (and perhaps dangerous). In her heart she knows she now faces the decision of whether or not to separate. With the children's support she plans a careful departure: using the money she has saved she finds an apartment for her and the children in a place kept secret from Bert; she discusses potential counterreactions with the children's teachers at school as well as with her family doctor and the police; and with her counselor's guidance she develops a safety plan with clear responses to anticipated risks.

When it comes time to leave she finds the process difficult and scary. Bert reacts strongly to her absence by interrogating friends, by destroying things belonging to her that remained in the house, and by phoning family members to verbally abuse them. At times she feels overwhelmed and contemplates returning, but collectively her family and friends help her stand firm and, somewhat shakily, she begins her long process of reintegration into a world without Bert and without his addictive relationship to alcohol.

Facilitative Meetings

In a social paradigm, rather than seeing the expertise of the practitioner as the primary source of wisdom and guidance for change, expertise is seen as emerging from within the social environment itself. Addiction practitioners can contribute to this process as long as they recognize that their role is to facilitate opportunities for reconnection rather than generating the solutions.

Practitioners contribute by facilitating reconnection but avoid imposing solutions

Practitioner Abilities

Social inclusive practice is not the same as family therapy. While family therapy shares a focus on relationships and systems, the application of its methods tends to operate in a particle frame, with the particle expanded to a family (see the discussion of family therapy in Chapter 11). In traditional family therapy the social system becomes something that is worked on, something that is observed, analyzed, and to some extent managed. For example, I was taught over many years in techniques involving co-therapists and observation rooms behind one-way mirrors to analyze the structure and interactional processes of a family and to look for opportunities to rechannel processes and perhaps shift unproductive alliances. Working within a social orientation is different. It views the practitioner as entering into the social system as a participant working to facilitate the family's own process, with the expectation that wisdom will emerge in a negotiated fashion from the experience and understanding of people present within the system. Taking up the role of an expert—a person who has the answers—instantly changed the dynamics of the interaction. Attention swings away from capacities within the family and focuses on what the relationship with the practitioner has to offer. The practitioner is thereby unable to continue in the role of a social facilitator. To maintain this role, practitioners need to actively reinforce that they do not have the answers, that responses can vary, and that the appropriate response will emerge from the collective group.

Meetings with Many People

The most direct and effective way for practitioners to develop their facilitatory abilities in social approaches is through participation in meetings with several people from an addictive system. At first practitioners who have worked primarily with individual clients may perhaps find it somewhat disconcerting to have more people present in the room; conversations are less easily directed and conflicts can erupt at any point. Over time the complexities of meeting with many people at once get easier and the advantages soon become obvious: intimates can provide radically different perspectives on an issue, they often come up with different ideas, and their participation is more likely to lead to enduring change. These meeting can happen in a variety of ways depending on the service setting, and the following subsections briefly discuss three common variants.

Facilitating meetings with multiple people becomes easier with practice

Meetings with Couples

Often the pivotal intimacy in an addictive system is that between spouses; consequently, the task of running a meeting with couples involves establishing a set of common understandings. It is critical in these meetings for all attending to appreciate that the spouse is not there primarily to support changes for the person in the addictive relationship but rather to enable the focus on relationships—both the addictive relationship and its interactions with the marital relationship. The focus varies according to the stage each partner is at on the twin cycles of fragmentation and crisis. For example, the intimate may be attending sessions as part of an initial attempt at collective action, or may be already well engaged into the process of reintegration.

Meetings with Families

Family meetings are more complex than meeting with individuals or couples; they take more time to arrange, they typically last longer, and they involve more complex assessment and planning processes. However, as discussed in Chapters 6 and 11, family sessions are worth the effort in that they are more likely to address the issues of all those affected and to engage the whole system in a pathway for change. In facilitating meetings with three or more clients, it helps to involve another colleague particularly in managing the meetings

> **Beginning a family meeting**
> - *Ensure all present have had early opportunities to speak:* talk briefly with each person in turn, connect on minor aspects such as school location, neighborhood characteristics
> - *Discuss some meeting boundaries:* people can leave when they wish, allow others to finish what they are saying, no abuse or put downs
> - *Acknowledge different reasons for coming:* "Some of you may not have wanted to be here"
> - *Explain the social orientation:* "What matters here is how you interact as a family"; "It is the quality of your relationships that will matter in the long run"
> - *Clarify facilitatory role:* "I don't have the answers"; "My task is to help you work things through in your own way"

and attending to the needs of all those present. One facilitator is then freed up to attend primarily to managing the session while the other can focus on responses to issues as they arise. The first meeting usually sets out to ensure each person is adequately engaged in ways as outlined in the inset box above. Once these processes are complete, social assessment can proceed in a similar way as described in previous sections. The presence of more people from the family system ensures the goals identified in the session are both more realistic and more inclusive of wider needs.

Community Meetings

The service practitioner can also facilitate opportunities for engaging other people from the layers of neighborhood and community. Such meetings might bring in other people in the broader network who may play a role in the reintegration process. For instance, an employer or a physician could attend meetings with intimates to assist in their planning for collective action.

Multiple Family Groups

Another common and useful strategy for a service to explore are multiple family groups. These typically involve weekly evening meetings with six to ten families together for 2 to 3 hours in a large meeting room. Such meetings form the basis of the Croatian/Italian club approach; they are also often used to connect families to residential rehabilitation programs, and they can function as a strong adjunct to community outpatient addiction services.

Meetings typically begin with tea and coffee and people talking informally with one another. When all participants have arrived and have settled down, the meeting proper begins with a reporting-in round during which issues for particular families begin to surface. The facilitator might then invite one of these families to explore relationship issues in more detail. Other families are likely to connect with many of the issues that one family explores, and members of other families contribute with common identifications and alternative strategies. Multiple family groups are particularly strong in equipping families with different perspectives on common issues. Single-family sessions miss out on this wealth of multiple perspectives and risk the narrower views of past approaches or limiting options to the practitioner's perspectives.

One-to-One Sessions

Practitioners may not always work in contexts where their team or the broader service accepts the importance of social inclusion. This will limit the opportunities for meeting in groups. Furthermore, for reasons such as a history of abuse, transportation issues, and lost contact, it may prove impractical to meet with groups. Although in social terms, meeting one-to-one has less social facilitation potential, there is still a range of activities in a meeting that could contribute to implementing reintegration as long as practitioners maintain a focus on relationships and not on individuals. The following subsections describe three techniques than can shift the orientation in one-to-one meetings from particles to social issues.

Empty Chairs

Working with empty chairs provides a handy way in one-to-one sessions to bring into the room a person's social involvements. Clients are invited to use their imagination to place a key intimate in the empty chair. This could be done by first asking for a description of the person sitting there, or by asking clients to describe what they would say and how they would act in the relationship. Alternatively, clients can leave their own chair and take on the role of this other person, with the practitioner asking them to swap chairs back and forth between themselves and the other person, thereby acting out a typical interchange. The technique can

---

Cathy/Dion: Empty chairs

In a session in which Dion was unable to attend, the practitioner establishes an empty chair to represent his presence:

"Okay, now we have your son, Dion, in that chair and heroin sitting in that chair. What would Dion want to say to the heroin?"

"Umm. He doesn't say anything to it. He says it all to me. He says 'heroin takes you away every evening, you love your heroin more than me, and when you're out if it you're really disgusting'... I feel stuck between two squabbling children."

"So, what does heroin say to you?"

"It just says, 'ignore him, he doesn't understand; he's always at you; he wants you to have no fun and lose all your friends.' Things like that."

"So... What do you want to do?"

"I want to keep going with both heroin and Dion, but it's so tiring attending to both. They constantly fight; Dion wants me to talk and connect, heroin wants me to get out of it..." Cathy is quiet for a moment.

"He must find it hard too."

"I guess. He can't really control what I do with my drugs. All he can do is try to work on me and make me feel bad."

be adapted in a variety of ways. For example, one empty chair could be allocated to the addictive substance/process, thereby depicting the addictive relationship. Other empty chairs can be added to represent other relationships. During the session the insert box above, Dion was absent, which gave the practitioner a chance to explore Cathy's perceptions of their relationship using empty chairs.

Picture Work

Pictorial depictions of relationships can assist a client in seeing the interactional nature of an addictive social system and in exploring projected consequences of changes. The practitioner invites clients (including the children) to make use of colored pens and large pieces of paper to create drawings that identify intimates and characterize their interconnections. Alternative materials could include blackboards or even objects in the room (chairs, pillows, pens). The closeness of objects could depict the strength of an intimacy, and colors, arrows, and pictures could depict qualities in the relationship (fear, unpredictability, compassion). Clients are then asked to explore changes to arrangements and to draw in what they anticipate would be obstacles and facilitators to such changes.

Relationship Homework

Practitioners typically set goals with the expectation that the agreed-on "homework" activities will be done. Relationship homework focuses specifically on tasks associated with the strength of intimacies and changes in connectedness. Accordingly, sessions function as reporting-in meetings on what happens outside sessions. The meetings themselves then become viewed as secondary events, where obstacles and progress in the real job of relationship building are discussed and changes planned as required. Typical activities could include establishing routines for talking and sharing each evening, taking 10-minute turns at listening without interrupting the other speaker, writing down issues in an open journal that then provides an agenda for evening discussions, and communicating in special formats such as "I feel __ because __ and I would like __."

Meetings provide an opportunity to "report in" on relationship work that is happening at home

Enhancing Network Capacity

An alternative way for practitioners to enhance reintegration is by working with the whole social environment in which the addictive relationship is occurring. This would involve moving out from office settings and linking

Community into neighborhoods and communities and working on projects that improve
oriented the infrastructures that lead to socially enriched environments into which
services are reintegrating families can connect. This could involve allocating a proportion
active in of the practitioner's time to projects that develop supportive networks, or
fostering alternatively employing people who focus specifically on social development
opportunities projects. Here are some examples of projects:
for
reintegration

Volunteer Networks

Volunteer networks are used to assist families with a variety of challenges
to health and well-being. Networks of volunteers form the basis for both the
club and twelve-step movements. But these types of networks do not suit
everyone, and an addiction service could provide a focal point for other types
of networks linking current with past clients, families with other families or
simply providing a place and support for groupings to meet (see the description of forming volunteer networks in Chapter 12).

Community Liaison

Practitioners and their services do not operate in isolation; they invariably
are positioned in a community and are responding to the needs of specific
populations. The nature of the communities might vary: for some (particularly in rural communities) the community might be a neighborhood or provincial town; for others it might be a suburb or an urban region; for others
it might be an institution such as a hospital or a workplace. Practitioners and
collections of practitioners can therefore be seen as positioned to play an
active role in setting up the types of linkages and support networks that
could both assist intimates in collective action and help family systems in
pursuing reintegration. To fulfill this role, services need to develop a visible
presence in their communities, and practitioners need to participate in helping the community improve its capacity in responding to addictive relationships in its midst. The resources practitioners provide could include logistic
support (a place to meet, stationery and printing), advice (access to knowledge and links to what is going on elsewhere), and assistance with those who
are ready for collective action or reintegration.

Occupational Supports

Another networking possibility is through practitioners helping workplaces develop their responsiveness to families affected by addictive relationships. For example, systems of training and referral could be established
through employee well-being programs that assist in identifying people at

risk and linking them into appropriate services and support networks. These networks could also play a crucial role in reestablishing occupational connectedness during a reintegration.

Telecommunication Opportunities

These opportunities have mainly been exploited in the particle- and expert-oriented forms of delivery. For example, telephone help lines are often available to provide advice and counseling to individuals. With the emergence of new telecommunication and Internet technologies, a number of possibilities could be developed to link multiples of people. For example, an emerging network of families might extend their support to other families through the use of an Internet site or an Internet chat room. Once relationships are established, contact could be reinforced using text messaging (see inset box).

> **Telecommunication Options**
> - *Telephone conferencing*: a way of connecting people who otherwise could not make meetings (e.g., physicians, distant relatives) or to conduct distant meetings for a whole family
> - *Text messaging*: distribution lists could be used for simple daily messaging with reminders of agreed strategies
> - *Internet chat rooms*: also could be used to connect people within families or to connect between families
> - *Web sites, blogs, and list serves*: could also assist in connecting and providing a base for sharing experiences

While the primary focus of this book is on the social potential in families and communities, this chapter has endeavored to highlight some of the potential for addiction practitioners to participate in supporting collective action with addictive relationships. The brief overview provided by this chapter admittedly does little justice to what is a large topic in its own right. Since few other socially oriented guides for practitioners are available, I hope to develop this material in more detail in a future book.

Chapter

Looking Ahea

> *"Possession" they call it.... Sometimes an entity jumps in the body—outlines*
> *waver in orange jelly.... As if I was usually there but subject to goof now and*
> *again.... Wrong! I am never here.... Never that is fully in possession, but*
> *somehow in a position to forestall ill-advised moves.... Patrolling is, in fact, my*
> *principal occupation.... No matter how tight Security, I am always somewhere*
> *Outside giving orders and Inside this strait jacket of jelly that gives and stretches*
> *but always reforms ahead of every movement, thought, impulse, stamped with the*
> *seal of alien inspection.*
>
> *(William Burroughs, "Naked Lunch"[1])*

When I first sat down to write this book I was unsure how it would unfold. Ideas had been swirling around in my head off and on for the 20 years since I first began working with people affected by addictive relationships, but for various reasons I had not been in the position to commit them to paper[2]. While on study leave for the first half of 2006 I began writing these ideas down and to my surprise they emerged with more coherence than I had anticipated. Looking back, what appears to have held the work together is the focus on intimacy. The impact of addictive relationships on intimacy can be observed at every level: when people enter addictive relationships they take on an alternative form of intimacy, when they struggle to change they are struggling with very strong interpersonal processes, when they attempt to reintegrate they are faced with the challenge of rebuilding and mending intimate connections, and, most importantly, addictive relationships create distortions and asymmetries for surrounding intimates. This I find is the most disturbing aspect of addictive contexts. Those who live with a person in an addictive relationship are invariably affected and, for many, affected in profound ways that persist through their lives. The addictive relationship appears to cut through the connections between intimates, impoverishing the lives of most of those involved and leaving behind them a trail of alienation, hurt, and shame. In contrast to this destructive potential, I have also watched many people rally all the strength and courage they possess to take on the enormous task of disengaging from an addictive relationship and reforming their connections into a world of multiple intimacies. Their journey invariably involves the ups and downs of hope and disappointment and the heartbreak of separations and reversions. What's more, the forming and reforming of intimacies is a very slow and fickle process and, as illustrated throughout this book, requires support at the level of individuals, family, community, and society.

P.J. Adams, Fragmented Intimacy: Addiction in a Social World
© Springer 2008

Where It Fits

Part of the challenge of exploring an alternative interpretation of addiction is the struggle with language—how to think in one zone without resorting in misleading ways to meanings from another zone. This is impossible when one interpretation dominates the other. While a number of new terms were developed in the book, it has still relied on many of the words and concepts derived from more traditional understandings. In an attempt to skirt and perhaps subvert this reliance, the argument in the book has sought to outline this alternative understanding through conceptual play embellished with reference to literature, metaphors, vignettes, and diagrams.

The book began with the dominance of the biological and psychological explanations for addiction that focus on the person as an isolated individual or "particle". The dominance of this particle orientation was seen as restricting development of other perspectives, especially the opportunities offered in viewing addictions as a social event. In a social world, addiction can be interpreted as one relationship among other relationships, a relationship that intensifies as other relationships deteriorate. A social perspective views personal identity as building up from diverse connections with people and other objects (both internal and external). This connectedness provides the raw material for interpretations of selfhood. As the addictive relationship intensifies, personal identity is gradually transposed from a broad circle of multiple and symmetrical (two-way) connections to a social world structured around one pivotal axis. Accordingly, the person's social identity becomes steadily oriented around the addictive substance/process, and other relationships are relegated to secondary and supportive roles. As a result relationships with other people become distorted and increasingly unidirectional.

In a social world addiction can be interpreted as one relationship among others

When the observer's gaze moves from the vantage point of looking down on addictive relationships to a position inside the addictive social system, its distorting action on intimacies is drawn into sharper focus. The strength of an intimacy can be seen as built up from a combination of emotionally laden interconnecting strands. In this book, these strands were identified as closeness, compassion, commitment, and accord. In normal contexts these strands occur in roughly symmetrical ways, with both parties to each relationship experiencing similar benefits and similar levels of power and control. The presence of addictive processes changes this balance. As the addictive relationship intensifies, other relationships are downgraded, and relationships with intimates become increasingly unidirectional and asymmetrical. Intimates may not be fully aware of these asymmetries, but following a series of disappointments they begin to appreciate the reduced status of their involvement. They begin to see that while they maintain closeness and commitment to their relationships, this is becoming less and less reciprocated by the person in the addictive relationship. Meanwhile the addictive relationship gathers in intensity to a point that the person within becomes increasingly committed to its survival. Since the main threats to its survival are located within the immediate social system, the person resorts increasingly to the use of intimacy management strategies that aim to weaken potential challenges from surrounding intimates. For many intimates these strategies will involve the use of violence and other controlling tactics; for others it may only extend as far as strategic noninvolvement or absences. Whatever strategies are used to maintain these asymmetrical relationships, the social system continues to build its single-axis focus around the addictive relationship.

The outcome of these processes is that intimates (in most case family members) find themselves living in an isolated and fragmented social world, with difficulties trusting others and difficulties maintaining links to broader networks. Intimates working in isolation make attempts to change the situation, but they encounter strong counterreactions instigated by the person in the addictive relationship. These reinforce their sense of isolation. An alternative way of responding that this book advocates begins with the opportunities to resist fragmentation through intimate reconnection and collective action. The initial attempts at collective action are unlikely to fully unsettle the strength of an addictive relationship but they can form the basis for pro-

Collective action targets the oppressive power of addictive relationships

gressive reconnections both to other intimates in the family and to layers of friends, extended family, work colleagues, and community professionals. This collective power is mobilized in repeated challenges to the dominance of the addictive relationship, all along making sure that the collective is not fragmented by any counterreactions. Eventually people in an addictive relationship may reach a point where protection is no longer viable and they embrace the prospect of change and join forces with intimates in the process of reintegration. Reintegration involves the progressive reformation of multiple and symmetrical connections in the domains of intimacy, occupational, physical, communal, and inner connectedness. This process, by its very nature, is slow, and to sustain momentum requires support at multiple levels.

The final part of the book explores places where a social understanding of addiction can assist in understanding and supporting the longer term processes of reintegration. First, a variety of approaches currently available for equipping families for change were examined and included the twelve-step movement, which provides a simple and practical guide to reforming communal and inner connectedness, and approaches in addiction services with an accent on family involvement. Second, the book examined ways family members can combine their strengths in reducing fragmentation in addictive systems. This involved highlighting the importance for family members of maintaining a realistic and pragmatic outlook on the possible long-term outcomes and to engage with one another in building sufficient strength to withstand the fragmenting power of counterreactions. Third, the effectiveness of collective action can be enhanced by harnessing the power of communities and neighborhoods to support both challenges to the addictive relationship and ongoing reintegration. This was illustrated in a Canadian volunteer network, the Croatian/Italian club movement, and an indigenous (Māori) approach to addiction. Finally, the book examined the part addiction professionals could play in facilitating (rather than "treating") the layered social potential of intimates, neighborhoods, and communities to initiate and support change.

Can Social and Particle Paradigms Work Together?

From the beginning, this book has emphasized how the particle and social paradigms offer quite different ways of looking at addictions. The inset box summarizes the key orientation differences between the two paradigms as they are applied to understandings of addiction. The primary focus for the particle paradigm is on people as individuals; in the social paradigm the focus is on people in relationships. Knowledge in the particle paradigm is valued for being universal and objective; in the social paradigm knowledge is derived from social contexts through interaction and negotiation. As a consequence expertise in the particle paradigm is held by specialized professionals such as practitioners, researchers, and teachers; in a social world expertise emerges collectively within a social context. Accordingly the particle frame for responding to addictions involves experts meeting one-to-one with individuals in socially isolated clinic settings, while the social frame involves interacting with many people at once within their social environment.

Contrasting Addiction Paradigms		
	Particle	Social
Focus	Individual	Relationships
Frame	Clinic	Environment
Knowledge	Objectivist	Interactional
Expertise	Practitioner	Collective

From both theoretical and practical standpoints there are strong reasons for asking whether it is possible for social and particle worldviews to work side by side. The threat to theory concerns whether the emergent paradigm would be submerged and disappear into the dominant paradigm. The threat to practice concerns whether strong differences in viewpoint could lead to misunderstandings and conflict between professionals in ways that negatively affect those they service.

The possibilities for an amicable coexistence take three forms: integration, separation, and complementation. In the first possibility, integration, viewing addiction as a social event can be subsumed or integrated into the dominant particle orientation. To some extent the biopsychosocial model has already proceeded down this track, and, as pointed out previously in Chapter 2 the value of a social orientation is lost by it being subsumed into the hostile environment of particle assumptions. In the second possibility, separation, a social paradigm operates entirely separately from contexts based on particle assumptions. This is theoretically the cleanest way for an emerging paradigm to progress because it develops unimpeded by the values and beliefs of adherents to the dominant paradigm. It could be implemented by adherents to the two paradigms cutting off from one another into two separate environments, which then enables them to sustain a high level of purity and integrity with their primary assumptions. While theoretically attractive, in practice such an arrangement is difficult to implement and may in the long term amplify differences and conflict. It is further impractical because in the field of addictions it would be practically impossible to find an environment that is not to some extent influenced by particle orientations.

In the third possibility, complementation, there is some degree of separation between the two paradigms, but at the same time opportunities are created to connect between the paradigms and the strengths of strategies belonging to each are implemented as appropriate. An example of this is observed in physics with the study of light. Some aspects of light can be explained as a series of particles, and other aspects (such as light refraction) can be explained as a series of waves. In physics, the particle and wave interpretations have managed to stand side by side without an unnecessary clash while contributing variously to explanations and at the same time maintaining their independence. For a complex, multilayered and dynamic field such as addictions, the option of complementary approaches (rather than integrative or separatist approaches) is more realistic than other alternatives and more likely to be supported by research. The challenge is to foster linkages between the perspectives while at the same time maintaining their independence. One way of imagining how this complementarity might be achieved is to think of the two paradigms as separate strands in a double helix similar to that of DNA. The two paradigms are intertwined but separate. Small links are made at different points, but as a whole they function in distinct spaces, thereby maintaining their independence and integrity.

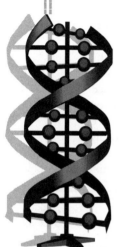

Figure 14.1 DNA double helix

Important Issues

The book offers a different way of interpreting addictions, but in so doing it raises a range of new issues and leaves many questions unanswered. The following subsections address five such issues.

What Happens with Complex Needs?

Addictive relationships are often combined with other life issues, particularly those that threaten mental well-being. People in addictive relationships are highly likely to experience significant periods of depression and anxiety,

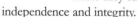

and they are more likely than nonaddicted people to experience psychotic episodes, personality problems, and other addiction problems.[3] How are these addictive relationships to be interpreted in social terms? How do they complicate the processes of fragmentation and intimacy distortions? Are the social dynamics of depression parallel to those of addiction or do they interact with them? Because these interactions are so common, these questions are important to address in the future development of a social approach to addictions.

How Do Biological and Social Dimensions Interact?

Chapter 4 briefly referred to the biological dimensions of addiction in terms of enhancing the initial intensification of an addictive relationship. This brief mention does little justice to the importance of biological processes, particularly for addictive relationships to mood-altering drugs (and arguably to mood enhancing processes such as gambling). A considerable amount of particle-oriented research has gone into the interplay between brain mechanisms and the psychology of addictions, but this effort has not extended to its interplay with social processes. For example, inquiry could explore how with different drugs (e.g., heroin versus cannabis) varying rates of tolerance interact with social contexts to produce unique features such as the need to resort to crime and the need for different levels of family control and secrecy.

What Is Quality Intimacy?

The question of how to identify quality intimacy is problematic. An assumption made here is that the asymmetry of relationships in an addictive system means they are of lower quality than those in normal multiconnected social systems. This assumption is difficult to fully justify. For example, many children who have been raised within these systems, while experiencing some difficulties at the time, move on to live balanced and fulfilling lives with little sign of ongoing problems with intimacy.[4] Furthermore, many people value intimacy in addictive relationships in spite of its fragmenting effects (see inset box, above). This book has proposed that the quality of these relationships is compromised by the presence of fragmenting intimacy management strategies. But the basis for making this claim needs to be developed. What criteria might be used to clarify and perhaps refine this position in the future? How maladaptive is the

> ### Leaving Las Vegas
> *Leaving Las Vegas*, a film by Mike Figgis, seriously challenges the notion that relationships in addictive relationships are devoid of quality. A man in an addictive relationship to alcohol has lost his wife, home, and job. He resolves that life is not worth continuing so he travels to a motel in Las Vegas to drink himself to death. While there he meets a prostitute who cares for him during this final period. What is perplexing about their relationship is that despite the late stage of his addictive relationship to alcohol, he is still capable of forming this intimacy and that she appears genuinely accepting of both his relationship to alcohol and his intention to die. While the man's deterioration is obvious, the depiction of meaningful intimacy in this context is still perplexing.

rigidity of the single-axis structure of addictive social systems? What indicators can be developed that identify the severity of fragmentation in order to estimate the time and effort a reintegration will take?

What Is Meant by "Symmetry"?

One question about intimacy addresses the degree of symmetry occurring between the intimates and the person in the addictive relationship. As explored in Chapter 5, intimates encounter increasing discrepancies between the level of closeness, compassion, commitment, and accord they put in to the relationship compared to what they receive back. At first, many fail to detect this is happening, but as time goes on they become increasingly dismayed and confused by the hard and brutal behavior of their loved ones. This book looked at these asymmetries in terms of one-sided power, unreciprocated closeness and compassion, and uncertain commitment. The effect of these processes needs closer examination, particularly in terms of tighter definition and the way they are experienced by people in addictive social systems.

The asymmetries in addictive systems require further investigation

Does High Connectedness Make Communities More Resilient?

A critical question for the future is the extent to which socially connected environments contribute to the strength and resilience of people affected by addictive relationships. Social connectedness has been identified as an important determinant of well-being in other areas, and some evidence is emerging for its role with addictions. For example, addictive relationships are more likely to thrive in fragmented social environments. But clarifying under what circumstances social connectedness is most likely to facilitate change is still in its early stages of exploration. For example, connecting into a community that has high levels of fear (due to factors such as poverty and crime) could potentially compromise rather than increase resilience.

Future Opportunities

One great advantage of a social orientation is its capacity to link up the disparate levels of intervention with addictive relationships. For example, there is currently a strong separation of those working in public health from those working in primary health and those working in specialist addiction services. This makes little sense when all three have a role in responding to addictive relationships. Social approaches are directly relevant to approaches taken with the individual, the community, and society as a whole; consequently, they can be seen as offering a bridging point that spans these three different levels of intervention.

Intervention Focal Points

A social perspective opens up a range of opportunities for building interventions with addictive systems. At one level it enables the emergence of
systems that support self-help initiatives. A thread through the current book
is the notion that collectives of people affected by addictions are better positioned than trained professionals to achieve change. Rather than focusing on
the weaknesses and limitations within families, a social approach seeks ways
to enable families to activate their own social strengths. This would entail
looking carefully at the availability to families of self-help resources that can
assist them both in working out what they are dealing with and in connecting
them into focal points of collective action. Communication strategies could
be implemented using publications, Web sites, and media campaigns promoting reintegration approaches.

A second intervention focal point relates to the opportunities for community development. A key opportunity here relates to strategies and
resources that better equip people in addictive contexts to counter fragmentation. These will primarily concentrate on improving connectedness within
neighborhoods and communities. The long-term challenge for communities
is the dual-pronged task of creating environments that are not supportive of
addictive relationships as well as fostering environments that are conducive
of reintegration. Both tasks require efforts at enhancing overall social coherence and connectedness within the community. Approaches to addictions in
the future could turn more from responding to isolated individuals to participating in initiatives that target the strength and vitality of communities.

A third focal point for intervention concerns the emerging contribution
of both social and health practitioners with a commitment to social responses
to addictive systems. Reviews of research into practice interventions are
beginning to note how intervention methods that incorporate social dimensions are proving to be more effective.[5] These methods remain enmeshed in
particle thinking and have as yet to unleash the full potential of a social orientation. Another key area for service development is in primary health care.
General practitioners and community nurses comprise a sizable part of the
health care work force and are in an excellent position to mediate relationships between families and other community resources, and between families
and other specialist services. Their regular contact with family members
makes them key players in the addictive family system, which enables them
to participate in a variety of potentially helpful ways, such as facilitating
meetings with key parties, liaising with services, and providing ongoing
support for reintegration. At yet another level, addictive relationships also
need to be seen as a major public health concern. Over recent decades the
contribution of addiction services to general social well-being has become
blurred in many countries where the driving force for policy (particularly
alcohol, drug, and gambling policy) is propelled by a focus on managing
consumption. Despite this preoccupation, addictive relationships remain a

A social approach opens up opportunities for public health, health promotion & primary health major contributor to the harm associated with dangerous consumptions, and public health and health promotion professionals could play a critical role in relevant strategies, such as improvements in local and national health services, public education, and community capacity building.[6] The roles of these professionals, in addiction services, primary health, and public health, could be improved by providing programs in basic and ongoing training in social understanding and social approaches to addictive relationships.

Research

Understanding addictive relationships in a social paradigm is partly hampered by the lack of a solid research base. This means that in contrast with particle paradigm research, there is a wide open field for researchers to explore social applications. To illustrate this potential, the following briefly outlines several different projects that could be undertaken in the near future and that capture the potential for different forms of research to contribute to further exploration within this paradigm.

First, it is particularly important to find out more about the social dynamics of addictive systems. One project could involve comparison of cultural interpretations of addictive relationships. Mariana Valverde's historical study of interpretations of addiction in European traditions made a start here by exploring the cultural meanings of addictions in different cultural settings. In a similar vein, the ideas in this book would link well with further historical and ethnographic work seeking to study the layers of meaning associated with the action of addictive relationships in a social world. For example, a study could contrast the interactions and meanings between particular migrant populations and a dominant culture. Another project could involve qualitative interview studies focusing on family members' accounts of their experience within addictive systems. A series of studies could invite intimates exposed to addictive relationships to relate their stories of fragmentation. How did they interpret the increasing asymmetry? What helped them in reconnecting with others and in moving toward collective action? Methods could include multiple interviews with the same families, checking interpretations as they develop, and inviting families to elaborate on key issues. As these rich descriptions emerge, subsequent projects could invite families who have successfully reintegrated to describe the types of collective action that they see having contributed to their success.

With an eye to community contexts, another set of research projects could focus on identifying the opportunities for collective and community responses to addictive relationships. Community participatory action research aims to foster the inner potential and expertise within communities to develop responses to major challenges in their own way and on their own terms. This approach to research is consistent with the social empowerment philosophy inherent to social approaches. A project in this area could begin by engaging with a community that

Research will play an important role in developing social approaches in the future

expresses concern about the impact addictive relationships, then by proceeding to work alongside it in finding ways to enhance environments of connectedness as a means of building strength to prevent, resist, and contain the impact of addictive relationships. This initial work could lead to developing a social intervention demonstration project when a community has opted to take on a more systematic and coordinated response to addictive relationships. Those involved might choose to undertake a club network, similar to the Croatian/Italian clubs, to support families in change. Such large-scale projects are likely to require funding, particularly for coordinating links and for documentation and evaluation.

Finally, as identified in the previous section, the benefits of taking a social approach to addictive relationships require the cooperation and support of addiction professionals. The development of social approaches therefore requires professionals to develop an understanding of the principles and application of its methods. Training initiatives could be provided at a number of levels—first as part of the basic training of key professionals (addiction counselors, health promoters, social workers), then as courses and supervision for qualified addiction professionals already practicing, and finally as courses for general health care professionals. Each of these training initiatives would need to be carefully documented and evaluated.

Final Thoughts

Chapter 2 described this book as an invitation to switch to a social paradigm. It is hoped that the book's various excursions into the depths of addictive systems, looking at them from both inside and outside, has gone some way in persuading the reader of the potential of approaching addiction as a social event. Realistically, it is unlikely that a switch into a social interpretation of addictions will attract all players in the field, particularly those with a strong investment in particle orientations. Furthermore, the invitation to switch might also prompt some observers to challenge and contest the assumptions of a social orientation. Such a response would be difficult to rebuff when particle orientations are so deeply entrenched in ways of thinking and behaving. What makes the new paradigm additionally vulnerable is the absence of significant inquiry on social approaches and particularly as it applies to intimacy. In order to explore these areas this book needed to develop alternative language and alternative conceptual tools to present its position. While these new resources are fragile and in need of credentialing, the invitation still stands and I am confident those who openly embrace this orientation will be rewarded with a range of new and helpful insights into this perplexing area.

Many people interested in addictions will have difficulty embracing a social perspective

Finally, I find it incomprehensible that governments continue to invest the majority of their funding and people resources into particle approaches to addictions; these approaches have for some time completely dominated research, training, book publications, and service interventions. I often wonder where it might lead if we were to invest only a small proportion of these resources into developing a social approach to addictions. For instance, what would happen if some funding was put aside for family and community projects that target support for collective action? I am convinced that should we apply social principles correctly, such as the approaches outlined in the latter part of this book, we will succeed in increasing services for those most affected by addictive relationships, and in providing greater coverage than is possible with the exclusive reliance on one-to-one counseling strategies that are currently the norm. The adoption of social intervention strategies will result in more people in addictive social systems receiving guidance and support, more people entering reintegration earlier, and more intimates living in contexts that were improved by intimacy management strategies. Maybe it is a pipe dream, but as the range and availability of dangerous consumptions spread and as they are increasingly commercialized, it seems likely that the number of addictive contexts will outstrip the capacity of our current approaches to respond. I am hoping that others who read this book will share my enthusiasm for their potential.

Notes

Chapter 1: Addiction in Perspective

[1]   This poem was attributed to Edgar Allan Poe by Thomas Ollive Mabbott in 1939, and again in 1969. The original manuscript supposedly hung on the wall of the Washington Tavern in Lowell, Massachusetts, for many years. It was apparently last seen around 1892. It was recalled from memory by a former bartender there about 1939. Although of questionable origin, the attribution has some merit and has not been seriously opposed. See www.eapoe.org/works/poems/alea.htm (accessed March 2007).

[2]   C. Kasl, *Women, Sex and Addiction: A Search for Love and Power* (Ticknor & Fields, 1989). B. Killinger, *Workaholics: The Respectable Addicts* (Simon and Schuster, 1992). P. Mellody and A. Miller, *Facing Love Addiction: Giving Yourself the Power to Change the Way You Love* (Harper, 1992). A helpful bibliography on codependency is available on: www.project-cork.org/bibliographies/data/Bibliography_Co-Dependency (accessed March 2007).

[3]   These estimates are usually reported as "current prevalence," which refers to the percentage of people who respond positively to questions about their use "over the last year" or sometimes "over the last 6 months." These figures are taken from J. Welte, G. Barnes, et al. (2001) "Alcohol and gambling pathology among U.S. adults: prevalence, demographic patterns and comorbidity" *Journal of Studies on Alcohol, 62*(5), 706–712 (the figures exclude addictions to tobacco). Prevalence estimates outside the U.S. can vary; for example, European studies indicate lower prevalence of around 0.5 percent for addictions to drugs; see C. Furr-Holden and J. Anthony (2003) "Epidemiologic differences in drug dependence—a US-UK cross-national comparison" *Social Psychiatry and Psychiatric Epidemiology, 38*(4), 165–172, and L. Kraus, R. Augustin, et al. (2003) "Estimating prevalence of problem drug use at national level in countries of the European Union and Norway" *Addiction, 98*(4), 471–485.

[4]   See reviews of gambling prevalence studies in H. Shaffer, M. Hall, et al. *Estimating the Prevalence of Disordered Gambling Behaviour in the United States and Canada: A Meta-Analysis* (Presidents and Fellows of Harvard College, 1997). In these studies addictions to gambling have been conservatively interpreted as "pathological" rather than the broader category of "problem gambling."

[5]   The Australian Productivity Commission's report *Australia's Gambling Industries: Final Report* (Productivity Commission, 1999, p. 7.33) examined the evidence of how many people can be significantly affected by one problem gambler and concluded that it could vary between 7 and 10 people.

[6]   Mariana Valverde in *Diseases of the Will: Alcohol and the Dilemmas of Freedom* (Cambridge University Press, 1998, pp. 50–51) traces the origins of the concept of addiction back to 1887 when a Dr. Norman Kerr of the British Society for the Scientific Study of Inebriety referred to habitual inebriates as "alcoholics."

[7]   Marc Schuckit, *Drug and Alcohol Abuse: A Clinical Guide to Diagnosis and Treatment,* 4th ed. (Plenum Medical, 1995, p. 5).

[8]   From R. Morse and D. Flavin (1992) "The definition of alcoholism." *Journal of the American Medical Association, 268*, p. 1013. Also adopted and quoted in H. Doweiko, *Concepts of Chemical Dependency,* 5th ed. (Brooks/Cole, 2002, p. 13).

[9]   World Health Organization (1952). *Technical Report, Series No. 48* (Expert Committee on Mental Health, 1952) quoted in J. Orford, *Excessive Appetites: A Psychological View of Addictions* (Wiley, 1985, p. 12).

10 As presented in A. Blume (2005) *Treating Drug Problems* (Wiley, 2005, pp. 5–11).

11 As described in their main book *Narcotics Anonymous*, 5th ed. (NA World Service Office, 1988, pp. 3–4).

12 As presented to clients and family members attending the Betty Ford Center in its Informational Brochure (1990).

13 Cognitive behavioral therapy approaches to treating addictions are the best example of a widely used approach that focuses on the capacity of thinking to influence changes in behavior. For a review see J. Morgenstern and R. Longabaugh (2000) "Cognitive-behavioral treatment for alcohol dependence: a review of evidence for its hypothe-sized mechanisms of action" *Addiction, 95*(10), 1475–1490.

14 From a public health perspective the impact of alcohol and other dangerous consumptions incorporates a wide range of harms that are not necessarily linked to addictions. For exam-ple, in P. Davies and D. Walsh, *Alcohol Problems and Alcohol Control in Europe* (Croom Helm, 1983), they stated "even fairly moderate levels of drinking may be transformed into alcohol problems if combined with the exacting demands of driving a car, handling machinery at work, or maintaining normal family and social relations" (pp. 19–20). See also G. Edwards, P. Anderson, et al., *Alcohol Policy and the Public Good* (Oxford University Press, 1994) and T. Babor, R. Caetano, et al., Alcohol: No Ordinary Commodity. *Research and Public Policy* (Oxford University Press, 2003).

15 To cite a few who adopt a broad brush approach, see R. Coombs (ed.), *Handbook of Addictive Disorders: A Practical Guide to Diagnosis and Treatment* (Wiley, 2004); H. Shaffer (1997) "The most important unresolved issue in the addictions: conceptual chaos" *Substance Use & Misuse, 32*(11), 153–158; and J. Orford, *Excessive Appetites: A Psychological View of Addictions* (Wiley, 1985).

16 Ibid. p. 323.

17 This widening of the term addiction to apply to consumptions that may only have minimal negative impacts has been criticized by a range of writers, who include M. Valverde, *Diseases of the Will* (Cambridge University Press, 1998); C. DiClemente, *Addiction and Change: How Addictions Develop and Addicted People Recover* (Guilford, 2003); and Helen Keane, *What's Wrong with Addiction* (Melbourne University Press, 2002).

18 Keane (2002), Ibid. p. 189.

19 From P. Carnes, R. Murray, et al. (2004) "Addiction interaction disorder" in R. Coombs (ed.), *Handbook of Addictive Disorders: A Practical Guide to Diagnosis and Treatment* (Wiley, 2004, pp. 57–58).

20 From Miller (1999), cited in H. Doweiko, *Concepts of Chemical Dependency*, 5th ed. (Brooks/Cole, 2002, p. 8).

21 From George DuWors, *White Knuckles and Wishful Thinking: Breaking the Chain of Compulsive Reaction in Alcoholism and Other Addictions* (Hogrefe & Huber, 1992, p. 3).

22 The descriptions of all four relationships and the people in them have been con-structed as composite scenarios based on multiple situations and aggregated from my own exposure to people affected by addictions. The characters and their situations are therefore all fictional and any unintended reference to particular people or contexts is entirely coincidental.

Chapter 2: A Social World

1 From Jean Francois Lyotard (1993) *Political Writings*. (University College London, 1993, p33). In compiling this chapter, I am strongly indebted to Lyotard's writings, particu-larly his book *The Postmodern Condition: A Report on Knowledge* (Minnesota University

Press, 1984[1979]), as well as Thomas Kuhn's seminal work in *The Structure of Scientific Revolutions* (University of Chicago, 1970) along with my early exposures to lectures by Paul Feyerabend and his wonderful book *Against Method: Outline of an Anarchistic Theory of Knowledge* (Verso, 1970).

2   Quoted in A. Salmond *The Trial of the Cannibal Dog: Captain Cook in the South Seas* (Allen Lane/Penguin 2003, p41). Although as master of the *Dolphin* William Robertson arrived in Tahiti shortly before Captain Cook, his reaction is typical of the strong impression these earlier visitors had to the bounteous nature of life on these islands.

3   The impact of Cook's voyages on the European imagination is discussed in A. Frost "New geographical perspectives and the emergence of the romantic imagination" in R. Fisher and H. Johnston (Eds.) *Captain Cook and His Times* (Australian National University Press, 1979, 5-20).

4   While Thomas Kuhn championed recognition of "paradigms" in the modern era, the term has a far longer presence in European thought that can be traced back to Aristotle's use in ancient Greece in his very influential book on *Physics*.

5   I have opted for the term *assumptions* over other contenders (such as *meta-theories, discourses, grand narratives* etc.) because it is a more familiar term. Its use risks encouraging reductionist and structuralist perspectives which tend to flatten basic understandings to one level, whereas the realm of assumptions is more accurately understood to function in multileveled, fluid and highly interactional ways.

6   Paul Feyerabend in *Against Method* (Verso, 1970) provides an excellent account of the irrationality of this paradigm switch.

7   Feyerabend, Kuhn and Lyotard all emphasized the critical importance of incommensurability between paradigms and highlight the confusion created when a person working on one platform of assumptions interprets what is happening on another platform.

8   Here I have opted for the term "objectivism" to characterize a set of assumptions that place knowledge as "out there", solid, ready to be discovered. This theory of knowledge emerged strongly during the European Enlightenment and reached is strongest expression in the logical positivism of the "Vienna Circle". It is also commonly referred to as "empiricism" and "naïve realism".

9   In Lyotard's *The Postmodern Condition* (Minnesota University Press, 1984[1979]) he describes this interpretation of knowledge as one genre of scientific discourse involving language games with their own rules and protocols. Both Lyotard and Feyerabend emphasize the importance of diversity in facilitating movement both within and across these language games.

10   One important philosopher of science Imre Lakatos "Falsification and the methodology of scientific research programmes" in I. Lakatos and A. Musgrave *Criticism and the Growth of Knowledge* (Cambridge University, 1970) argued that research based on one paradigm can run its course and eventually run out of steam (or "positive heuristic"). New paradigms can then attract adherents because they offer new territories for discovery.

11   Thomas Kuhn *The Structure of Scientific Revolutions* (University of Chicago, 1970, p158).

12   Classic periods of pluralism, such as classical Athens, Moorish Spain and Vienna in the 1900s, were transitory phenomenon. For discussions of the pluralism of these periods see A. Janik and S. Toulmin's *Wittgenstein's Viena.* (Simon & Schuster, 1973), R. Fletcher *Moorish Spain* (University of California Press,1993) and S. Pomeroy *Ancient Greece: A Political, Social, and Cultural History* (Oxford University Press, 1999).

13   My strongest experience of paradigm dominance in academic environments occurred in psychology departments during the 1970 until 1990 where operant behaviourism and related objectivist psychologies maintained virtually exclusive dominance over competing traditions.

14   A critical literature on the wholesale application of illness metaphors to mental wellbeing is available and exemplified in books such as Thomas Szasz's *The Myth of Mental Illness: Foundations of a Theory of Personal Conduct* (Harper & Row, 1974) and Michel Foucault's *Madness and Civilization* (Pantheon, 1965).

15   This total form of dominance is often referred to as "hegemony" and is a critical concept for many post-modern thinkers including Derrida, Lyotard, Foucault, Bourdieu etc., see I. Burkitt *Bodies of Thought: Embodiment, Identity and Modernity* (Sage 1999).

16   See Mariana Valverde's excellent book on *Diseases of the Will: Alcohol and the Dilemmas of Freedom* (Cambridge University, 1998).

17   Ibid 43-67.

18   Provided by the WHO Expert Committee on Mental Health (1957) on *Addiction Producing Drugs,* pp17-25.

19   World Health Organisation Expert Committee on Mental Health (1957). *Addiction Producing Drugs: 7th Report of the WHO Expert Committee.* Geneva, World Health Organisation: 17-25.

20   For example, see discussions in S. Shaw "The disease concept of dependence" in N. Heather, I. Robertson, et al. (Eds.) *The Misuse of Alcohol: Crucial Issues in Dependence, Treatment, and Prevention* (University Press, 1985) and N. Heather and I. Robertson *Problem Drinking: Third Edition* (Oxford Medical Publications, 1997).

21   Particle thinking is adopted by many of the specialist approaches to research on addictions that include sub-disciplines such as: biomedicine, pharmacology, behavioral and cognitive psychology, social psychology.

22   The increasing recognition of social influences such as culture, class and community environments are explored in books such as Mac Marshall (Ed.) *Beliefs, Behaviors and Alcoholic Beverages in Cross Cultural Survey.* (University of Michigan, 1979), Stan Einstein's (Ed.) *The Community's Response to Drug Use* (Pergamon 1980) and John Davies' *The Myth of Addiction* (Harwood Academic, 1992).

23   For example, applications of the biopsychosocial model can be found in D. Lende and E. Smith (2002). "Evolution meets biopsychosociality: an analysis of addictive behaviour, *Addiction, 97*(4), 470-1 and P. Rogers and H. Smit (2000) "Food craving and food "addiction": a critical review of the evidence from a biopsychosocial perspective" *Pharmacology, Biochemistry and Behavior, 66*(1), 3-14.

24   See this discussed in A. Blume *Treating Drug Problems* (Wiley, 2005, p21). The biopsychosocial model is also championed by Marlatt and VandenBos's (Eds.) "Introduction" in *Addictive Behaviours: Readings on Etiology, Prevention and Treatment* (American Psychological Association, 1997).

25   C. DiClemente (2003). *Addiction and Change: How Addictions Develop and Addicted People Recover* (Guilford Press, 2003, p18).

26   Translated by Gilmour in F. Nietzsche (1989 [1873]) "On Truth and Lying in an Extramoral Sense" in *Friedrich Nietzsche on Rhetoric and Language* (Harper & Row, 1989).

27   For excellent summaries of post-modernism see D. R. Dickens and A. Fontana (Eds.) *Postmodernism & Social Inquiry* (Guilford 1994), and H. Bertens and J. Natoli (Eds.) *Postmodernism: Key Figures* (Blackwell, 2002).

28   Since 2003 I and a group of colleagues began hosting an annual two day *Dangerous Consumptions Colloquium* for academics in Australia and New Zealand interested in applications of social theory to alcohol, drugs, gambling and other dangerous consumptions. In November 2006 we held our fourth event ("DC4") in Canberra, and we

plan to continue running them for the foreseeable future. For an overview see P. Adams, J. Fitzgerald, et al., (Eds.) (2005) "Special Issue: Dangerous Consumptions" *Addiction Research and Theory, 13*(6).

[29] For example, some of his most well known students include Helmut Wagner, Peter Berger and Thomas Luckmann, and he had a profound influence on the ethnomethodology of Harold Garfinkel. For more detail see G. Psathas (2004). "Alfred Schutz's influence on American sociologists and sociology." *Human Studies, 27*(1), 1-35.

[30] Alfred Schutz *The Phenomenology of the Social World* (Heinemann Educational, 1972).

[31] R. Wilkinson and M. Marmot *Social determinants of health: The solid facts* (WHO European Office, 2003).

[32] See D. Fergusson and M. Lynskey (1996). "Adolescent resiliency to family adversity." *Journal of child psychiatry, 37*(3), 281-292 and C. Olsson, L. Bond, et al. (2003). "Adolescent resilience: a concept analysis." *Journal of Adolescence, 26,* 1-11. In an article by S. Fergus and M. Zimmerman (2005). "Adolescent resilience: A framework for understanding healthy development in the face of risk." *Annual Review of Public Health, 26,* 399-419 they discuss three models of resilience: compensatory, protective and challenge models, where each involves a different type of research strategy.

[33] Ron Labonte (1990). "Empowerment: Notes on Professional and Community Dimensions." *Canadian Review of Social Policy, 26,* 64-75, and G. Laverack (2001). "An identification and interpretation of the organisational aspects of community empowerment." *Community Development Journal, 36*(2), 40-50.

[34] See K. Rubin, K. Dwyer, et al. (2004). "Attachment, friendship, and psychosocial functioning in early adolescence." *Journal of Early Adolescence, 24*(4), 326-356.

[35] See discussions of the effectiveness in of community capacity building approaches in G. Laverack *Health Promotion Practice: Power and Empowerment* (Sage, 2004) and demonstrated in the large community development projects led by Barbara Israel and colleagues (2006) in "Challenges and facilitating factors in sustaining community-based participatory research partnerships: lessons learned from the Detroit, New York City and Seattle Urban Research Centers" *Journal of Urban Health, 83*(6), 1022-40.

[36] Summaries of the various practice applications of systems theory can be found in Lynn Hoffman's *Family Therapy: An Intimate History* (Norton & Co, 2001) and P. C. Rosenblatt's *Metaphors of Family Systems Theory: Toward New Constructions* (Guilford, 1997).

[37] Te Taniwha in Whitianga describing her first sighting of Cook and his crew as cited by Anne Salmond in *Two Worlds: First Meetings between Maori and Europeans 1642-1772* (Penguin/Viking, 1991, p87). The complexities of the varying interpretations of civilization and savagery are contrasted in G. Obeyesekere *The Apotheosis of Captain Cook: European Mythmaking in the Pacific* (Princeton University Press, 1992).

[38] Quoted in A. Salmond *Between Worlds: Early Exchanges Between Maori and Europeans 1773-1815* (Viking, 1997, p78).

[39] As argued by T. Kuhn *The Structure of Scientific Revolutions* (University of Chicago, 1970, p115) and by I. Lakatos "Falsification and the methodology of scientific research programmes" in I. Lakatos and A. Musgrave (Eds.) *Criticism and the Growth of Knowledge* (Cambridge University, 1970, pp91-196).

[40] Quoted in A Salmond *Two Worlds* (Penguin/Viking, 1991, p112).

[41] Quoted in A. Salmond *The Trial of the Cannibal Dog* (Allen Lane/Penguin, 2003, p385).

[42] Ibid. p232. Description provided by Johann Forster on board Captain Cook's voyage in the ship *Resolution* to Antarctica.

Chapter 3: Addiction and Connecting

1   Jack London *John Barleycorn of Alcoholic Memoirs* (Arco, 1967, p. 15). The book tells the
     tale of London's own addictive relationship to alcohol, with "John Barleycorn" named
     as a person but in reality representing alcohol.

2   There is an expanding literature on social connection, particularly in the
     human development literature on its contribution to resiliency. An overview is
     provided by H. Kaplan, "Toward an understanding of resilience" in M. Glantz
     and J. Johnson, *Resilience and Development: Positive Life Adaptations* (Kluwer/Plenum,
     1999, pp. 17–83); C. Olsson, L. Bond, et al. (2003), "Adolescent resilience: a con-
     cept analysis." *Journal of Adolescence, 26*, 1–11; and K. Rubin, K. Dwyer, et al. (2004)
     "Attachment, friendship, and psychosocial functioning in early adolescence."
     Journal of Early Adolescence, 24(4), 326–356.

3   George Lakoff has discussed the processes involved in forming categories and
     argues they do not function like Venn diagrams, or pigeonholes, but are con-
     ceptually based on what he calls "idealised cognitive models". See his book
     Women, Fire, and Dangerous Things: What Categories Reveal about the Mind (University of
     Chicago, 1987).

4   This is discussed in more detail in Chapter 2, but briefly it has emerged from the
     related disciplines of sociology, social anthropology, and critical social psychology. Key
     works in its emergence include Gregory Bateson, *Steps in an Ecology of Mind* (Granada,
     1972); Alfred Schutz, *The Phenomenology of the Social World* (Heinemann, 1972); and
     Elizabeth Bott, *Family and Social Network,* 2nd ed (Basic Books, 1971).

5   In his book on addictions, Jim Orford *Excessive Appetites: A Psychological View of Addictions*
     (Wiley, 1985) also includes what we have termed process addictions, including gambling,
     eating, and sexuality. Applying the concept of addictions beyond substance addictions is
     controversial and has generated considerable debate. For example, see coverage of the
     debate over gambling in Howard Shaffer (1999), "Strange bedfellows: a critical view of
     pathological gambling and addiction." *Addiction, 94*(10), 1445–1448.

6   The term *addictive substance/process* is used throughout the book to signal that addictive
     relationships can form with a variety of objects, including "substances" such as heroin,
     alcohol, cocaine, and food, as well as "processes" such as gambling and sex.

7   There is a sizable literature on aspects in which alcohol is embedded in European,
     indigenous and other cultures. For a summary of these, see D. Heath (ed.), *International
     Handbook on Alcohol and Culture* (Greenwood, 1995).

8   Gerda Reith's revealing book, *The Age of Chance: Gambling in Western Culture* (Routledge,
     1999), explores in detail the evolution of cultural meanings around gambling within
     European culture, tracing it back to early civilizations such as Mesopotamian
     and Egyptian cultures.

9   The sociocultural dynamics of illicit drug use has received less attention than alcohol,
     but ethnographic and discourse work is emerging in works such as N. Zinberg, *Drug,
     Set, and Setting: The Basis for Controlled Intoxicant Use* (Yale University, 1984), and J. B.
     Davies, Drugspeak: *the Analysis of Drug Discourse* (Harwood, 1997).

10   The main North American manual used for diagnosing mental disorders, the
     Diagnostic and Statistical Manual of Mental Disorders, 4th ed. (DSM-IV; American
     Psychiatric Association, 1994), identifies "dependent substance use" with one
     of its seven key criteria involving "a great deal of time … spent in activities
     necessary to obtain the substance (e.g., visiting multiple doctors or driving
     long distances), use the substance (e.g., chain smoking), or recover from its
     effect."

¹¹ Another of the seven criteria for dependency in the DSM-IV refers to "important social, occupational, or recreational activities are given up or reduced because of substance use." This progressive narrowing of lifestyle refers to progressive deterioration or disconnection from other previously active parts of a person's life.

¹² In their book *The Alcoholic Marriage: Alternative Perspectives* (Grune & Stratton, 1977), T. Paolino and B. McCrady point out that for every excessive drinker there are at least five others who suffer directly or indirectly from this involvement.

¹³ Many factors influence the rate at which addictions emerge. The type of addictive substance/process affects rates, with those with biological enhancement tending to emerge faster (e.g., heroin and tobacco). Age can affect the rate, with an intense relationship at a younger age more likely to lead to addiction.

¹⁴ People attempting to reintegrate from an addictive relationships to opioids have often talked to me of how difficult it was adjusting and accepting a normal lifestyle. For them the whole concept of a life without the danger, irregularity, even the romance of the drug subculture was difficult to accept.

¹⁵ The links between trauma and addictions are well documented. For example, for a summary on sexual abuse, see the introductory chapter to B. Veysey and C. Clark (eds.), *Sexual Abuse in Women with Alcohol and Other Drug and Mental Disorders: Program Building* (Haworth, 2004, pp. 1–39).

¹⁶ The impacts of colonization and subsequent oppression is most acutely observed by the elevated levels of addictive relationships formed by rapidly colonized indigenous populations, such as Australian aboriginal, Maori and North American Indian. For a summary on gambling, see V. McGowan, J. Droessler, et al. *Recent Research in the Socio-Cultural Domain Of Gaming and Gambling: An Annotated Bibliography And Critical Overview* (Alberta Gaming Research Institute, 2000), and for substance use, see F. Beauvais, E. Oetting, et al. (1989), "American Indian youth and drugs, 1976–87: a continuing problem." *American Journal of Public Health, 79,* 634–636.

Chapter 4: Responding to Addiction

¹ First verse of a poem "The Cold Hub" by the New Zealand poet James K. Baxter from his collection, *The Rock Woman: Selected Poems* (Oxford University Press, 1969, p. 52).

² In George Vaillant, *The Natural History of Alcoholism Revisited* (Harvard University, 1995), he provides an interesting account of the long-term progression with addictive relationships to alcohol. In long-term studies of cohorts of people with addictive relationships to alcohol, he identified the difficulties faced in achieving long-term change and the threats of premature death. He provides a summary of alcoholism and morbidity and mortality (pp. 200–215).

³ Vaillant also explores the important functions of abstinence in a reintegration process. He writes, "it must be remembered that abstinence is a means, not an end. It is a puritanical goal that removes but does not replace. It is justifiable as a treatment goal only if moderate drinking is not a viable alternative and only if sight is not lost of the real goal—social rehabilitation" (Ibid., p. 277).

⁴ Otto Neurath's stated his metaphor as, "We are like sailors who must rebuild their ship on the open sea, never able to dismantle it in dry dock, and to reconstruct it there out of the best materials," quoted on p. 205 in P. Roth (1984), "On missing Neurath's Boat," *Synthese, 61,* 205–231.

⁵   See George DuWors, *White Knuckles and Wishful Thinking: Breaking the Chain of Compulsive Reaction in Alcoholism and Other Addictions* (Hogrefe & Huber, 1992) for a more detailed discussion of the nature of "white-knuckling," particularly his discussion of it in the context of relapse (reversion) (pp. 53–80).

⁶   Most residential addiction treatment programs strongly emphasize the importance of avoiding closely intimate and particularly sexual relationships during the first couple of years of change. Their reasons for this include both the danger of static replacement and the risk of it diverting from the slower process of forming multiple attachments.

⁷   In fact, the research evidence suggests that the majority of those attending programs are unlikely to succeed in maintaining abstinence for over 1 year, as discussed in M. Berglund, S. Thelander, et al. (2003), "Treatment of alcohol abuse: An evidence-based review," *Alcoholism: Clinical and Experimental Research, 27*(10), 1645–1656.

⁸   Stephanie Brown in her model of recovery from alcoholism identifies "transition" as key phase in what she describes as "the alcohol axis" leading onto the phase of "early recovery". See her book, *Treating the Alcoholic: A Development Model of Recovery* (Wiley, 1985) pp. 37–54.

⁹   Vaillant argues that the first years of attempting change are difficult to discern from fluctuations in the relationship. In the natural history of addictive relationships with alcohol a short time frame may dupe people into seeing a fluctuation as evidence of change. See discussions in his article (1988), "What can long-term follow-up teach us about relapse and prevention of relapse in addiction?" *British Journal of Addiction, 83*, 1147–1157, as well as in his book *The Natural History of Alcoholism Revisited* (Harvard University, 1995).

¹⁰ The range of therapies currently employed by addiction practitioners vary widely from body and process oriented approaches (e.g., psychodrama and gestalt therapy), to thinking therapies (e.g., rational emotive therapy and cognitive behavioural therapy) to social approaches (e.g., family therapy and networking therapy). An overview of these is provided in A. Blume, *Treating Drug Problems* (Wiley, 2005), or T. Jarvis, J. Tebbutt, et al. *Treatment Approaches for Alcohol and Drug Dependence,* 2nd ed. (Wiley, 2005).

¹¹ Many countries have shifted their prescribing of opioid substitution from specialist addiction services to primary health. This is aimed to provide improved access, more personalized care and less stigmatization. For discussion of this switch, see M. Weinrich and M. Stuart (2000), "Provision of methadone treatment in primary care medical practices: a review of the Scottish experience and implications for US Policy," *Journal of the American Medical Association, 283*(10), 1343–1348.

¹² In V. Dole and M. Nyswander (1965), "Medical treatment for diacetylmorphine (heroin) addiction," *Ibid. 193*, 645–656.

¹³ For comprehensive coverage, see J. Ward, R. Mattick, et al. (eds.), *Methadone Maintenance Treatment and Other Opioid Replacement Therapies* (Harwood Academic, 2000).

¹⁴ There remains considerable debate regarding whether methadone maintenance merely maintains the status quo or whether it genuinely provides a pathway to reintegration. One group argues that it enables engagement in a process of change; others argue it merely substitutes an illegal with a legal drug. The issues are discussed in N. Seivewright, and J. Greenwood (1996), "What is important in drug misuse treatment?" *Lancet, 347*, 373–376, and in H. Doweiko *Concepts of Chemical Dependency,* 5th ed. (Brooks/Cole, 2002, p. 396).

¹⁵ The term *reversion* has been chosen over the more familiar term *relapse*. Relapse belongs more squarely in a particle paradigm, with a focus on the struggles of

an individual person and implications of relapse from illness. In a social paradigm, the critical focus is on the complex of relationships and when a person "reverts" they are returning to an already established configuration of connections, with the addictive relationship as the central axis.

[16] The results of Project Match have been published in a variety of papers, but a good summary can be found in F. Glaser, N. Heather, et al. (1999) ,"Comments on Project Match: matching alcohol treatments to client heterogeneity" *Addiction, 94*(1), 31–70.

[17] The three conditions were protocolized forms of cognitive behavioral therapy, twelve-step facilitation therapy, and motivational enhancement therapy. The project was not set up to compare the effectiveness of the different therapies, more to investigate which people are more likely to benefit from which type of therapy.

[18] Reviews of controlled studies find similarly that improvements of up to a third of people attending well-structured therapeutic interventions will change but this leaves the large proportion of them reverting back. See W. Miller and P. Wilbourne (2002), "Review: Mesa Grande: a methodological analysis of clinical trials of treatments for alcohol use disorders" *Addiction*, 97, 265–277, and M. Berglund, S. Thelander, et al. (2003), "Treatment of alcohol abuse: an evidence-based review," *Alcoholism: Clinical and Experimental Research, 27*(10), 1645–1656.

[19] In their influential book, *Motivational Interviewing: Preparing People to Change Addictive Behaviour* (Guilford, 1991), William Miller and Steve Rollnick identified reversion (or "relapse") as a common part of what they refer to as the "cycle of change." For example, while giving up smoking, people frequently relapse because they are inadequately prepared for maintenance of the change, mainly because they have underestimated what it might involve to continue and need to be better prepared next time round.

[20] The term *recovery* is more commonly used, both for rehabilitation from addictions and from mental health issues. In mental health it is being increasingly linked to a resiliency or strength building approach to mental health concerns, with emphasis particularly on raising quality of life by building a network of strong connections. See wider discussion of this in J. Russo, *Applying a Strengths Based Approach in Working with People with Developmental Disabilities and their Families* (Manticore, 1998). However, since the term *recovery* emphasizes the psychological rather than the social dimensions of this process, it is better described as "reintegration."

[21] In M. Stanton, T. Todd, et al., *The Family Therapy of Drug Abuse and Addiction* (Guilford, 1982), the authors point out that for adults with addictive relationships to illicit drugs, contrary to what their disorderly and transient lifestyles suggest, "there is a preponderance of evidence... that, despite their protestations of independence, the majority of addicts maintain close family ties" (p. 9).

Chapter 5: Becoming Intimate

[1] From F. Scott Fitzgerald's novel (1934) *Tender Is the Night: A Romance* (Charles Scribner, 1934, p389). This novel is relevant to Fitzgerald's own troubled history with alcohol and depicts the ongoing deterioration in relationships for someone with a similar involvement with intoxication.

[2] Through working as a practitioner I became accustomed to hearing about the negative impact of addictions, such as drunken and offensive behavior, accidents and injuries, repeated court involvements, and work crises. But the one area I found hardest to accept was hearing about the troubles people

experience in their homes. It comes in many forms: parents arguing, children witnessing violence, sexual abuse, emotional neglect, destructive mind games, and so on. It is in the home, in family relationships that addictions do most harm, and yet to the outside world these appear the least visible impacts.

3   The terms *subjectivity* and *phenomenology* are relevant to the perspective adopted throughout this book but have been avoided in the interest of keeping the language accessible to as many readers as possible.

4   I have searched the literature on intimacy and addiction for a suitable framework for this book. While there is some relevant and important pieces (such as Anthony Gidden, *The Transformation of Intimacy: Sexuality, Love, and Eroticism in Modern Societies* (Polity, 1992), and Helen Keane, (2004) "Disorders of desire: addiction and problems of intimacy," *Journal of Medical Humanities, 25*(3), 189–204), I found little available that would support the type of analysis being undertaken in this book. For that reason this chapter uses an original and relatively simple framework for talking about the link between intimate relationships and addictive relationships.

5   Wittgenstein's influential theory of "language as use" and "family resemblances" is developed in his *Philosophical Investigations* (Blackwell, 1974[1953]).

6   George Lakoff, in *Women, Fire, and Dangerous Things: What Categories Reveal About the Mind* (University of Chicago Press, 1987), has explored Wittgenstein's ideas further in arguing that most words we use refer to categories rather than things and that in turn these categories require imaginative reference to concepts (which he calls "idealized cognitive models") that in turn call on social and cultural associations.

7   Wittgenstein's *Philosophical Investigations* (Blackwell, 1974[1953], p. 32).

8   The extensive literature on the effectiveness of counseling and psychotherapy has consistently indicated that the qualities of the practitioner and the relationship with the client matter more that the type of psychotherapeutic methods. For example, Bruce Wampold, in *The Great Psychotherapy Debate: Models, Methods, and Findings* (Lawrence Erlbaum, 2001), summarizes this issue by concluding that psychotherapy can be more effective than placebo, that no particular approach can claim consistently greater effectiveness than another, and that key factors relate to whether or not the therapist has established a positive working alliance with the client, and that this accounts for much more of the variance in outcomes than specific approaches.

9   In recognition of this response, most stars, such as Michael Jackson, will repeatedly emphasize how important their fans are to them.

10 The key importance of a "continuum of risk" perspective in thinking about risks to health was championed by Geoffrey Rose in *The Strategy of Preventive Medicine* (Oxford University Press, 1992) and has been used in a variety of areas in addiction studies where binary conceptions have limited options (such as normal/dependent drinking, social/pathological gambling, and ethical/unethical funding); see J. Gerevich (2005) "Binarisms, regressive outcomes and biases in the drug policy interventions: a theoretical approach," Substance Use and Misuse, 40(4), 451–472; S. Ioannou (2005) "*Health logic and health-related behaviours*" *Critical Public Health*, 15(3), 263–273; and P. J. Adams (1997) "Assessing whether to receive funding support from tobacco, alcohol, gambling and other dangerous consumption industries," *Addiction 102*, 1027–1033.

Chapter 6: Intimacies in Addictive Contexts

1   From Anne Bronte's novel *The Tenant of Wildfell Hall* (Oxford University Press, 1993[1848] p. 245). It is based on her experiences of her brother Branwell's addictive relationship to alcohol and centers on Helen's marriage to Arthur and how his addiction led her and her son to leave him—an unusual response by women in those times.

2   It is possible to conceive of the person personifying the addictive substance/process and constructing an emotional life around it in ways that engage compassion and commitment. For example, the person might conceive of the gambling machine as a personal friend. But this would also require high levels of imagination in ways that might be difficult to sustain.

3   I am grateful to Ken, a person reintegrating from an addictive relationship to alcohol, who many years ago first explained to me some of these feelings. I have since explored these with other people pursuing their paths of reintegration and they identify strongly with these descriptions. They have helped me adapt them into the present configuration.

4   People in addictive relationships have a high likelihood of experiencing anxiety as well as a broad range of other mental health concerns. For example, F. Lotufo-Neto and V. Gentil (1994), "Alcoholism and phobic anxiety: a clinical-demographic comparison," *Addiction, 89*(4), 447–453 examined the effects of phobic anxiety between people both in and not in addictive relationships to alcohol and found that those with more phobic anxiety tended to have more intense addictive relationships with a lower likelihood of change. Also S. Maynard (1997), "Growing up in an alcoholic family system: The effect on anxiety and differentiation of self," *Journal of Substance Abuse, 9*(1), 161–170, examined the interactions between anxiety and growing up in an addictive system.

5   High rates for people in addictive relationships also experiencing severe depression have been reported in studies of both the general population and with people who present to services, see R. Kessler, C. Nelson, et al. (1996), "The epidemiology of co-occurring addictive and mental disorders: implications for prevention and service utilization," *American Journal of Orthopsychiatry, 66*(1), 17–31, and N. Miller, D. Klamen, et al. (1996), "Prevalence of depression and alcohol and other drug dependence in addictions treatment populations," *Journal of Psychoactive Drugs, 28*(2), 111–124.

6   Several of these emotions are described in a study of the lived experience of men attending Alcoholics Anonymous, R. Zakrzewski and M. Hector (2004), "The lived experiences of alcohol addiction: men of Alcoholics Anonymous" *Issues in Mental Health Nursing, 25*: 61–77. Examinations of specific emotions include: on fear, F. Thorberg and M. Lyvers (2006), "Attachment, fear of intimacy and differentiation of self among clients in substance disorder treatment facilities," *Addictive Behaviors, 31*(4), 732–737, and for shame, R. Potter-Efron and D. Efron (1993), "Three models of shame and their relation to the addictive process," *Alcoholism Treatment Quarterly, 10*(1–2), 23–48.

7   In P. Steinglass, L. Bennett, et al. *The Alcoholic Family* (Basic Books, 1987), they point out how addictive systems can attain their own character and equilibrium, which enables them to continue for long periods of time (see discussion later in the chapter).

8   The influence of social norms and their relationship to social surveillance are central to Michelle Foucault's concept of "disciplinary power" as discussed in M. Foucault, *Discipline and Punish: The Birth of the Prison* (Pantheon, 1977). Here norms of belief and behavior become internalized to the extent that a person monitors their own behavior in relation to those norms, so in a sense they become their own jailer.

⁹   Attachment theory is a central approach in developmental psychology that looks at the family processes that influence emergence of personal identity and behavior patterns. It has been applied in many ways to understanding addictive relationships, particularly in the formation and responses by younger people to addictive systems; see R. Finzi-Dottan, Cohen, et al. (2003), "The drug-user husband and his wife: attachment styles, family cohesion, and adaptability." *Substance Use and Misuse 38*(2): 271–292, and A. McNally, T. Palfai, et al. (2003), "Attachment dimensions and drinking-related problems among young adults: the mediational role of coping motives" *Addictive Behaviors, 28*(6), 1115–1127.

¹⁰ P. Steinglass, L. Bennett, et al. *The Alcoholic Family* (Basic Books, 1987).

¹¹ Ibid., p. 49.

¹² Ibid., p. 100.

Chapter 7: Intimacy and Power

¹   Mark Twain's Huckleberry Finn (Whitman, 1955[1890]) p. 38.

²   The impacts of a systematic program of violence typically lead to global effects on the recipients with effects that include impacts on their physical well-being (through stress, neglect of health care), impacts on their mental well-being (high anxiety, depression, posttraumatic effects), impacts on their emotional functioning (low self-esteem, hyperreactivity), and impacts on their social functioning (isolation, low social confidence, deceptive practices). See L.E.A. Walker, *The Battered Woman Syndrome* (Springer, 1984), and M. Bograd, "Power, gender and the family: feminist perspectives on family systems theory," in M. Dutton-Douglas and L. Walker (eds.) *Feminist Psychotherapies: Integration of Therapeutic and Feminist Systems* (Ablex, 1988, pp. 118–133).

³   See H. Johnson, *Dangerous Domains: Violence Against Women in Canada* (Nelson, 1996), and K.E. Leonard, "Alcohol use and marital aggression in newlywed couples," in X. Arriaga and S. Oskamp (eds.), Violence in Intimate Relationships (Sage, 1999, pp. 113–135).

⁴   I have practiced extensively in both the violence and the addiction fields and, thinking back, I find it difficult to recall many families affected by addictive relationships where violence, abuse, or neglect was not happening in some form or at some level. It may not always take the form of strong tactics such as violence or ongoing emotional abuse, but often can take the form of less obvious but more draining strategies such as the unilateral withdrawal of attention and affection and the neglect of the other's needs.

⁵   As described in various papers in J. J. Collins Jr (ed.), *Drinking and Crime: Perspectives on the Relationship between Alcohol Consumption and Criminal Behavior* (Tavistock, 1982). Also see D. G. Saunders, *Violence Against women: Synthesis of Research on Offender Interventions* (National Institute of Justice, 2003).

⁶   In the ten years I was a facilitator in stopping violence programs, at least half of the participants in our programs admit alcohol and drug abuse is associated with their violence, and similar high rates have been reported in other programs, such as F. Fitch and A. Papantonio (1983), "Men who batter: some pertinent characteristics," *Journal of Nervous and Mental Disease, 171*(3), 190–192; P. Kivel, *Men's Work: How to Stop the Violence that Tears Our Lives Apart* (Ballantine, 1992); and M. Testa (2004), "The role of substance use in male-to-female physical and sexual violence: a brief review and recommendations for future research," *Journal of Interpersonal Violence*, 19(12), 1494–1505. Further evidence of a link between substance misuse and male partner in many controlled studies, see E. Gondolf (1995), "Alcohol abuse, wife assault and power needs," *Social Service Review, 69*(2), 274–284; T. O'Farrell

and C. Murphy (1995), "Marital violence before and after alcoholism treatment," *Journal of Consulting and Clinical Psychology, 63*, 256–262; and S. Boles and K. Miotto (2003), "Substance abuse and violence: a review of the literature." *Aggression and Violent Behavior, 8*(2), 155–174.

7   Summaries of research can be found in R. Ackerman (1988), "Complexities of alcohol and abusive families," *Focus on Chemically Dependent Families, 11*(3), 15; and J. Smith (2000), "Addiction medicine and domestic violence," *Journal of Substance Abuse Treatment, 19*(4), 329–338. For example S. Stith, R. Crossman, et al. (1991), "Alcoholism and marital violence: a comparative study of men in alcohol treatment programs and batterer treatment programs," *Alcoholism Treatment Quarterly, 8*(2), 3–20, compared men attending violence intervention programs with those attending alcohol treatment programs and found very little difference between them, and thus they recommended screening men who are both violent and addicted for tailored interventions.

8   For example, Jerry Flanzer states in "Alcohol and other drugs are key causal agents of violence" in R. Gelles and D. Loseke, *Current Controversies on Family Violence* (Sage, p. 178), "An individual harboring intense underlying anger that has been contained by psychological defence mechanisms can become physically aggressive and intimidating as a result of the of the disinhibiting effects of alcohol".

9   The literature on the biological processes associated with alcohol and violence is quite large. For fuller discussion, see S. Boles and K. Miotto (2003), "Substance abuse and violence: a review of the literature," *Aggression and Violent Behavior, 8*(2), 155–174, and P. Hoaken and S. Stewart (2003), "Drugs of abuse and the elicitation of human aggressive behavior," *Addictive Behaviors, 28*(9), 1533–1554.

10 Neurotransmitters are chemicals that enable transfer of electrical pulses between neurons and thereby relaying signals across the nervous system.

11 See an overview in A. Badawy (2003), "Alcohol and violence and the possible role of serotonin," *Criminal Behaviour and Mental Health, 13*(1), 31–44.

12 Richard Gelles challenges the relevance of the notion of disinhibition with respect to violence and supports this with reference to research on culture, laboratory experiments, blood tests on men arrested, and survey research. See R. Gelles, "Alcohol and other drugs are associated with violence: they are not its cause." *Current Controversies on Family Violence* (Sage, 1993, pp. 182–196). Kai Pernanen (1997), "Uses of 'disinhibition' in the explanation of intoxicated behavior," *Contemporary Drug Problems, 24*, 703–729, examines the various senses of "disinhibition" and concludes that while in some formal senses alcohol acts as a disinhibitor, this is different than claiming a causal link. Along similar lines, Sarah Galvani (2004), "Responsible disinhibition: alcohol, men and violence to women," *Addiction Research and Theory, 12*(4), 357–371, argues for the notion of "responsible disinhibition" where the intoxicated man is still held accountable for his violent behavior.

13 In considering the relationship between alcohol and violence against women, R. Tolman and L. Bennett (1990), "A review of quantitative research on men who batter," *Journal of Interpersonal Violence, 5*(1), state: "The widely held belief that drinking directly causes woman abuse is questionable in the light of experimental evidence that expectancy of alcohol-related aggression is a better predictor of aggressive behaviour than is the consumption of alcohol.... Although acute alcohol intoxication has proven to be a better predictor of general crimes of violence... it is chronic alcohol abuse that better predicts woman abuse" (p. 90).

14 The significance of the closeness of intoxication is hotly contested. See the introduction by C. Wekerle and A. Wall (eds.) in *The Violence and Addiction Equation: Theoretical*

and Clinical Issues in Substance Abuse and Relationship Violence (Brunner/Mazel, 2002). See also discussion of the complexities in C. Humphreys, L. Regan, et al. (2005). "Domestic violence and substance use: Tackling complexity" *British Journal of Social Work, 35*(8), 1303–1320.

[15] For example, the relationship of cannabis to violence is well documented. Summaries of the literature are in T. Brown, A. Werk, et al. (1999), "Violent substance abusers in domestic violence treatment," *Violence and Victims, 14*, 179–190, and T. Moore and G. Stuart (2005), "A review of the literature on marijuana and interpersonal violence," *Aggression and Violent Behavior*, 10(2), 171–192.

[16] The literature here is relatively new, but research is beginning to appear on gambling: V. Lorenz and R. Yaffee (1988), "Pathological gambling and psychosomatic, emotional and mental difficulties as reported by the spouse," *Journal of Gambling Behavior*, 4, 13–26, and R. Muelleman, T. DenOtter, et al. (2002), "Problem gambling in the partner of the emergency department patient as a risk factor for intimate partner violence," *Journal of Emergency Medicine, 23*(3), 307–312. On work, B. Robinson and P. Post (1997), "Risk of addiction to work and family functioning," *Psychological Reports*, 81(1), 91–95. The research on addictive relationships to sex has yet to get underway, but a number of practitioner and self-help books have been published such as E. Griffin-Shelley, *Sex and Love: Addiction Treatment and Recovery* (Praeger/ Greenwood, 1997).

[17] I have often worked with families where partners and children who were exposed for long periods to an addictive system, even though they have left long before, still fear talking about their experiences 20 or 30 years later. Some women remain in severely violent relationships for decades. This contrasts, in my experience, with what happens with nonaddictive violent contexts where women often attempt to escape their relationships within 5 to 10 years.

[18] See C. MacAndrew and R. Edgerton, *Drunken Comportment: A Social Explanation* (Aldine, 1969).

[19] Ibid., p. 165.

[20] This perspective also connects with the "alcohol expectancies" literature in psychology, which argues that if people believe they will be violent when they drink, then they will probably act violently; see J. Collins and P. Messerschmidt (1993), "Epidemiology of alcohol-related violence," *Alcohol Health and Research World, 17*(2), 93–99. In a survey of over 1000 students, R. Lindman and A. Lang (1994), "The alcohol-aggression stereotype: a cross-cultural comparison of beliefs," *International Journal of the Addictions, 29*(1), 1–13, found student expectations of what intoxicated aggression meant varied according to different cultural backgrounds. Furthermore, Holly Johnson (2000), "The role of alcohol in male partners' assaults on wives," *Journal of Drug Issues, 30*(4), 725–740, analyzed a large Canadian sample (12,300) of woman and found that once negative attitudes to women were factored out, the relationship between alcohol and violence became nonsignificant.

[21] See R. L. Sexton, "Ritualized inebriation, violence, and social control in Cajun Mardi Gras," *Anthropological Quarterly, 74*(1), 37.

[22] A feminist interpretation of violence is sometimes referred to as "profeminist" as a way of including men who support the primary assumptions of feminism. For discussion of this, see E. Gondolf (1985), "Anger and oppression in men who batter: empiricist and feminist perspectives and their implications for research," *Victimology: An International Journal, 10*, 311–324, E. Pence and M. Paymar, *Education Groups for Men Who Batter: The Duluth Model* (Springer, 1993). Alternatively it is referred to as a "sociological" approach, see R. Dobash, R. Dobash, et al., "Confronting violent men," in J. Hanmer and C. Itzin (eds.), *Home Truths About Domestic Violence: Feminist Influences on Policy and Practice: A Reader* (Routledge, 2000). In this approach male partner violence is interpreted as a sociopolitical problem as described by D. Adams, "Feminist based

interventions for battering men," in P. Caesar and L. Hamberger, *Treating Men Who Batter: Theory, Practice and Programs* (Springer, 1989, p. 3), where controlling behavior needs to be understood in the context of the whole social ecology that provides support for violence. As also described in J. Edleson and R. Tolman, *Intervention for Men Who Batter: An Ecological Approach* (Sage, 1992).

[23] Further examination of the social and political utility of violence can be found in Z. Eisikovits and J. Edleson (1989), "Intervening with men who batter: a critical review of the literature," *Social Services Review,* (September), 384–414, and in K. Yllö, "Through a feminist lens: gender, power, and violence," in R. Gelles and D. Loseke, *Current Controversies on Family Violence* (Sage, 1993, pp. 47–60).

[24] The broader social supports have been tracked back to male entitlement beliefs, see P. Adams, A. Towns, et al., "Dominance and entitlement: the rhetoric men use to discuss their violence towards women," in M. Talbot et al. *Language and Power in the Modern World* (Edinburgh University, 2003, pp. 184–198). Violence supporting beliefs based on male privilege are described in M. Russell, "Wife assault theory, research, and treatment: a literature review," *Journal of Family Violence, 3*, 193–208, and institutional beliefs on the overriding importance of protecting marriages in N. Robertson (1999), "Stopping violence programmes: enhancing the safety of battered women or producing better-educated batterers?" *New Zealand Journal of Psychology, 28*(2), 88–78, which also points out how stopping violence programs themselves can be used as a means of furthering the repertoire of justifications and potentially up-skilling abusers.

[25] Key works in this area include: on responsibility, see A. Jenkins, *Invitations to Responsibility: The Therapeutic Engagement of Men Who Are Violent and Abusive* (Dulwich Centre Publications, 1990). On beliefs that support violence, see E. Pence and M. Paymar, *Education Groups for Men Who Batter: The Duluth Model* (Springer, 1993), and on broader supports, see S. Schechter and L. Gary, "A framework for understanding and empowering battered women," in M. Straus, *Abuse and Victimization Across the Lifespan* (John Hopkins, 1988, pp. 240–253).

[26] In a series of articles, my colleagues and I have argued that feminist approaches move beyond particle interpretations and include the social and political dynamics of abuse. See Adams, P. J. (in press), "Interventions with men who are violent to their partners: strategies for early engagement," *Journal of Marital and Family Therapy*, and A. Towns and P. Adams (2000), "'If I really loved him enough, he would be okay': Women's accounts of male partner violence," *Violence Against Woman, 6*(6), 558–585.

[27] For instance, in a U.K. interview study with 2027 participants, K Graham, M. Plant, et al. (2004), "Alcohol, gender and partner aggression: a general population study of British adults," *Addiction Research and Theory, 12*(4), 385–401, reported that heavier alcohol use increased the level of reported interpersonal violence and that in these circumstances slightly more women than men admitted to being violent

[28] For a comprehensive discussion on silencing, see the editor's introduction in L. Thiesmeyer (ed.), *Discourse and Silencing: Representation and the Language of Displacement* (John Benjamins, 2003), and the chapter in the same book by my colleagues and I entitled "Silencing Talk of Men's Violence Towards Women."

[29] This is, of course, the central idea behind Foucault's notion of "disciplinary power," where surveillance strategies lead people to become in a sense their own jailer, monitoring their own behavior with regard to imposed or evolved societal norms. For broader discussions of this in relation to violence, see N. Gavey, *Just Sex? The Cultural Scaffolding of Rape* (Routledge, 2004), and A. Towns and P. Adams (2000), "'If I really loved him enough, he would be okay': women's accounts of male partner violence," *Violence Against Woman, 6*(6), 558–585.

Chapter 8: Fragmented Lives

[1] From Frank McCourt's autobiographical account of his early childhood, *Angela's Ashes: A Memoir of a Childhood* (Flamingo, 1997, p. 207).

[2] The surprising paucity of research in this area is highlighted in reviews such as R. Velleman and J. Orford, *Risk and Resilience: Adults Who Were the Children of Problem Drinkers* (Harwood Academic, 1999), and S. Harter (2000), "Psychosocial adjustment of adult children of alcoholics: a review of the recent empirical literature," *Clinical Psychology Review, 20*(3), 311–337.

[3] See K. Sher, K. Walitzer, et al. (1991), "Characteristics of children of alcoholics: Putative risk factors, substance use and abuse, and psychopathology," *Journal of Abnormal Psychology, 100*, 427–448.

[4] See R. Mathew, W. Wilson, et al. (1993), "Psychiatric disorders in adult children of alcoholics: Data from the Epidemiologic Catchment Area project," *American Journal of Psychiatry, 150*, 793–800.

[5] See P. Steinglass, L. Bennett, et al., *The Alcoholic Family* (Basic Books, 1987, p. 18).

[6] For example, S. Harter (2000), "Psychosocial adjustment of adult children of alcoholics: a review of the recent empirical literature" *Clinical Psychology Review, 20*(3), 311–337, argues that the research is inadequate as yet to draw conclusions; methodological weaknesses include small sample sizes and lack of comparison groups.

[7] These factors are covered in reviews by J. Ritter, M. Stewart, et al. (2002), "Effects of childhood exposure to familial alcoholism and family violence on adolescent substance use, conduct problems, and self-esteem," *Journal of Traumatic Stress, 15*(2), 113–122, and A. Barrett and R. Turner (2006), "Family structure and substance use problems in adolescence and early adulthood: examining explanations for the relationship," *Addiction, 101*(1), 109–120.

[8] For example, using a general measure of mental health concerns, A. Fulton and W. Yates (1990), "Adult children of alcoholics: a valid diagnostic group?" *Journal of Nervous and Mental Disease, 178*, 505–508, failed to find significant differences in the frequency of mental disorders for people in addictive relationships than for other populations. These included depressive and anxiety disorders.

[9] In a long-term study of 500 heavy drinkers in the English West Midlands, J. Orford, and S. Dalton (2005), "A four-year follow-up of close family members of Birmingham untreated heavy drinkers," *Addiction Research and Theory, 13*(2), 155–170, they followed 25 close family members over 4 years and found, surprisingly, that as time went on, the family members considered the drinking in more benign terms.

[10] As resilience research has established itself more strongly in studying risks to youth well-being, the approach is becoming more frequently applied to dangerous consumptions as illustrated in K. Griffin, G. Botvin, et al. (2003), "Effectiveness of a universal drug abuse prevention approach for youth at high risk for substance use initiation," *Preventive Medicine, 36*(1), 1–7; C. Olsson, L. Bond, et al. (2003), "Adolescent resilience: a concept analysis," *Journal of Adolescence, 26*, 1–11; and A. Carle and L. Chassin (2004), "Resilience in a community sample of children of alcoholics: its prevalence and relation to internalizing symptomatology and positive affect," *Applied Developmental Psychology, 25*, 577–595.

[11] For example, J. Ritter, M. Stewart, et al. (2002), "Effects of childhood exposure to familial alcoholism and family violence on adolescent substance use, conduct problems, and self-esteem," *Journal of Traumatic Stress, 15*(2), 113–122, examined three domains of adolescent functioning in a high-risk community sample of 109 families and found that the combination of childhood exposure to addictive family systems plus exposure to family violence were associated with their psychosocial functioning as adolescents.

[12] For example, S. Harter and T. Taylor (2000), "Parental alcoholism, child abuse, and adult adjustment," *Journal of Substance Abuse, 11*(1), 31–44, explored exposures to parents in addictive relationships to alcohol and abuse for 333 college students. They found that symptom distress and social maladjustment was more pronounced for those who had experienced both addictive home contexts and abuse.

[13] A range of factors can play a role, for example, the age for intimates when the addictive relationship emerged, their developmental stage, the nature of the way they left home, the stage at which they try to reform their own intimacies; see R. Ackerman and E. Gondolf (1991), "Adult children of alcoholics: the effects of background and treatment on ACOA symptoms," *International Journal of Addictions, 26*, 1159–1171.

[14] In the absence of other material I have devised these examples from my experience with addictive systems through my work as an addiction practitioner. The intention behind presenting so many examples is to highlight the wide diversity and complexity in intimate responses in addictive family systems.

[15] The processes of early parental attachments have a strong influence over how intimacy is approached in later life. Developmental literature on attachment is extensive. A good overview is provided by R. Karen, *Becoming Attached: First Relationships and How they Shape our Capacity to Love* (Oxford University Press, 1998).

[16] These issues in addictive family systems are explored in M. Stanton, T. Todd, et al., *The Family Therapy of Drug Abuse and Addiction* (Guilford, 1982).

[17] Ibid. Stanton and colleagues provide many illustrations of how adults and children in addictive systems end up taking on inappropriate roles that lead onto forming enmeshed alliances across the parental divide that have negative impacts on all involved.

[18] In their review M. West and R. Prinz (1987), "Parental alcoholism and childhood psychopathology," *Psychological Bulletin, 102*(2), 204–218, the authors outlined how children in addictive systems, particularly boys, display outwardly hostile behaviors that can develop into conduct disorders and other behavioral problems.

[19] The research on the long-term impacts of childhood exposure to addictive family systems is still emergent and is coming up with inconsistent findings. Until research methods improve, all we can say generally is that many such children grow up with issues associated with antisocial behavior, mental health issues (such as anxiety and depression), and relationship difficulties. See the review by S. Harter and T. Taylor (2000), "Parental alcoholism, child abuse, and adult adjustment," *Journal of Substance Abuse, 11*(1), 31–44.

[20] While attachment theory has found applications to understanding the effects of growing up in an addictive system, such as N. El-Guebaly, M. West, et al. (1993), "Attachment among adult children of alcoholics," *Addiction, 88*, 1405–1411, a specific focus on adolescents has yet to be fully explored. See also J. Ritter, M. Stewart, et al. (2002), "Effects of childhood exposure to familial alcoholism and family violence on adolescent substance use, conduct problems, and self-esteem," *Journal of Traumatic Stress, 15*(2), 113–122.

[21] Resilience theory has been extensively applied to a wide range of issues associated with adolescent development. For instance, in S. Fergus and M. Zimmerman (2005), "Adolescent resilience: a framework for understanding healthy development in the face of risk," *Annual Review of Public Health, 26*, 399–419, the authors identify three models of resilience—compensatory, protective, and challenge—with each involving different types of research. The approach has been applied to adolescent substance use, violence, and sexual risk, and this is discussed in A. Carle and L. Chassin (2004), "Resilience in a community sample of children of alcoholics: its prevalence and relation to internalizing symptomatology and positive affect," *Journal of Applied Developmental Psychology, 25*, 577–595. In this article the authors stated that "resilience has not been adequately studied in the children of alcoholic parents literature and little information exists regarding this group" (p. 579). It is a promising area for future research.

[22] Proactive employee assistance programs (EAPs) develop workplace systems where a potentially troubled employee is identified via documented evidence of impaired job performance and then referred to peer referral officers who assist them in accessing appropriate counseling, which, in the case of troubles associated with addictive substances/processes might involve brief motivational counseling or constructive confrontation. Descriptions of these approaches are provided in T. Blum and P. Roman (1992), "A description of clients using employment assistance programs," *Alcohol Health & Research World, 16,* 120–127, and S. Milne, T. Blum, et al. (1994), "Factors influencing employees' propensity to use an employee assistance program," *Personnel Psychology, 47,* 123–145.

[23] In an upcoming article on relapse, P. Adams and H. Warren (in press), "Responding to the risks associated with the relapse of recovering staff members within addiction services," *Substance Use and Abuse,* we explore the widespread impacts on addiction services when employees and managers with historical addictive relationships experience a reversion. They can have strong impact on clients, colleagues, and services.

[24] A World Health Organization (WHO)-sponsored analysis of alcohol and public health mainly in European countries, G. Edwards, P. Anderson, et al., *Alcohol Policy and the Public Good* (Oxford University Press, 1994, p. 35), outlines how countries such as Spain and France, which consume high amounts of alcohol, also had to contend with high health, justice system, and social costs.

[25] The reluctance of medical practitioners to enter into discussions about addictive relationships with people affected is well documented with people in addictive relationships. For example, in the United States a national survey of 648 primary care physicians found 94 percent failed to include substance abuse among five diagnoses they offered when presented with early symptoms of alcohol abuse in an adult patient. See CASA National Center on Addiction and Substance Abuse, *Missed Opportunity: National Survey of Primary Care Physicians and Patients on Substance Abuse* (Columbia University, 2000). Similar concerning findings are noted in M. Fleming (2004), "Screening and brief intervention in primary care settings," *Alcohol Research and Health, 28*(2), 57–62, and in our own work with WHO, P. Adams, A. Powell, et al. (1997), "Incentives for general practitioners to provide brief interventions for alcohol problems," *New Zealand Medical Journal, 110,* 291–294.

[26] This is also undoubtedly related to privileges enjoyed by men in terms of higher access (customary and economic) to most dangerous consumptions. For example, in a comparison of addictive relationships to drugs between the U.S. and U.K., in both countries higher prevalence was associated with "being male, non-married, of a low socio-economic status (SES), and living in an urban setting," in C. Furr-Holden and J. Anthony (2003), "Epidemiologic differences in drug dependence—a US-UK cross-national comparison," *Social Psychiatry and Psychiatric Epidemiology, 38*(4), 165–172.

[27] Various studies have found varying impacts on a child depending on whether the parent is the father or the mother. For example, in a long-term study of 85,000 children in Denmark, M. Christoffersena, and K. Soothill (2003) ,"The long-term consequences of parental alcohol abuse: a cohort study of children in Denmark," *Journal of Substance Abuse Treatment, 25,* 107–116, the authors found that the range of negative effects were worse when the mother rather than the father was in the addictive relationship. They concluded, "A mother's alcohol abuse may have somewhat different consequences from a father's alcohol abuse" (p. 115) and that future research needs to improve our understanding of these gender relationships.

[28] Women's options in leaving partner's in addictive relationships are arguably influenced by factors such as fewer educational and economic opportunities, the needs for child care, and social expectations of women to remain devoted to their partners.

[29] In S. Greenfield, A. Brooks, et al. (2007), "Substance abuse treatment entry, retention, and outcome in women," *Drug and Alcohol Dependence, 86,* 1–21, the authors reviewed the

literature examining characteristics associated with treatment outcome in women with substance use disorders, and concluded that while gender specific treatment programs do not necessarily improve treatment retention or outcome, they are better suited for women with specific issues (such as co-occurring issues with sexual abuse or eating disorders). Other reviews of gender dynamics include D. Heath (1991), "Women and alcohol: cross-cultural perspectives," *Journal of Substance Abuse 3*(2): 175–185, and D. Gefou-Madianou (ed.), *Alcohol, Gender and Culture* (Routledge, 1992).

30 Arguably this also applies to illicit drugs, where state policy on customs and law enforcement significantly influence supply and cost.

31 Prior to the modern proliferation of gambling in Western-style democracies, traditional forms of gambling such as track betting and poker were dominated by men. With the rise of continuous forms of gambling (e.g., electronic gambling machines and casino tables), the participation of women and their levels of problem gambling have quickly risen and are approaching male rates, see J. Hraba and G. Lee (1996), "Gender, gambling and problem gambling," *Journal of Gambling Studies, 12*(1), 83–101, and R. Desai, P. Maciejewski, et al. (2006), "Gender differences among recreational gamblers: association with the frequency of alcohol use," *Psychology of Addictive Behaviors, 20*(2), 145–153.

32 An overview of the diverse ways alcohol is incorporated into cultural practices is provided in D. Heath, *Drinking Occasions: Comparative Perspectives on Alcohol and Culture* (Brunner/Mazel, 2000).

33 See essay collections by D. Gefou-Madianou (ed.), *Alcohol, Gender and Culture* (Routledge, 1992), and D. Heath, *Drinking Occasions: Comparative Perspectives on Alcohol and Culture* (Brunner/Mazel, 2000), and a special issue edited by M. Marshall, G. Ames, et al. (2001), "Anthropological perspectives on alcohol and drugs at the turn of the new millennium," *Social Science and Medicine, 53*(2), 153–64.

34 A description of this sequence is provided in S. Tse, J. Wong, et al. (2004), "A public health approach for Asian people with problem gambling in foreign countries," *Journal of Gambling Issues, 12*, 1–15, and C. Jiacheng (1995), "China," in D. Heath (ed.), *International Handbook on Alcohol and Culture* (Greenwood, 1995, pp. 42–50).

35 Mac Marshall's most influential work on drinking and Pacific culture is his *Weekend Warriors: Alcohol in Micronesian Culture* (Mayfield, 1979). His notion of "weekend warriors" could also be extended into understanding customary drinking practices in modern Western societies. Also his edited book, *Beliefs, Behaviors and Alcoholic Beverages in Cross Cultural Survey* (University of Michigan Press, 1979), provides another detailed look into the interrelationships between alcohol use and changes in Pacific culture.

36 In a detailed study of Niuean men in Auckland, Vili Nosa interviewed them about their changes in their drinking practices since migrating to New Zealand. While binge drinking was a common pattern, he found many of their practices differentiated strongly from their heavy drinking European contemporaries. V. Nosa, *The Perceptions and Use of Alcohol Among Niuean Men Living in Auckland* (Unpublished PhD dissertation, University of Auckland, 2005).

37 The interactions between colonization and addiction issues is summarized in M. Gracey (1998), "Substance misuse in Aboriginal Australians," *Addiction Biology, 3*, 29–46, and L. French (2004), "Alcohol and other drug addictions among Native Americans: the movement toward tribal-centric treatment programs," *Alcoholism Treatment Quarterly, 22*(1), 81–91.

38 In D. Heath, "An anthropological view of alcohol and culture in international perspective," in his *International Handbook on Alcohol and Culture* (Greenwood 1995, pp. 328–347), he provides an overview of using anthropological methods in understanding the interactions of alcohol use with culture.

Chapter 9: Collective Opportunities

[1] Quoted in A. Sinclair, *Dylan Thomas: No Man More Magical* (Holt, Rinehart & Winston, 1975, p.172) from letters from Laugharne in early 1950s shortly before his death.

[2] An academic exploration of the inner power dimensions relating to addictions cannot be adequately done within either the particle or social paradigm. We need a third critical paradigm, an "experiential" or "existential" paradigm, which involves assumptions that equip the study of the complexities in this area. This third paradigm and its application to addictions will be a key focus of my work and writing over the next few years.

[3] The importance of the concept of empowerment for community development is reviewed by N. Wallerstein (2006) for the World Health Organization in What Is the Evidence on Effectiveness of Empowerment to Improve Health? (*WHO Regional Office for Europe's Health Evidence Network*, 2006). The review highlights how empowering initiatives can lead to positive health outcomes and reduce disparities in health. Also the thinking on community empowerment is outlined by Ron Labonte. (1990), "Empowerment: Notes on Professional and Community Dimensions," *Canadian Review of Social Policy, 26*, 64–75.

[4] For a review of how the health of communities can be improved using the principles of community empowerment, see G. Laverack, *Health Promotion Practice: Power and Empowerment* (Sage, 2004, pp. 60–72).

[5] Community development literature in both developed and developing countries provides many examples where organizations in positions of power (governments, aid agencies, international bodies) impose their ideas of how a particular community should develop. Their efforts often falter because communities have difficulties owning the initiatives. For critical discussion of this, see N. Wallerstein (1992), "Powerlessness, empowerment, and health: implications for health promotion program," *American Journal of Health Promotion, 6*, 197–205, and R. Labonte and G. Laverack (2001), "Capacity building in health promotion, Part 1: for whom? And for what purpose?" *Critical Public Health, 11*(2), 111–127.

[6] Considerable research on youth has focused on the various ways in which social connectedness (connectedness to school, parents, and peers) contributes to strength and resilience. For discussion on this literature, see R. Baumeister, and M. Leary (1995), "The need to belong: desire for interpersonal attachments as a fundamental human motivation," *Psychological Bulletin, 117*(3), 497–529, and A. Masten, H. Gest, et al. (1999), "Competence in the context of adversity: pathways to resilience and maladaptation from childhood to late adolescence," *Development and Psychopathology, 11*, 143–169.

[7] The relationship between resilience and social involvement with alcohol issues is outlined in R. Velleman, and J. Orford, *Risk and Resilience: Adults Who Were the Children of Problem Drinkers* (Harwood Academic, 1999), and in A. Carle and L. Chassin (2004), "Resilience in a community sample of children of alcoholics: its prevalence and relation to internalizing symptomatology and positive affect," *Applied Developmental Psychology, 25*, 577–595.

[8] I have opted for the term *social capacity* because it can be used more flexibly than other equivalent terms such as community capacity and social capital.

[9] The different experiences between men and women in addictive systems and accessing services are being increasingly researched. See T. Brown, M. Kokin, et al. (1995), "The role of spouses of substance abusers in treatment: gender differences," *Journal of Psychoactive Drugs 27*(3): 223–229, and S. Greenfield, A. Brooks, et al. (2007), "Substance abuse treatment entry, retention, and outcome in women: a review of the literature," *Drug and Alcohol Dependence, 86*, 1–21.

10   This is a weakness in motivational interviewing approaches, which rely heavily on psychological theory such that the responsibility for moving through each stage of change and actually changing is still located with the individual, without acknowledging the wider context and the other layers of responsibility. For example, the structural influences on change (class, poverty, colonization) are de-emphasized.

11   This is most obvious in individual treatment approaches, but also reflected in motivational and brief intervention approaches, which locate the responsibility for change almost exclusively on the individual.

12   The concept of "community" is complex and multidimensional, as illustrated in B. Israel, B. Checkoway, et al. (1994), "Health education and community empowerment: conceptualizing and measuring perceptions of individual, organisational and community control," *Health Education Quarterly, 21*(2), 149–170.

13   As will be discussed more fully in Chapter 11, several current interventions aim to engage family members as a means of later engaging the person in the addictive relationship. For example, J. Barber, and B. Crisp (1995), "The 'pressures to change' approach to working with the partners of heavy drinkers," *Addiction, 90*, 269–276, developed procedures for engaging family members as a means of putting pressure on the person in the addictive relationship to change. A summary of these strategies is provided in A. Copello, R. Velleman, et al. (2005), "Family interventions in the treatment of alcohol and drug problems," *Drug and Alcohol Review, 24*, 369–385.

14   A further complication related to the ownership of change centers on where the intent for change first arises, in other words, identifying who really wants the change. This is not always easy, particularly in a social world where motives are interconnected across many layers. Nonetheless, in some circumstances the key instigators are obvious and where they clearly operate with their own agendas from more powerful positions, they have a reduced capacity for engaging ownership and consequently are less likely to be effective. For example, government research may detect a rise in marital violence associated with alcohol use, and health department officials decide to invest in appropriate harm reduction strategies. Part of their plan includes deploying addiction counselors to work alongside physicians to engage referrals in considering change. Since the counselors' performance is appraised according to how many clients they engage, they become highly motivated in pursuing the government's agenda. Through interactions, the top-down intentions of the counseling soon become obvious and to the counselors' dismay clients become reluctant to attend sessions. What such strategies failed to take into account is that each client is likely to be at a different point on the twin cycles of social fragmentation in which change is only a fleeting possibility, and even if the timing is right, the engagement is likely to be minimal if it is seen as somebody else's idea.

Chapter 10: Reintegration

1   From *The Collected Poems of Theodore Roethke* (Faber & Faber, 1966, p. 19). Roethke faced his own ongoing struggles with an addictive relationship to alcohol.

2   See the excellent discussion of this in G. Lakoff and M. Johnson, *Metaphors We Live By* (University of Chicago Press, 1979).

3   In a detailed exploration of the rhetoric used in modern economics, Don (Dierdre) McCloskey in *The Rhetoric of Economics* (Harvester Press, 1985) explores how heavily rhetorical devices are used in academic literature to generate a sense of neutrality and objectivity.

4   See this discussed in D. Massaro (1986), "The computer as a metaphor for psychological inquiry: considerations and recommendations," *Behaviour Research Methods, Instruments*

and Computers, 18, 73–92. This type of metaphor is also discussed by J. Searle, *Minds, Brains and Science* (Harvard University Press, 1984).

5   Together AA, NA and Al-Anon have generated a vast number of self-help brochures, booklets, and books. For example, a GSO archive of brochures, books, and other material is available at: http://www.alcoholics-anonymous.org/en_gso_archives.cfm (accessed Feb 2007).

6   Books written as self-help guides for reintegrating families and couples include C. Patterson-Sterling, *Rebuilding Relationships in Recovery: A Guide to Healing Relationships Impacted by Addiction* (Xlibris, 2004), and C. Nakken, *Reclaim Your Family from Addiction: How Couples and Families Recover Love and Meaning* (Hazelden, 2000).

7   The importance of the body and spatiality is increasingly seen as playing a role in social identity and social relating. Summaries of this literature can be found in I. Burkitt, *Bodies of Thought: Embodiment, Identity and Modernity* (Sage, 1999), and C. Shilling (2003), *The Body and Social Theory* (Sage, 1999).

8   Self-help guide books on recovery provide strong emphasis on attention to physical well-being, relaxation strategies, and reducing stress. See N. Denzin, *The Alcoholic Society: Addiction and Recovery of the Self* (Transaction, 1993), and B. Ley-Jacobs, *Nature's Road to Recovery: Nutritional Supplements for the Recovering Alcoholic, Chemical-dependent and the Social Drinker: A Health Learning Handbook* (BL Publications, 1999).

9   Discussions of AA and spirituality can be found in *Alcoholics Anonymous,* 4th ed. (AA World Services, 1976), and also summaries in C. Cook (2004), "Addiction and spirituality," *Addiction, 99*(5), 539–551, and A. Morjaria and J. Orford (2002), "The role of religion and spirituality in recovery from drink problems: a qualitative study of Alcoholics Anonymous members and South Asian men," *Addiction Research and Theory, 10*(3), 225–256.

10   I have completed a detail study of these experiences and how they communicate them in *A Rhetoric of Mysticism* (unpublished PhD dissertation, University of Auckland, 1991).

Chapter 11: Family Resources

1   From Marian Keyes's novel, *Rachel's Holiday* (Penguin 1997, p. 578), about a woman's reluctant experiences in an addiction rehabilitation program.

2   There are also more drug specific groups such as Marijuana Anonymous and Cocaine Anonymous. See discussion in R. Room and T. Greenfield (1993), "Alcoholics anonymous, other 12-step movements and psychotherapy in the US population, 1990," *Addiction, 88*(4), 555–562, and M. Peyrot (1985), "Narcotics anonymous: its history, structure, and approach" *International Journal of Addictions,* 20(10), 1509–1522.

3   For example, the concept of codependency has been criticized for the way it overextends understanding of addiction and pathologizes women. See articles by S. Anderson (1994), "A critical analysis of the concept of codependency," *Social Work, 39*(6), 677–685, and L. Stafford (2001), "Is codependency a meaningful concept?" *Issues in Mental Health Nursing, 22*(3), 273–286.

4   A breakdown of attendance is available on AA General Service Office, *AA Fact File* (AA Publishing, 1956 [2006], p. 7).

5   Mariana Valverde's (1998), *Diseases of the Will: Alcohol and the Dilemmas of Freedom* (Cambridge University Press, 1998, p. 122).

6   As outlined in Chapter 4, at the start of a reintegration process the reformation of connections will take time, and in the meantime a person may need to seek transitional replacement of the addictive relationship using a potent involvement, which in the twelve-step context could include an inner connectedness with a higher power, or

simply social connectedness with people in the meetings and with people in the movement as a whole.

[7] See, for example, overviews provided by C. Whitfield (1989), "Co-dependence: our most common addiction—some physical, mental, emotional and spiritual perspectives," *Alcoholism Treatment Quarterly, 6,* 19–36, and M. Hands and G. Dear (1994), "Co-dependency: a critical review," *Drug and Alcohol Review, 13,* 437–445.

[8] The publications are many, but leading books include M. Beattie, *Codependent No More* (Collins Dove, 1989); R. Norwood, *Women Who Love Too Much* (Arrow Books, 1990); and P. Mellody, *Facing Codependence* (Harper & Row, 1989).

[9] This view is echoed in criticisms by Eve Sedgewick in her influential essay "Epidemics of the Will" in *Tendencies* (Duke University Press, 1998, 130–142), and in M. Valverde, *Diseases of the Will* (Cambridge University Press, 1998, pp. 34–35, 128).

[10] The literature on the effectiveness of family approaches has been summarized in A. Copello, R. Velleman, et al. (2005), " Family interventions in the treatment of alcohol and drug problems," *Drug and Alcohol Review, 24,* 369–385, as well as in W. Miller and P. Wilbourne (2002), "Review: Mesa Grande: a methodological analysis of clinical trials of treatments for alcohol use disorders," *Addiction, 97,* 265–277.

[11] Ibid., p. 276, and quoted by A. Copello, R. Velleman, et al. (2005), "Family interventions in the treatment of alcohol and drug problems," *Drug and Alcohol Review, 24,* 369–385.

[12] More familiarly called the therapeutic community or TC movement, but the term "micro-" has been included to differentiate it from the more macro-community approaches that are discussed in the next chapter.

[13] Pauline O'Flaherty, Being Strong: *An Exploration of Discourses Concerning Transition to Life Beyond Residential Drug and Alcohol Treatment* (unpublished thesis, University of Auckland, 1999).

[14] The Johnson intervention, named after the Johnson Institute, is described in detail in G. Loneck, J. Garret, et al. (1996), "The Johnson intervention and relapse during outpatient treatment," *American Journal of Drug and Alcohol Abuse, 22,* 233–246.

[15] Ibid. pp 233–246. See also in the same journal, pp. 1421–1440.

[16] See M. Liepman, "Using family influence to motivate resistant alcoholics to enter treatment: the Johnson Institute approach," in T. O'Farrell, *Treating Alcohol Problems: Marital and Family Interventions* (Guilford Press, 1993, pp. 54–77).

[17] Outlined in J. Garrett, J. Landau, et al. (1998), "The ARISE intervention-using family and network links to engage addicted persons in treatment," *Journal of Substance Abuse Treatment, 15,* 333–343.

[18] Described in detail in their book, R. Meyers and W. Miller (eds.), *A Community Reinforcement Approach to Addiction Treatment* (Cambridge University Press, 2001).

[19] As outlined by G. Hunt, and N. Azrin (1973), "A community-reinforcement approach to alcoholism," *Behavior Research and Therapy, 11,* 91–104. The approach was originally developed in Illinois as a treatment package involving a range of treatment strategies that included job-finding, marital therapy, social/leisure counseling, and social clubs.

[20] R. Meyers and W. Miller (eds.), *A Community Reinforcement Approach to Addiction Treatment* (Cambridge University Press, 2001, pp. 46–61).

[21] In a randomized controlled trial comparing CRA alone with CRAFT, R. Sisson and N. Azrin (1986), "Family-member involvement to initiate and promote treatment of problem drinkers," *Journal of Behavior Therapy and Experimental Psychiatry, 17,* 15–21, found the family component of craft led to more improved outcomes.

[22] R. Meyers, W. Miller, et al., "Community Reinforcement and Family Training (CRAFT)" in their *A Community Reinforcement Approach to Addiction Treatment* (Cambridge University Press, 2001, p. 150).

[23] Ibid. A lay version of this approach is provided in R. Meyers and B. Wolfe, *Get Your Loved One Sober: Alternatives to Nagging, Pleading, and Threatening* (Hazelden, 2004).

[24] The focus on the person in the addictive relationship rather than the potential in the family system is clear in their book, J. Smith and R. Meyers, *Motivating Substance Abusers to Enter Treatment: Working with Family Members* (Guilford Press, 2004).

[25] Recent reviews on family oriented interventions (including family therapy) are available in articles such as H. Liddle (2004), "Family-based therapies for adolescent alcohol and drug use: research contributions and future research needs," *Addiction, 99*(suppl 2), 76–92, and A. Copello, L. Templeton, et al. (2006), "Family interventions for drug and alcohol misuse: Is there a best practice?" *Current Opinion in Psychiatry, 19*(3), 271–276.

[26] See M. Stanton, T. Todd, et al., *The Family Therapy of Drug Abuse and Addiction* (Guilford, 1982).

[27] As described in Marc Galanter, *Network Therapy for Alcohol and Drug Abuse* (Guilford, 1993), and M. Galanter and D. Brook (2001), "Network therapy for addiction: bringing family and peer support into office practice," *International Journal of Group Psychotherapy, 51*(1), 101–122.

[28] As described in J. Combs and G. Freedman, *Narrative Therapy: The Social Construction of Preferred Realities* (Norton, 1996).

[29] Colleagues and I have attempted for over 20 years to incorporate family approaches into addiction services. Early on we used standard family therapy practices that included one-way mirrors, videos telephones, and letter writing. We adopted theories and approaches based on strategic, structural, conjoint, psychoanalytic, cybernetic, and narrative understandings. We set up couples groups, multiple family groups, family education days, and family session times. We developed staff training in family approaches, we set up community liaison initiatives, and we developed guidelines and other materials for practitioners on family inclusion. What was both disheartening and fascinating was how little impact these efforts had in shifting the focus of services in favor of families. In effect, family approaches have been more consistently adopted in situations in which an adolescent in an addictive relationship, as illustrated in J. Szapocznik, A. Perez-Vidal, et al. (1988), "Engaging adolescent drug abusers and their families in treatment: a strategic structural systems approach," *Journal of Consulting and Clinical Psychology, 56*, 552–557.

[30] P. Steinglass, L. Bennett, et al., *The Alcoholic Family* (Basic Books, 1987, p.47).

[31] Ibid., pp. 47–48.

[32] See review by B. Brook, "Adolescents who abuse substances," in P. Kymissis and D. Halperin (1996), *Group Therapy with Children and Adolescents* (American Psychiatric Press, 1996, pp. 243–264).

[33] See R. Cronkite, J. Finney, et al., "Remission among alcoholic patients and family adaption to alcoholism: a stress and coping perspective," in R. Collins, K. Leonard, and J. Searles, *Alcohol and the Family: Research and Clinical Perspectives* (Guilford, 1990, pp. 309–337).

[34] See R. Moos, J. Finney, et al., *Alcoholism Treatment: Context, Process and Outcome* (Oxford University Press, 1990).

[35] See R. Cronkite, J. Finney, et al., "Remission among alcoholic patients and family adaption to alcoholism: a stress and coping perspective," in R. Collins, K. Leonard, and J. Searles, *Alcohol and the Family: Research and Clinical Perspectives* (Guilford, 1990, p. 327).

[36] Barbara McCrady, in "The marital relationship and alcoholism treatment" in R. L. Collins, K. E. Leonard & J. S. Searles (Eds.), *Alcohol and the Family: Research and Clinical Perspectives* (Guildford, 1190, pp. 338–355). looked at three different models of marital relationship and treatment; family disease, family systems and social learning. She advocated a combination of systems and social learning

approaches. Other couple approaches are discussed in Jim Orford, "The coping perspective," in R. Velleman, A. Copello and J. Maslin, *Living with Drink: Women Who Live with Problem Drinkers* (Longman, 1998, pp. 128–149), and in E. Epstein, B. McCrady, et al., "Couple therapy in the treatment of alcohol problems," in A. Gurman and N. Jacobson, *Clinical Handbook of Marital Therapy*, 3rd ed. (Guilford, 2002, pp. 597–628).

[37] For example as described in J. Dittrich (1993), "Group programs for wives of alcoholics," in T. O'Farrell, *Treating Alcohol Problems: Marital and Family Interventions* (Guilford, 1993, pp. 78–114).

[38] See R. Velleman and L. Templeton (2003), "Alcohol, drugs and the family: a UK research programme," *European Addiction Research, 9*, 103–112.

[39] The willingness to engage with others also included involvement with the person in the addictive relationship and with other associates such as GPs as described by A. Copello, J. Orford, et al. (2000), "Methods for reducing alcohol and drug related family harm in non-specialist settings," *Journal of Mental Health, 9*, 319–333, and in a primary care package of treatment involving brief psycho-social interventions described in A. Copello, L. Templeton, et al. (2000), "A treatment package to improve primary care services for relatives of people with alcohol and drug problems," *Addiction Research, 8*(5), 471–484.

[40] This approach was developed into a manual for a controlled trial the UK Alcohol Treatment Trial (UKATT) comparing this approach with motivational enhancement therapy, A. Copello, J. Orford, et al. (2002), "Social behavior and network therapy: basic principles and early experiences," *Addictive Behaviors, 27*, 345–366.

[41] Sources of information vary enormously. More socially oriented material can be found in books such as R. Meyers and B. Wolfe, *Get Your Loved One Sober: Alternatives to Nagging, Pleading, and Threatening* (Hazelden, 2004), and C. Patterson-Sterling, *Rebuilding Relationships in Recovery: A Guide to Healing Relationships Impacted by Addiction* (Xlibris Corporation, 2004), or on Web sites such as Kina Families and Addiction Trust www.kinatrust.org.nz, or Addiction and Family Resource Group, www.addictionandfamily.org

[42] The importance of writing as a means of processing difficult and traumatic experiences has been highlighted in the work of James Pennebaker, whose research has spawned a wide variety of other research programs looking at the effects of traumatic writing on both psychological and physical well-being. See reviews in B. Esterling, L. L'Abate, et al., (1999) "Empirical foundations for writing in prevention and psychotherapy: mental and physical health outcomes," *Clinical Psychology Review, 19*(1), 79–96, and J. Pennebaker (1999), "The effects of traumatic disclosure on physical and mental health: the values of writing and talking about upsetting events," International *Journal of Emergency Mental Health*, 1(1), 9–18.

Chapter 12: Mobilizing Communities

[1] Quoted in K. Tamasese, C. Peteru, et al., *O le Taeao Afua The New Morning: A Qualitative Investigation into Samoan Perspectives on Mental Health and Culturally Appropriate Services* (The Family Centre and New Zealand Health Research Council, 1997).

[2] The Greater Toronto Area is a moderately large urban area amalgamating five sprawling suburbs into a combined population of around six million people. Its well-educated and predominantly European middle class contrasts with its significantly less wealthy influxes of recent immigrants from all over the world leading to about half its population being born outside Canada, belonging to over 70 different ethnicities, and speaking over 100 different languages. The Donwood has provided the main residential treatment services for this area.

3   I am grateful for information on these programs through discussions with David Korn, Jim Mulligan, Penny Pattinson, Dennis James, and Wayne Skinner, all of whom worked in association with the volunteer program at the Donwood at the time.

4   Initially it was stated as a requirement that program graduates attend these groups, but in later years it was merely recommended. Nonetheless, the majority of clients participated and usually for the whole period of 2 years.

5   A major concern is the inappropriate promotion of rigid approaches to addiction based on the volunteers' own personal experiences or the dogmatic literature to which they maintain a primary allegiance. Understanding needs to emerge for the participants from multiple sources and in ways that they can devise strategies independently.

6   As many as sixty recruits might attend the information sessions, and would then be divided into about ten groups.

7   The unexpected amalgamation of the Addiction Research Centre, the Clark Institute (for research in biological psychiatry), the Donwood, and hospital-based mental health services into the large new organization of the Centre for Addiction and Mental Health (CAMH), by the accounts of many I talked to came as a shock and resulted in a painful adjustment, particularly for the addiction branches where people were forced to contend with large and dominant mental health structures.

8   The network won several awards.

9   In a book translated into English on the clubs, V. Hüdolin, P. Gosparini, et al. (eds.), *Clubs of Treated Alcoholics: A Guide for the Work in the Clubs of Treated Alcoholics (Social-Ecological Approach)* (European School of Alcohology and Ecologica Psychiatry, 2001), the authors have opted consistently for the term treated alcoholics. My impression is that the terms treated and *alcoholic* may for them have different connotations and less medicalized overtones than in Anglo-American contexts. For that reason I have chosen to refer to them here simply and more neutrally as "clubs."

10 I did not realize this was Francesco Piani, who I was later to visit several times in San Daniele (50 km north of Trieste). Six months later I was at a WHO collaborators meeting in Liverpool and managed to speak with two Italian collaborators, Franco Marcomini and Valentino Patussi, who discussed their involvement in clubs in Padua and Florence. They also urged me to contact Pieroluigi Morisini in Rome because he had been trying to evaluate the effectiveness of the clubs. I later visited him and he then directed me to Francesco Piani in San Danielle.

11 My first visit occurred in 1997 to the clubs in Rome and Udine. During a subsequent visit in 1999 I participated in a 1-week (50-hour) "sensibilization" program on the clubs run for the first time in English. The last time I visited was in 2006 mainly to check their progress and confirm the content in this book.

12 See V. Hüdolin, P. Gosparini, et al. (eds.), *Club of Treated Alcoholics: A Guide for the Work in the Clubs of Treated Alcoholics* (European School of Alcohology and Ecological Psychiatry, 2001).

13 Ibid., pp. 112–113.

14 Giovanni Pitacco, living in Trieste, was treated in Zagreb for his addictive relationship to alcohol and grew tired of traveling across the boarder to attend clubs in Croatia. In 1979, with the support of others, he set up the first club in Trieste. The Italians were initially skeptical about the chances of adapting clubs because they saw Italian culture as very different (and perhaps more modern) than those in the former Yugoslavia. These reservations were found to have little substance. Over the next two decades, this first club in Trieste multiplied many times as clubs spread rapidly throughout Italy.

15 The CTA (Italian Club) Web site can be found at: www.aicat.net.

16 One of the WHO collaborators, Dr Pierluigi Struzzo, works as a general practitioner (GP) in Udine and trained as a *servant teacher* in the first Italian clubs. I talked with him in detail about his involvement in clubs during a WHO meeting in France. He emphasized

the great potential clubs have at a local level in linking addiction services with primary health care.

[17] Dr. Struzzo has explored the potential for local clubs and GPs to work together on a variety of levels. He envisages an opportunity for cooperative linkages between GPs with an understanding of clubs and local servant teachers, and providing family referrals and supporting their ongoing reintegration.

[18] Based on material in L. Musso, *Handbook for Setting Up a Local Introductory Course: How to Do It?* (Turin, Clubs of Treated Alcoholics, 2001, p. 53).

[19] In V. Hüdolin, P. Gosparini, et al. (eds.), *Club of Treated Alcoholics: A Guide for the Work in the Clubs of Treated Alcoholics* (European School of Alcohology and Ecological Psychiatry, 2001, p. 223). The left box has been abbreviated from "The area of alcohology programmes (Area alcohology schools, Interclub, Congresses etc.)" to "The Club Network."

[20] Ibid., pp. 211–237.

[21] In L. Musso, *Handbook for Setting Up a Local Introductory Course: How to Do It?* (Clubs of Treated Alcoholics, 2001, p.38) the handbook describes the concept of the net as needing to be "fine mesh," "dynamic," and all inclusive.

[22] Various attempts (such as Project MATCH) have looked at evaluating the effectiveness of a simplified and protocolized form of twelve-step counseling, but to my knowledge a major evaluation of the twelve-step groups as they occur in the community has not been undertaken mainly because of the complexities of recruitment and follow-up, regional variations, and concerns about confidentiality.

[23] In Croatia the numbers have dropped to about 140 clubs, a response to more basic priorities following the physical and social devastation of 1991; see discussion in V. Hüdolin, P. Gosparini, et al. (eds.), *Club of Treated Alcoholics* (European School of Alcohology and Ecological Psychiatry, 2001, pp. 42–49).

[24] Ibid., pp. 88–110.

[25] It was initially funded in 1993 by a grant from the Italian Minister of Health of approximately US$300,000. Ibid., pp. 309–318.

[26] Asian colleagues emphasize the importance of collective unity over the individualism they observe in Western contexts. See discussion in S. Tse, J. Wong, et al. (2004), "A public health approach for Asian people with problem gambling in foreign countries," *Journal of Gambling Issues, 12,* 1–15.

[27] I am very grateful to my friend and colleague Pam Armstrong, who has provided me with access through our various contacts to what will be described in the following section. Since very little is written on a Māori interpretation of addictive relationships, I have relied heavily on the way she presents the material.

[28] This is discussed more fully in Steven Fischer, *A History of the Pacific Islands* (Palgrave, 2002).

[29] As described by Michael King in his overview in *The Penguin History of New Zealand* (Penguin, 2003).

[30] James Bellich in his landmark *Making Peoples: A History of the New Zealanders from Polynesian Settlement to the End of the Nineteenth Century* (Penguin, 1996) describes in detail how in the early years up until the 1850s Māori and European relationships were fairly intertwined, with Māori vastly outnumbering the settlers. Then as emigration from the British Isles increased on a more systematic basis and with Māori deaths from European diseases, European settlers soon outnumbered Māori and land confiscations became widespread.

[31] Care will also be taken to use quotations as much as possible and content will be checked with Māori active in the field.

[32] Of course, the word people (He tangata) is not understood here to refer to a particle; it refers to people as interconnecting beings.

[33] From a presentation by Pam Armstrong on *The Dynamics of Whanaungatanga* (Ngati Wai, 2003, slide 4).

[34] Ibid., slide 15.

[35] Stated by Pa (Father) Henare Tate and quoted in Pam Armstrong, *The Dynamics of Whanaungatanga* (unpublished report, 2003, p. 9).

[36] Ibid., p. 9.

[37] Michael Shirres quoted in Pam Armstrong *The Dynamics of Whanaungatanga* (unpublished report, 2003, p. 12).

[38] From Michael Shirres, *Te Tangata: The Human Person*. (Auckland, Accent, 1997 pp. 44–45).

[39] From Mason Durie, *Maui Ora: The Dynamics of Maori Health*. (Oxford University Press, 2001, p. 203).

[40] Ibid., Chapter 7, "Whanau and Community," p. 206.

[41] Described in Pam Armstrong, *The Dynamics of Whanaungatanga* (unpublished report, 2003, p. 13).

[42] Ibid., p. 6.

[43] Pa Henare Tate (unpublished report) quoted in Ibid., p. 4.

[44] Pa Henare Tate (unpublished report) quoted in Ibid., p. 6.

[45] A range of different Maori health models have been used to support the development of physical, social, psychological, and spiritual connectedness, and their use has been extended to work with mental health issues including addictive relationships; see T. Huriwai, P. Armstrong, et al. (2001), "Whanaungatanga: A process in the treatment of Mâori with alcohol and drug problems," *Substance Use and Misuse, 36*(8), 1033–1052, and M. Durie, *Mauri Ora: The Dynamics of Maori Health* (Oxford University Press, 2001).

[46] In H. Moewaka-Barnes (2000), "Collaboration in community action: a successful partnership between indigenous communities and researchers," *Health Promotion International 15*(1): 17–25, the author argues that unlocking the power of connectedness is more likely to occur in a Māori cultural framework than in European contexts.

[47] We were grateful for 3-year funding support from the Alcohol Advisory Council (ALAC) of New Zealand.

[48] The original group consisting of Pam Armstrong, Delaraine Armstrong, Catherine Clark, Lil George, and myself, with the wisdom and support of the kaumatua (authoritative elder) Titari Pitama. Pam and I had visited the Italian clubs and were keen to use their framework to develop something for Māori. The others in the group were more cautious and wanted to base the network on Māori protocols. Their caution proved well-founded because the network emerged stronger in locations in which Māori approaches were encouraged.

[49] As outlined in Wendy Henwood's process evaluation of the early stages of the project in *Evaluation of "He Ope Awhina Ia Tatou"* (Unpublished report, Nga Manga Puriri, 2000).

[50] The difficulties experienced here and with other family projects prompted a small group of like-minded practitioners (including myself) to form a national trust, *Kina: Families and Addiction Trust,* which aimed to promote family inclusion in alcohol and drug services.

[51] Funded by the New Zealand Ministry of Health as a joint project between Massey University's unit Social Health Outcomes Research Evaluation (SHORE) and Whariki together with the participating communities.

[52] As outlined in K. Conway, M. Tunks, et al. (2000), "Te Whanau Cadillac—a Waka for change," *Health Education & Behavior, 27,* 339–350.

[53] The cultural independence of Maori services is identified as a significant issue by P. Robertson, T Haitana, et al. (2006), "A review of work-force development literature for the Maori addiction treatment field in Aotearoa/New Zealand," *Drug & Alcohol Review, 25,* 233–239. They point out how kaupapa Maori services provide the opportunity

for individuals and *whanau* (family/extended family) to work with ethnically matched health workers in ways that increase service accessibility and improve treatment outcomes.

54 As described in a booklet produced by the Kina Families and Addiction Trust, *Family Inclusive Practice in the Addiction Field: A Guide for Practitioners Working with Couples, Families and Whanau.* (Napier, NZ, Kina Families and Addiction Trust, 2005), p. 60.

Chapter 13: Applications to Practice

1 This quotation comes from an important editorial in the leading journal on addiction in which the case was made for a stronger focus on family. A. Copello and J. Orford (2002), "Editorial: addiction and the family: Is it time for services to take notice of the evidence?," *Addiction, 97,* p. 1362.

2 I tried for many years to engage addiction practitioners in working with families. In early years I worked with family therapy approaches, refined my own skills, and then attempted to engage other staff in the techniques. Fellow practitioners were interested, but their use of the methods did not sustain long beyond the training. Later I was involved in training all staff in units (counselors, receptionists) in what we termed "family inclusive practice." Participants listened patiently but again their interest did not translate to sustained application. Later I was part of a widespread community initiative to support families affected by addiction. We tried to link services with the project, but again, while they were sympathetic, they did not actually engage in practice. It now appears to me that whatever the factors in services that discourage family inclusion, they must be very strong and they will need to be addressed in a wider and stronger way than training and encouragement.

3 Most addiction services in nations with developed economies link into health services that are predominantly medical, and consequently they tend to focus primarily on delivering to individuals where the involvement of others is a secondary issue.

4 For example, even recent texts place a heavy emphasis on primarily psychological and to some extent biological dimensions of addiction. This is clear in Carlos DiClemente, *Addiction and Change: How Addictions Develop and Addicted People Recover* (Guilford, 2005), and Arthur Blume, *Treating Drug Problems* (Wiley, 2005).

5 The best studies of service counseling interventions indicate that only one third of clients improve, and since the interventions' effectiveness is typically only tracked for 18 months to 3 years, the studies may not address the long-term outcomes. George Vaillant argues that the effect of these interventions should be monitored for 5 to 10 years; see G. Vaillant (1988), "What can long-term follow-up teach us about relapse and prevention of relapse in addiction?," *British Journal of Addiction, 83,* 1147–1157.

6 Over a 20-year period I pursued many different attempts to promote family inclusion in addiction services (see Note 2 above). These tended to last only as long as I and other similarly committed colleagues were willing to push it. The services themselves did not sustain the initiatives. We concluded that the whole environment was not conducive to social approaches and shifted tactics by forming a national trust to promote and support family inclusion. Information on *Kina Family and Addictions Trust* can be accessed at www. kinatrust.co.nz.

7 Most government health ministries and major mental health services have developed guidelines and protocols regarding the management of risk associated with violence, self-harm, and suicide.

8 The colonization of women's experience in violent relationships is a topic that my colleagues and I have examined for some time. For example, see A. Towns and P. Adams (2000), "'If I really loved him enough, he would be okay': women's accounts of male

partner violence," *Violence Against Woman, 6*(6), 558–585; P. Adams, A. Towns, and N. Gavey, "Dominance and entitlement: the rhetoric men use to discuss their violence towards women," in M. Talbot, K. Atkinson and D. Atkinson (eds.), Language and *Power in the Modern World* (Edinburgh University Press, 2003) pp. 184–198; and A. Towns, P. Adams, & N. Gavey (2003), "Silencing talk of men's violence towards women," in L. Theismeyer (ed.), *Discourse and Silencing: Representation and the Language of Displacement* (John Benjamins, 2003).

9   The work of postmodern writers is placing increasing emphasis on the symbolic importance of how people interact with space and how the body plays an instrumental role in identity and social meaning. For summaries of this literature, see I. Burkitt, *Bodies of Thought: Embodiment, Identity and Modernity* (Sage, 1999), and C. Shilling, *The Body and Social Theory* (Sage, 2003).

10   In my doctoral dissertation I researched the various rhetorical strategies people without religious affiliations use to convey their mystical and religious experiences. See P. Adams, *A Rhetoric of Mysticism* (Unpublished dissertation, University of Auckland, 1991).

Chapter 14: Looking Ahead

1   From William Burroughs' *Naked Lunch* (Flamingo, 1993, p. 174).

2   For example, the importance of coexistent concerns is summarized in a review article by P. Buckley (2006), "Prevalence and consequences of the dual diagnosis of substance abuse and severe mental illness," *Journal of Clinical Psychiatry, 67*(suppl 7), 5–9; the authors found that one quarter of people with severe mental illness have issues with addictive relationships and half of those in addictive relationships also struggle with major mental health concerns.

3   Research suggests the presence of abuse may be a critical factor. See summaries in J. Ritter, M. Stewart, et al. (2002), "Effects of childhood exposure to familial alcoholism and family violence on adolescent substance use, conduct problems, and self-esteem," *Journal of Traumatic Stress, 15*(2), 113–122, and C. Humphreys, L. Regan, et al. (2005), "Domestic violence and substance use: tackling complexity," *British Journal of Social Work, 35*(8), 1303–1320.

4   Alex Copello in particular has been pointing this out as described in A. Copello and J. Orford (2002), "Editorial: addiction and the family: is it time for services to take notice of the evidence?," *Addiction, 97*, 1361–1363, and A. Copello, R. Velleman, et al. (2005), "Family interventions in the treatment of alcohol and drug problems," *Drug and Alcohol Review, 24*, 369–385.

5   See N. Wallerstein (2006), *What is the Evidence on Effectiveness of Empowerment to Improve Health?* (WHO Health Evidence Network, 2006).

Glossary

The following describes the meaning of key terms as they are used in this book.

Addictive relationship: A strong and long-term relationship between a person and an addictive substance/process (alcohol, drugs, gambling, work) that, as it intensifies, leads to deteriorations in other relationships. It refers specifically to the relationship with the addictive object and should not be confused with relationships with intimates.

Addictive substance/process: An object or an activity with mood-altering potential with which a person can develop a high level of focus and reliance to such an extent that it can take on a dominant position in that person's life. The main variants include alcohol and other illicit and prescribed mood-altering drugs, gambling, work, sex, and binge eating.

Addictive system: The multilayered network of relationships to which the person in the addictive relationship belongs. Other members of the system include immediate intimates, other family members or friends, neighbors, or community residents.

Assumptions: Fundamental understandings of the nature of reality and how we access that reality. They comprise unavoidable elements of a paradigm and simultaneously limit and enable what a paradigm is about.

Circle of intimates: The array of relationships with people who care about a person. It is used interchangeably with the term *family*.

Collective action: A planned and coordinated response to the social fragmentation that has been imposed on a family system by a person in an addictive relationship. It is used to describe both a phase within the cycle of intimate responses and a general social-oriented approach to addictive relationships that can include neighborhoods and communities.

Connectedness: The meaningful involvement a person has with other people, things, and activities. In this book social connectedness (relationships with family, friends, and colleagues) are emphasized, but important forms of connectedness also occurs in relation to spiritual, environmental, and imaginary domains.

Connecting strands of intimacy: The experiential elements to a relationship that enable a sense of being connected or bonded to other people (or other objects). The book identifies four main strands (the "four C's") as closeness, compassion, commitment, and accord.

Controlling tactics: Strategies and techniques used for the primary purpose of controlling the thoughts, beliefs, emotions, and behavior of other intimates. They can vary in intensity from subtle strategies (such as judgmental comments and ignoring a person) to violent and controlling behavior (such as hitting, restricting freedoms, and ongoing surveillance).

Counterreactions: Active responses by the person in the addictive relationship to perceived threats to that relationship. These responses can take a wide variety of forms and can include violence and other strong intimacy management strategies.

Crisis: The phase affecting both the person in the addictive relationship and surrounding intimates during which fragmentation within the addictive system accumulates to a point where it causes major disruptions. These disruptions could take the form of marital conflicts, separations, violence, court involvements, job losses, and major mental health issues.

Cycle of response phases: The cyclical sequence of phases that people commonly experience in relation to an addictive relationship. Two interlinked cycles were identified: those pertaining to the person in the addictive relationship and those pertaining to surrounding intimates. The sequences of phases differ between the two but they both share the phases of fragmentation, crisis, and reappraisal.

Family: A group of people participating in a network or system of close personal relationships. This may or may not include blood relatives, and in most circumstances refers to the small group of people who care most for each other.

Fragmentation: Process that involves the progressive deterioration in the strength of relationships. Within an addictive system it leads people to feel cut off, alienated, and isolated from each other and from sources of strength and validation.

Initiation: The phase during which an addictive relationship initially emerges. The processes that contribute to initiation are often assisted by enhancing factors such as "biological enhancers" (e.g., craving and tolerance) and "social enhancers" (e.g., availability, normalized consumption).

Intensification: The phase during which a forming (or reforming) addictive relationship is strengthened as a function of both increasing reliance on the addictive substance/processes and deteriorations in alternative relationships.

Intimacy management strategies: A wide range of strategies deployed by the person in an addictive relationship to control surrounding relationships in order to minimize the opportunity for threats to the addictive relationship.

Intimates: People who are in close personal relationships with a person in an addictive relationship.

Paradigm: A complex and multilayered network of assumptions that provide the conceptual framework for seeing, thinking, and communicating about what is experienced in a particular world.

Particle paradigm: A cluster of assumptions that revolve around the idea that the self is primarily an individual object and that this object, or particle, is the appropriate focal point for understanding addictive processes. The paradigm is most clearly articulated in medical and psychological approaches to addictive relationships.

Person in the addictive relationship: person addicted to a substance or a process (alcohol, gambling, sex); this should not be confused with surrounding intimates who have close relationships with that person.

Power within: The strength a person derives from within their inner being, such as those associated with spiritual connectedness, ethical beliefs, or other forms of inner resilience. It differs from strength derived from other external social or societal forms of power such as those derived from access to positions involving money, prestige, or physical force.

Reappraisal: The phase immediately following a period of crisis when both the person in the addictive relationship and other intimates are in a position to reevaluate their stance on the addictive system and their involvement in the cycles of response phases.

Reconnection: The phase in the intimate's response cycle during which intimates seek to reestablish relationships with others in the addictive system whose connections have been fragmented by the intimacy management strategies of the person in the addictive relationship.

Reformation: A central phase in reintegration where the person in an addictive relationship or other intimates seek to establish (or reestablish) multiple and symmetrical relationships within their social world.

Reintegration: The long-term process of reconstructing multiple and symmetrical relationships with people and activities other than the addictive relationship. This involves simultaneously dismantling the dominance of the addictive relationships while slowly enhancing the number and strength of other relationships.

Replacement: This involves the substitution of one addictive substance/process for another; for example, replacing alcohol with gambling or work. Since the single-focus structure of the social system remains intact, during replacement the person can easily revert to the original substance/process. Two types of replacement are "static substitution," where no changes occur to the social system, and "transitional replacement," where a temporary bridge is provided while the first stages of a reintegration are undertaken.

Response phases: Periods occurring in sequence that involve personal and systemic responses to the fluctuating strength of an addictive relationship.

Four key phases are shared both by the person in the addictive relationship and by other intimates: fragmentation, crisis, reappraisal, and reintegration.

Reversion: Occurs when a person who had previously set out to reduce the strength of an addictive relationship opts to return to the addictive system.

Social empowerment: The sense that emerges within a group of people when they collectively make choices and take action to overcome obstacles that they would have difficulty managing as individuals.

Social paradigm: A cluster of assumptions that revolve around the idea that much of the way people experience and behave can be understood in terms of their relationships. Accordingly, addiction is interpreted less in terms of the person as an individual particle and more in terms of relationships, both as he or she connects with the addictive substance/process and with other people/things. The paradigm is most clearly articulated in social science and humanities approaches that speak of people in terms of systems, networks, and communities.

Social world: The broader social environment that is grounded on a paradigm (and its network of assumptions) and within which people live, make sense of things, and share meanings. It also refers to a person's or a grouping of people's "social perspective" or "cultural orientation."

Bibliography

A.A. General Service Office. (1956 [2006]). *A.A. Fact File*. New York: A.A. Publishing.

A.A. (1976). *Alcoholics Anonymous*, 4th ed. New York: A.A. World Services, Inc.

Ackerman, R. J. (1988). Complexities of alcohol and abusive families. *Focus on Chemically Dependent Families, 11*(3), 15.

Ackerman, R. J., & Gondolf, E. W. (1991). Adult children of alcoholics: the effects of background and treatment on ACOA symptoms. *International Journal of Addictions, 26*, 1159–1171.

Adams, P. J. (1991). A Rhetoric of Mysticism. Unpublished PhD Dissertation, Auckland, University of Auckland.

Adams, P. J. (2007). Assessing Whether to Receive Funding Support from Tobacco, Alcohol, Gambling and other Dangerous Consumption Industries. *Addiction, 102*(7), 1027–1033.

Adams, P. J. (in press). Interventions with men who are violent to their partners: strategies for early engagement. *Journal of Marital and Family Therapy*.

Adams, P. J., Fitzgerald, J., & Livingstone, C. (Eds.). (2005). Special Issue: Dangerous Consumptions. *Addiction Research and Theory, 13*(6).

Adams, P. J., Powell, A., McCormick, R., & Paton-Simpson, G. (1997). Incentives for general practitioners to provide brief interventions for alcohol problems. *New Zealand Medical Journal, 110*, 291–294.

Adams, P. J., Towns, A., & Gavey, N. (2003). Dominance and entitlement: the rhetoric men use to discuss their violence towards women. In M. Talbot, K. Atkinson & D. Atkinson (eds.), *Language and Power in the Modern World* (pp. 184–198). Edinburgh: Edinburgh University Press.

Adams, P. J., & Warren, H. (in press). Responding to the risks associated with the relapse of recovering staff members within addiction services. *Substance Use and Abuse*.

Anderson, S. C. (1994). A critical analysis of the concept of codependency. *Social Work, 39*(6), 677–685.

American Psychiatric Association. (1994). *Diagnostic and Statistical Manual of Mental Disorders*, 4th ed. Washington, DC: American Psychiatric Association.

Armstrong, P. (1999). The Dynamics of Whanaungatanga (unpublished report). Ngungaruru: Ngati Wai.

Australian Productivity Commission. (1999). Australia's Gambling Industries: Final Report. Canberra: Productivity Commission.

Babor, T., Caetano, R., Casswell, S., Edwards, G., Giesbrecht, N., Graham, K., et al. (2003). *Alcohol: No Ordinary Commodity. Research and Public Policy*. Oxford: Oxford University Press.

Badawy, A. A. B. (2003). Alcohol and violence and the possible role of serotonin. *Criminal Behavior and Mental Health, 13*(1), 31–44.

Barber, J. G., & Crisp, B. R. (1995). The "pressures to change" approach to working with the partners of heavy drinkers. *Addiction, 90*, 269–276.

Barrett, A. E., & Turner, R. J. (2006). Family structure and substance use problems in adolescence and early adulthood: examining explanations for the relationship. *Addiction, 101*(1), 109–120.

Bateson, G. (1972). *Steps in an Ecology of Mind*. London: Granada.

Baumeister, R., & Leary, M. (1995). The need to belong: desire for interpersonal attachments as a fundamental human motivation. *Psychological Bulletin, 117*(3), 497–529.

Baxter, J. K. (1969). *The Rock Woman: Selected Poems.* London: Oxford University Press.

Beattie, M. (1989). *Codependent No More.* Victoria: Collins Dove.

Beauvais, F. B., Oetting, E. R., Wolf, W., & Edwards, R. W. (1989). American Indian youth and drugs, 1976–87: a continuing problem. *American Journal of Public Health, 79*, 634–636.

Bellich, J. (1996). *Making Peoples: A History of the New Zealanders from Polynesian Settlement to the End of the Nineteenth Century.* Auckland: Allen Lane: Penguin Books.

Berglund, M., Thelander, S., Salaspuro, M., Franck, J., Andréasson, S., & Öjehagen, A. (2003). Treatment of alcohol abuse: an evidence-based review. *Alcoholism: Clinical and Experimental Research, 27*(10), 1645–1656.

Bertens, H., & Natoli, J. (Eds.). (2002). *Postmodernism: Key Figures.* Malden, MA: Blackwell.

Betty Ford Center. (1990). Informational Brochure.

Blum, T. C., & Roman, P. M. (1992). A description of clients using employment assistance programs. *Alcohol Health & Research World, 16*, 120–127.

Blume, A. W. (2005). *Treating Drug Problems.* Hoboken, NJ: Wiley.

Bograd, M. (1988). Power, gender and the family: feminist perspectives on family systems theory. In M. A. Dutton-Douglas & L. E. A. Walker (Eds.), *Feminist Psychotherapies: Integration of Therapeutic and Feminist Systems* (pp. 118–133). Norwood, NJ: Ablex.

Boles, S. M., & Miotto, K. (2003). Substance abuse and violence: a review of the literature. *Aggression and Violent Behavior, 8*(2), 155–174.

Bott, E. (1971). *Family and Social Network,* 2nd ed. New York: Basic Books.

Bronte, A. (1993[1848]). *The Tenant of Wildfell Hall.* Oxford: Oxford University Press.

Brook, B. W. (1996). Adolescents who abuse substances. In P. Kymissis & D. A. Halperin (Eds.), *Group Therapy with Children and Adolescents* (pp. 243–264). Washington, DC: American Psychiatric Press.

Brown, S. (1985). *Treating the Alcoholic: A Development Model of Recovery.* New York: Wiley.

Brown, T. G., Kokin, M., Seraganian, P., & Shields, N. (1995). The role of spouses of substance abusers in treatment: gender differences. *Journal of Psychoactive Drugs, 27*(3), 223–229.

Brown, T. G., Werk, A., Caplan, T., & Seraganian, P. (1999). Violent substance abusers in domestic violence treatment. *Violence and Victims, 14*, 179–190.

Buckley, P. F. (2006). Prevalence and consequences of the dual diagnosis of substance abuse and severe mental illness. *Journal of Clinical Psychiatry, 67*(Suppl. 7), 5–9.

Burkitt, I. (1999). *Bodies of Thought: Embodiment, Identity and Modernity.* London: Sage.

Burroughs, W. (1993). *Naked Lunch.* London: Flamingo, Harper Collins.

Carle, A. C., & Chassin, L. (2004). Resilience in a community sample of children of alcoholics: its prevalence and relation to internalizing symptomatology and positive affect. *Journal of Applied Developmental Psychology, 25*, 577–595.

Carnes, P. J., Murray, R. E., & Charpentier, L. (2004). Addiction interaction disorder. In R. H. Coombs (Ed.), *Handbook of Addictive Disorders: A Practical Guide to Diagnosis and Treatment* (pp. 31–59). Hoboken, NJ: Wiley.

CASA National Center on Addiction and Substance Abuse. (2000). Missed Opportunity: National Survey of Primary Care Physicians and Patients on Substance Abuse Conducted by the Survey Research Laboratory, University of Illinois at Chicago. New York: Columbia University.

Christoffersena, M. N., & Soothill, K. (2003). The long-term consequences of parental alcohol abuse: a cohort study of children in Denmark. *Journal of Substance Abuse Treatment, 25*, 107–116.

Collins, J. J., & Messerschmidt, P. M. (1993). Epidemiology of alcohol-related violence. *Alcohol Health & Research World, 17*(2), 93–99.

Collins Jr, J. J. (Ed.). (1982). *Drinking and Crime: Perspectives on the Relationship between Alcohol Consumption and Criminal Behavior.* London: Tavistock.

Combs, J., & Freedman, G. (1996). *Narrative Therapy: The Social Construction of Preferred Realities.* New York: W. W. Norton.

Conway, K., Tunks, M., Henwood, W., & Casswell, C. (2000). Te Whanau Cadillac—a Waka for change. *Health Education & Behavior, 27*, 339–350.

Cook, C. C. H. (2004). Addiction and spirituality. *Addiction, 99*(5), 539–551.

Coombs, R. H. (Ed.). (2004). *Handbook of Addictive Disorders: A Practical Guide to Diagnosis and Treatment.* Hoboken, NJ: Wiley.

Copello, A., Orford, J., Hodgson, R., Tober, G., Barrett, C., & on behalf of the UKATT Research Team. (2002). Social behavior and network therapy: basic principles and early experiences. *Addictive Behaviors, 27*, 345–366.

Copello, A., Orford, J., Velleman, R., Templeton, L., & Krishnan, M. (2000). Methods for reducing alcohol and drug related family harm in non-specialist settings. *Journal of Mental Health 9*, 319–333.

Copello, A. G., & Orford, J. (2002). Editorial: Addiction and the family: Is it time for services to take notice of the evidence. *Addiction, 97*, 1361–1363.

Copello, A. G., Templeton, L., & Velleman, R. (2006). Family interventions for drug and alcohol misuse: Is there a best practice? *Current Opinion in Psychiatry 19*(3), 271–276.

Copello, A. G., Templeton, L. J., Krishnan, M., Orford, J., & Velleman, R. (2000). A treatment package to improve primary care services for relatives of people with alcohol and drug problems. *Addiction Research, 8*(5), 471–484.

Copello, A. G., Velleman, R. D. B., & Templeton, L. J. (2005). Family interventions in the treatment of alcohol and drug problems. *Drug and Alcohol Review, 24*, 369–385.

Cronkite, R. C., Finney, J. W., Nekich, J., & Moos, R. H. (1990). Remission among alcoholic patients and family adaption to alcoholism: A stress and coping perspective. In R. L. Collins, K. E. Leonard & J. S. Searles (eds.), *Alcohol and the Family: Research and Clinical Perspectives* (pp. 309–337). New York: Guilford Press.

Davies, J. B. (1992). *The Myth of Addiction: An Application of the Psychological Theory of Attribution to Illicit Drug Use.* Chur, Switzerland: Harwood Academic.

Davies, J. B. (1997). *Drugspeak: the Analysis of Drug Discourse.* Amsterdam: Harwood Academic.

Davies, P., & Walsh, D. (1983). *Alcohol Problems and Alcohol Control in Europe.* London: Croom Helm.

Denzin, N. K. (1993). *The Alcoholic Society: Addiction and Recovery of the Self.* New Brunswick, NJ: Transaction Publishers.

Desai, R. A., Maciejewski, P. K., Pantalon, M. V., & Potenza, M. N. (2006). Gender differences among recreational gamblers: Association with the frequency of alcohol use. *Psychology of Addictive Behaviors, 20*(2), 145–153.

Dickens, D. R., & Fontana, A. (Eds.). (1994). *Postmodernism and Social Inquiry.* New York: Guilford Press.

DiClemente, C. C. (2005). *Addiction and Change: How Addictions Develop and Addicted People Recover.* New York: Guilford Press.

Dittrich, J. (1993). Group programs for wives of alcoholics. In T. J. O'Farrell (ed.), *Treating Alcohol Problems: Marital and Family Interventions* (pp. 78–114). New York: Guilford Press.

Dobash, R. P., Dobash, R. E., Cavanagh, K., & Lewis, R. (2000). Confronting violent men. In J. Hanmer & C. Itzin (Eds.), *Home Truths about Domestic Violence: Feminist influences on Policy and Practice: A Reader.* London: Routledge.

Dole, V. P., & Nyswander, M. P. (1965). Medical treatment for diacetylmorphine (heroin) addiction. *Journal of the American Medical Association, 193*, 645–656.

Doweiko, H. E. (2002). *Concepts of Chemical Dependency*, 5th ed. Pacific Grove, CA: Brooks/Cole.

Durie, M. (2001). *Mauri Ora: The Dynamics of Maori Health.* Melbourne: Oxford University Press.

DuWors, G. M. (1992). *White Knuckles and Wishful Thinking: Breaking the Chain of Compulsive Reaction in Alcoholism and Other Addictions.* Seattle: Hogrefe & Huber.

Edleson, J. L., & Tolman, R. M. (1992). *Intervention for Men who Batter: An Ecological Approach.* Newbury Park, CA: Sage.

Edwards, G., Anderson, P., Babor, T. F., Casswell, S., et al. (1994). *Alcohol Policy and the Public Good.* Oxford: Oxford University Press.

Einstein, S. (Ed.). (1980). *The Community's Response to Drug Use.* New York: Pergamon Press.

Eisikovits, Z. C., & Edleson, J. L. (1989). Intervening with men who batter: A critical review of the literature. *Social Services Review,* September, 384–414.

El-Guebaly, N., West, M., Maticka-Tyndale, E., & Pool, M. (1993). Attachment among adult children of alcoholics. *Addiction, 88,* 1405–1411.

Epstein, E., McCrady, B., Epstein, E. E., & McCrady, B. S. (2002). Couple therapy in the treatment of alcohol problems. In A. Gurman & N. Jacobson (eds.), *Clinical Handbook of Marital Therapy,* 3rd ed. (pp. 597–628). New York: Guilford Press.

Esterling, B. A., L'Abate, L., Murray, E. J., & Pennebaker, J. W. (1999). Empirical foundations for writing in prevention and psychotherapy: Mental and physical health outcomes. *Clinical Psychology Review, 19*(1), 79–96.

Fergus, S., & Zimmerman, M. A. (2005). Adolescent resilience: a framework for understanding healthy development in the face of risk. *Annual Review of Public Health, 26,* 399–419.

Fergusson, D. M., & Lynskey, M. T. (1996). Adolescent resiliency to family adversity. *Journal of Child Psychiatry, 37*(3), 281–292.

Feyerabend, P. K. (1975). *Against Method: Outline of an Anarchistic Theory of Knowledge.* London: Verso.

Finzi-Dottan, R., Cohen, O., Iwaniec, D., Sapir, Y., & Weizman, A. (2003). The drug-user husband and his wife: Attachment styles, family cohesion, and adaptability. *Substance Use and Misuse, 38*(2), 271–292.

Fischer, S. R. (2002). *A History of the Pacific Islands.* Hampshire: Palgrave.

Fitch, F. J., & Papantonio, A. (1983). Men who batter: some pertinent characteristics. *Journal of Nervous and Mental Disease, 171*(3), 190–192.

Fitzgerald, F. S. (1934). *Tender Is the Night: A Romance.* New York: Charles Scribner's Sons.

Flanzer, J. P. (1993). Alcohol and other drugs are key causal agents of violence. In R. Gelles & D. Loseke (eds.), *Current Controversies on Family Violence* (pp. 171–181). Newbury Park, CA: Sage.

Fleming, M. F. (2004). Screening and brief intervention in primary care settings. *Alcohol Research and Health, 28*(2), 57–62.

Fletcher, R. (1993). *Moorish Spain.* Berkeley/Los Angeles, CA: University of California Press.

Foucault, M. (1965). *Madness and Civilization* (R. Howard, Trans.). New York: Pantheon.

Foucault, M. (1977). *Discipline and Punish: The Birth of the Prison* (A. Sheridan, Trans.). New York: Pantheon.

French, L. A. (2004). Alcohol and other drug addictions among Native Americans: the movement toward tribal-centric treatment programs. *Alcoholism Treatment Quarterly 22*(1), 81–91.

Frost, A. (1979). New geographical perspectives and the emergence of the romantic imagination. In R. Fisher & H. Johnston (eds.), *Captain Cook and His Times* (pp. 5–20). Canberra: Australian National University Press.

Fulton, A. I., & Yates, W. R. (1990). Adult children of alcoholics: a valid diagnostic group? *Journal of Nervous and Mental Disease, 178,* 505–508.

Furr-Holden, C. D. M., & Anthony, J. C. (2003). Epidemiologic differences in drug dependence—a US-UK cross-national comparison. *Social Psychiatry and Psychiatric Epidemiology, 38*(4), 165–172.

Galanter, M. (1993). *Network Therapy for Alcohol and Drug Abuse.* New York: Guilford Press.

Galanter, M., & Brook, D. (2001). Network therapy for addiction: Bringing family and peer support into office practice. *International Journal of Group Psychotherapy, 51*(1), 101–122.

Galvani, S. (2004). Responsible disinhibition: alcohol, men and violence to women. *Addiction Research and Theory, 12*(4), 357–371.

Garrett, J., Landau, J., Shea, R., Stanton, M. D., Baciewicz, G., & Brinkman-Sull, D. (1998). The ARISE intervention-using family and network links to engage addicted persons in treatment. *Journal of Substance Abuse Treatment, 15*, 333–343.

Gavey, N. (2004). *Just Sex? The Cultural Scaffolding of Rape.* London/New York: Routledge.

Gefou-Madianou, D. (Ed.). (1992). *Alcohol, Gender and Culture.* London: Routledge.

Gelles, R. J. (1993). Alcohol and other drugs are associated with violence: They are not its cause. In R. Gelles & D. Loseke (eds.), *Current Controversies on Family Violence* (pp. 182–196). Newbury Park, CA: Sage.

Gerevich, J. (2005). Binarisms, regressive outcomes and biases in the drug policy interventions: A theoretical approach. *Substance Use and Misuse, 40*(4), 451–472.

Giddens, A. (1992). *The Transformation of Intimacy: Sexuality, Love & Eroticism in Modern Societies.* Cambridge: Polity Press.

Glaser, F. B., Heather, N., Drummond, D. C., Finney, J. W., Lindstrom, L., Sutton, S., et al. (1999). Comments on Project MATCH: matching alcohol treatments to client heterogeneity. *Addiction, 94*(1), 31–70.

Gondolf, E. W. (1985). Anger and oppression in men who batter: empiricist and feminist perspectives and their implications for research. *Victimology: An International Journal, 10*, 311–324.

Gondolf, E. W. (1995). Alcohol abuse, wife assault and power needs. *Social Service Review, 69*(2), 274–284.

Gracey, M. (1998). Substance misuse in Aboriginal Australians. *Addiction Biology, 3*, 29–46.

Graham, K., Plant, M., & Plant, M. (2004). Alcohol, gender and partner aggression: a general population study of British adults. *Addiction Research and Theory, 12*(4), 385–401.

Greenfield, S. F., Brooks, A. J., Gordon, S. M., Green, C. A., Kropp, F., McHugh, R. K., et al. (2007). Substance abuse treatment entry, retention, and outcome in women: a review of the literature. *Drug and Alcohol Dependence, 86*, 1–21.

Griffin-Shelley, E. (1997). *Sex and Love: Addiction Treatment and Recovery.* Westport, CT: Praeger/Greenwood.

Griffin, K. W., Botvin, G. J., Nichols, T. R., & Doyle, M. M. (2003). Effectiveness of a universal drug abuse prevention approach for youth at high risk for substance use initiation. *Preventive Medicine, 36*(1), 1–7.

Hands, M., & Dear, G. (1994). Co-dependency: a critical review. *Drug and Alcohol Review, 13*, 437–445.

Harter, S. L. (2000). Psychosocial adjustment of adult children of alcoholics: a review of the recent empirical literature. *Clinical Psychology Review, 20*(3), 311–337.

Harter, S. L., & Taylor, T. L. (2000). Parental alcoholism, child abuse, and adult adjustment. *Journal of Substance Abuse, 11*(1), 31–44.

Heath, D. B. (1991). Women and alcohol: cross-cultural perspectives. *Journal of Substance Abuse, 3*(2), 175–185.

Heath, D. B. (1995a). An anthropological view of alcohol and culture in international perspective. In D. B. Heath (ed.), *International Handbook on Alcohol and Culture* (pp. 328–347). Westport, CT: Greenwood Press.

Heath, D. B. (2000). *Drinking Occasions: Comparative Perspectives on Alcohol and Culture.* Philadelphia: Brunner/Mazel.

Heath, D. B. (Ed.). (1995b). *International Handbook on Alcohol and Culture.* Westport, CT: Greenwood Press.

Heather, N., & Robertson, I. (1997). *Problem Drinking*, 3rd ed. New York: Oxford Medical Publications.

Henwood, W. (2000). *Evaluation of "He Ope Awhina Ia Tatou".* Whangarei: Nga Manga Puriri.

Hoaken, P. N. S., & Stewart, S. H. (2003). Drugs of abuse and the elicitation of human aggressive behavior. *Addictive Behaviors, 28*(9), 1533–1554.

Hoffman, L. (2001). *Family Therapy: An Intimate History.* New York: W. W. Norton.

Hraba, J., & Lee, G. (1996). Gender, gambling and problem gambling. *Journal of Gambling Studies, 12*(1), 83–101.

Hudolin, V., Piani, F., & Sforzina, M. (1998). Club of Treated Alcoholics: Social Ecological Approach (Hudolin's Method): Manual for the Work in Clubs of Treated Alcoholics. *Udine: European School of Alcohology and Ecological Psychiatry.*

Humphreys, C., Regan, L., River, D., & Thiara, R. K. (2005). Domestic violence and substance use: tackling complexity. *British Journal of Social Work, 35*(8), 1303–1320.

Hunt, G. M., & Azrin, N. H. (1973). A community-reinforcement approach to alcoholism. *Behavior Research and Therapy, 11,* 91–104.

Huriwai, T., Armstrong, P., Huata, P., Kingi, J., & Robertson, P. (2001). Whanaungatanga: a process in the treatment of Māori with alcohol and drug problems. *Substance Use and Misuse, 36*(8), 1033–1052.

Ioannou, S. (2005). Health logic and health-related behaviors. *Critical Public Health, 15*(3), 263–273.

Israel, B., Checkoway, B., Schultz, A., & Zimmerman, M. (1994). Health education and community empowerment: conceptualizing and measuring perceptions of individual, organizational and community control. *Health Education Quarterly, 21*(2), 149–170.

Israel, B., Krieger, J., Vlahov, D., Ciske, S., Foley, M., Fortin, P., et al. (2006). Challenges and facilitating factors in sustaining community-based participatory research partnerships: lessons learned from the Detroit, New York City and Seattle Urban Research Centers. *Journal of Urban Health, 83*(6), 1022–1040.

Janik, A., & Toulmin, S. (1973). *Wittgenstein's Vienna.* New York: Simon & Schuster.

Jarvis, T. J., Tebbutt, J., Mattick, R. P., & Shand, F. (2005). *Treatment Approaches for Alcohol and Drug Dependence,* 2nd ed. Chichester: Wiley.

Jenkins, A. (1990). *Invitations to Responsibility: The Therapeutic Engagement of Men Who Are Violent and Abusive.* Adelaide: Dulwich Centre Publications.

Jiacheng, X. (1995). China. In D. B. Heath (ed.), *International Handbook on Alcohol and Culture* (pp. 42–50). Westport, CT: Greenwood Press.

Johnson, H. (1996). *Dangerous Domains: Violence Against Women in Canada.* Toronto: Nelson.

Johnson, H. (2000). The role of alcohol in male partners' assaults on wives. *Journal of Drug Issues, 30*(4), 725–740.

Kaplan, H. B. (1999). Toward an understanding of resilience. In M. D. Glantz & J. L. Johnson (eds.), *Resilience and development: Positive life adaptations* (pp. 17–83). New York: Kluwer Academic/Plenum Publishers.

Karen, R. (1998). *Becoming Attached: First Relationships and How they Shape our Capacity to Love.* New York: Oxford University Press.

Kasl, C. D. (1989). *Women, Sex and Addiction: A Search for Love and Power.* New York: Ticknor & Fields.

Keane, H. (2004). Disorders of desire: addiction and problems of intimacy. *Journal of Medical Humanities, 25*(3), 189–204.

Kessler, R. C., Nelson, C. B., McGonagle, K. A., Edlund, M. J., Frank, R. G., & Leaf, P. J. (1996). The epidemiology of co-occurring addictive and mental disorders: implications for prevention and service utilization. *American Journal of Orthopsychiatry, 66*(1), 17–31.

Keyes, M. (1997). *Rachel's Holiday.* London: Penguin Books.

Killinger, B. (1992). *Workaholics: The Respectable Addicts.* London: Simon and Schuster.

Kina Families and Addiction Trust. (2005). *Family Inclusive Practice in the Addiction Field: A Guide for Practitioners Working with Couples, Families and Whanau.* Napier, NZ: Kina Families and Addiction Trust.

King, M. (2003). *The Penguin History of New Zealand.* Auckland: Penguin Books.

Kivel, P. (1992). *Men's Work: How to Stop the Violence that Tears our Lives Apart*. New York: Ballantine Books.

Kraus, L., Augustin, R., Frischer, M., Kummler, P., Uhl, A., & Wiessing, L. (2003). Estimating prevalence of problem drug use at national level in countries of the European Union and Norway. *Addiction, 98*(4), 471–485.

Kuhn, T. S. (1970). *The Structure of Scientific Revolutions*, 2nd ed., enlarged. Chicago: University of Chicago Press.

Labonte, R. (1990). Empowerment: Notes on Professional and Community Dimensions. *Canadian Review of Social Policy, 26*, 64–75.

Labonte, R., & Laverack, G. (2001). Capacity building in health promotion, Part 1: for whom? And for what purpose? *Critical Public Health, 11*(2), 111–127.

Lakatos, I. (1970). Falsification and the methodology of scientific research programmes. In I. Lakatos & A. Musgrave (eds.), *Criticism and the Growth of Knowledge* (pp. 91–196). Cambridge: Cambridge University Press.

Lakoff, G. (1987). *Women, Fire, and Dangerous Things: What Categories Reveal About the Mind*. Chicago: University of Chicago Press.

Lakoff, G., & Johnson, M. (1979). Metaphors We Live By. Chicago: University of Chicago Press.

Lambie, I., Seymour, F., Lee, A., & Adams, P. (2002). Resiliency in the victim-offender cycle in male sexual abuse. *Sexual Abuse: A Journal of Research and Treatment, 14*(1), 31–48.

Laverack, G. (2001). An identification and interpretation of the organisational aspects of community empowerment. *Community Development Journal, 36*(2), 40–50.

Laverack, G. (2004). *Health Promotion Practice: Power and Empowerment*. London: Sage.

Lende, D. H., & Smith, E. O. (2002). Evolution meets biopsychosociality: an analysis of addictive behavior. *Addiction, 97*(4), 470–471.

Leonard, K. E. (1999). Alcohol use and marital aggression in newlywed couples. In X. Arriaga & S. Oskamp (Eds.), *Violence in Intimate Relationships* (pp. 113–135). Thousand Oaks, CA: Sage.

Ley-Jacobs, B. M. (1999). *Nature's Road to Recovery: Nutritional Supplements for the Recovering Alcoholic, Chemical-dependent and the Social Drinker: A Health Learning Handbook*. Temecula, CA: BL Publications.

Liddle, H. A. (2004). Family-based therapies for adolescent alcohol and drug use: Research contributions and future research needs. *Addiction 99*(Suppl. 2), 76–92.

Liepman, M. (1993). Using family influence to motivate resistant alcoholics to enter treatment: the Johnson Institute approach. In T. J. O'Farrell (ed.), *Treating Alcohol Problems: Marital and Family Interventions* (pp. 54–77). New York: Guilford Press.

Lindman, R. E., & Lang, A. R. (1994). The alcohol-aggression stereotype: a cross-cultural comparison of beliefs. *International Journal of the Addictions, 29*(1), 1–13.

London, J. (1967). *John Barleycorn of Alcoholic Memoirs*. London: Arco.

Loneck, G., Garret, J., & Banks, S. (1996a). Comparison of the Johnson Interventions to four other methods of referral to outpatient treatment. *American Journal of Drug and Alcohol Abuse, 22*, 1421–1440.

Loneck, G., Garret, J., & Banks, S. (1996b). The Johnson Intervention and relapse during outpatient treatment. *American Journal of Drug and Alcohol Abuse 22*, 233–246.

Lorenz, V. C., & Yaffee, R. A. (1988). Pathological gambling and psychosomatic, emotional and mental difficulties as reported by the spouse. *Journal of Gambling Behavior, 4*, 13–26.

Lotufo-Neto, F., & Gentil, V. (1994). Alcoholism and phobic anxiety: a clinical-demographic comparison *Addiction, 89*(4), 447–453.

Lyotard, J.-F. (1984[1979]). *The Postmodern Condition: A Report on Knowledge* (G. Bennington & B. Massumi, Trans.). Minneapolis: Minnesota University Press.

Lyotard, J.-F. (1993). *Political Writings* (B. Hutchings & K. P. Geiman, Trans.). London: University College London Press.

MacAndrew, C., & Edgerton, R. B. (1969). *Drunken Comportment: A Social Explanation.* Chicago: Aldine Publishing.

Marlatt, G. A., & VandenBos, G. R. (Eds.). (1997). *Addictive Behaviors: Readings on Etiology, Prevention and Treatment.* Washington, DC: American Psychological Association.

Marshall, M. (1979a). *Weekend Warriors: Alcohol in Micronesian Culture.* Palo Alto, CA: Mayfield.

Marshall, M. (Ed.). (1979b). *Beliefs, Behaviors and Alcoholic Beverages in Cross Cultural Survey.* Ann Arbor, MI: University of Michigan Press.

Marshall, M., Ames, G. M., & Bennett, L. A. (2001). Anthropological perspectives on alcohol and drugs at the turn of the new millennium. *Social Science and Medicine, 53*(2), 153–164.

Massaro, D. W. (1986). The computer as a metaphor for psychological inquiry: considerations and recommendations. *Behavior Research Methods, Instruments and Computers, 18,* 73–92.

Masten, A. S., Gest, H. J., Tellegen, A., Garmezy, N., & Ramirez, M. (1999). Competence in the context of adversity: pathways to resilience and maladaptation from childhood to late adolescence. *Development and Psychopathology, 11,* 143–169.

Mathew, R. J., Wilson, W. H., Blazer, D. G., & George, L. K. (1993). Psychiatric disorders in adult children of alcoholics: data from the Epidemiologic Catchment Area project. *American Journal of Psychiatry, 150,* 793–800.

Maynard, S. (1997). Growing up in an alcoholic family system: The effect on anxiety and differentiation of self. *Journal of Substance Abuse, 9*(1), 161–170.

McCloskey, D. N. (1985). *The Rhetoric of Economics.* University of Wisconsin: Harvester Press.

McCourt, F. (1997). *Angela's Ashes: A Memoir of a Childhood.* London: Flamingo.

McGowan, V., Droessler, J., Nixin, G., & Grimshaw, M. (2000). *Recent Research in the Socio-Cultural Domain Of Gaming and Gambling: An Annotated Bibliography and Critical Overview* (Literature Review). Edmonton, AB: The Alberta Gaming Research Institute.

McNally, A. M., Palfai, T. P., Levine, R. V., & Moore, B. M. (2003). Attachment dimensions and drinking-related problems among young adults: the mediational role of coping motives. *Addictive Behaviors, 28*(6), 1115–1127.

Mellody, P. (1989). *Facing Codependence.* San Francisco: Harper & Row.

Mellody, P., & Miller, A. W. (1992). *Facing Love Addiction: Giving Yourself the Power to Change the Way You Love.* San Francisco: Harper.

Meyers, R. J., & Miller, W. R. (eds.). (2001). *A Community Reinforcement Approach to Addiction Treatment.* Cambridge: Cambridge University Press.

Meyers, R. J., Miller, W. R., & Smith, J. E. (2001). Community Reinforcement and Family Training (CRAFT). In R. J. Meyers & W. R. Miller (eds.), *A Community Reinforcement Approach to Addiction Treatment* (pp. 147–160). Cambridge: Cambridge University Press.

Meyers, R. J., & Wolfe, B. L. (2004). *Get Your Loved One Sober: Alternatives to Nagging, Pleading, and Threatening.* Center City, MS: Hazelden.

Miller, N. S., Klamen, D., Hoffmann, N. G., & Flaherty, J. A. (1996). Prevalence of depression and alcohol and other drug dependence in addictions treatment populations. *Journal of Psychoactive Drugs, 28*(2), 111–124.

Miller, W. R., & Rollnick, S. (1991). *Motivational Interviewing: Preparing People to Change Addictive Behavior.* New York: Guilford Press.

Miller, W. R., & Wilbourne, P. L. (2002). Review: Mesa Grande: a methodological analysis of clinical trials of treatments for alcohol use disorders. *Addiction, 97,* 265–277.

Milne, S. H., Blum, T. C., & Roman, P. M. (1994). Factors influencing employees' propensity to use an employee assistance program. *Personnel Psychology, 47,* 123–145.

Moewaka-Barnes, H. (2000). Collaboration in community action: a successful partnership between indigenous communities and researchers. *Health Promotion International, 15*(1), 17–25.

Moore, T. M., & Stuart, G. L. (2005). A review of the literature on marijuana and interpersonal violence. *Aggression and Violent Behavior, 10*(2), 171–192.

Moos, R. H., Finney, J. W., & Cronkite, R. (1990). *Alcoholism Treatment: Context, Process and Outcome.* New York: Oxford University Press.

Morgenstern, J., & Longabaugh, R. (2000). Cognitive-behavioral treatment for alcohol dependence: a review of evidence for its hypothesized mechanisms of action. *Addiction, 95*(10), 1475–1490.

Morjaria, A., & Orford, J. (2002). The Role of Religion and Spirituality in Recovery from Drink Problems: A Qualitative Study of Alcoholics Anonymous Members and South Asian Men. *Addiction Research and Theory, 10*(3), 225–256.

Morse, R. M., & Flavin, D. K. (1992). The definition of alcoholism. *Journal of the American Medical Association, 268*, 1012–1014.

Muelleman, R. L., DenOtter, T., Wadman, M. C., Tran, T. P., & Anderson, J. (2002). Problem gambling in the partner of the emergency department patient as a risk factor for intimate partner violence. *Journal of Emergency Medicine, 23*(3), 307–312.

Musso, L. (1999). *Handbook for Setting Up a Local Introductory Course: How to Do It?* Turin: Clubs of Treated Alcoholics.

Nakken, C. (2000). *Reclaim Your Family From Addiction: How Couples and Families Recover Love and Meaning.* Minnesota: Hazelden.

Narcotics Anonymous. (1988). *Narcotics Anonymous*, 5th ed. Van Nuys, CA: NA World Service Office.

Nietzsche, F. (1989 [1873]). On Truth and Lying in an Extra-moral Sense. In Gilman, Blair, & Parent (eds.), *Friedrich Nietzsche on Rhetoric and Language.* New York: Harper & Row.

Norwood, R. (1990). *Women Who Love Too Much.* London: Arrow Books.

Nosa, V. H. (2005). The Perceptions and Use of Alcohol Among Niuean Men Living in Auckland. Unpublished PhD, University of Auckland, Auckland.

O'Farrell, T. J., & Murphy, C. M. (1995). Marital violence before and after alcoholism treatment. *Journal of Consulting and Clinical Psychology, 63*, 256–262.

O'Flaherty, P. (1999). Being Strong: An Exploration of Discourses Concerning Transition to Life Beyond Residential Drug and Alcohol Treatment. Unpublished MA Thesis, University of Auckland, Auckland.

Obeyesekere, G. (1992). *The Apotheosis of Captain Cook: European Mythmaking in the Pacific.* Princeton, NJ: Princeton University Press.

Olsson, C. A., Bond, L., Burns, J. M., Vella-Brodrick, D. A., & Sawyer, S. M. (2003). Adolescent resilience: a concept analysis. *Journal of Adolescence, 26*, 1–11.

Orford, J. (1985). *Excessive Appetites: A Psychological View of Addictions.* Chichester: Wiley.

Orford, J. (1998). The coping perspective. In R. Velleman, A. Copello & J. Maslin (eds.), *Living with Drink: Women Who Live with Problem Drinkers* (pp. 128–149). London: Longman.

Orford, J., & Dalton, S. (2005). A four-year follow-up of close family members of Birmingham untreated heavy drinkers. *Addiction Research and Theory, 13*(2), 155–170.

Paolino, T. J., & McCrady, B. S. (1977). *The Alcoholic Marriage: Alternative Perspectives.* New York: Grune & Stratton.

Patterson-Sterling, C. (2004). *Rebuilding Relationships in Recovery: A Guide to Healing Relationships Impacted by Addiction.* Philadelphia: Xlibris Corporation.

Pence, E., & Paymar, M. (1993). *Education Groups for Men Who Batter: The Duluth Model.* New York: Springer.

Pennebaker, J. W. (1999). The effects of traumatic disclosure on physical and mental health: the values of writing and talking about upsetting events. *International Journal of Emergency Mental Health, 1*(1), 9–18.

Pernanen, K. (1997). Uses of "disinhibition" in the explanation of intoxicated behavior. *Contemporary Drug Problems, 24*, 703–729.

Peyrot, M. (1985). Narcotics anonymous: its history, structure, and approach. *International Journal of Addictions, 20*(10), 1509–1522.

Pomeroy, S. B. (1999). *Ancient Greece: a Political, Social, and Cultural History*. Oxford: Oxford University Press.

Potter-Efron, R. T., & Efron, D. E. (1993). Three models of shame and their relation to the addictive process. *Alcoholism Treatment Quarterly, 10*(1–2), 23–48.

Psathas, G. (2004). Alfred Schutz's influence on American sociologists and sociology. *Human Studies, 27*(1), 1–35.

Reith, G. (1999). *The Age of Chance: Gambling in Western Culture*. London: Routledge.

Ritter, J., Stewart, M., Bernet, C., Coe, M., & Brown, S. A. (2002). Effects of childhood exposure to familial alcoholism and family violence on adolescent substance use, conduct problems, and self-esteem. *Journal of Traumatic Stress, 15*(2), 113–122.

Robertson, N. (1999). Stopping violence programmes: enhancing the safety of battered women or producing better-educated batterers? *New Zealand Journal of Psychology, 28*(2), 88–78.

Robertson, P. J., Haitana, T. N., Pitama, S. G., & Huriwai, T. (2006). A review of work-force development literature for the Maori addiction treatment field in Aotearoa/New Zealand. *Drug and Alcohol Review, 25*, 233–239.

Robinson, B. E., & Post, P. (1997). Risk of addiction to work and family functioning. *Psychological Reports, 81*(1), 91–95.

Roethke, T. (1966). *The Collected Poems of Theodore Roethke*. London: Faber & Faber.

Rogers, P. J., & Smit, H. J. (2000). Food craving and food "addiction": a critical review of the evidence from a biopsychosocial perspective. *Pharmacology, Biochemistry and Behavior, 66*(1), 3–14.

Room, R., & Greenfield, T. (1993). Alcoholics anonymous, other 12–step movements and psychotherapy in the US population, 1990. *Addiction, 88*(4), 555–562.

Rose, G. (1992). *The Strategy of Preventive Medicine*. Oxford: Oxford University Press.

Rosenblatt, P. C. (1997). *Metaphors of Family Systems Theory: Toward New Constructions*. New York: Guilford Press.

Roth, P. A. (1984). Critical discussion: On missing Neurath's Boat: Some reflections on recent Quine literature. *Synthese, 61*, 205–231.

Rubin, K. H., Dwyer, K. M., Booth-LaForce, C., Kim, A. H., Burgess, K. B., & Rose-Krasnor, L. (2004). Attachment, friendship, and psychosocial functioning in early adolescence. *Journal of Early Adolescence, 24*(4), 326–356.

Russell, M. (1988). Wife assault theory, research, and treatment: a literature review. *Journal of Family Violence, 3*, 193–208.

Russo, J. (1998). *Applying a Strengths Based Approach in Working with People with Developmental Disabilities and their Families*. New York: Manticore Publishers.

Salmond, A. (1991). *Two Worlds: First Meetings between Maori and Europeans 1642–1772*. Auckland: Penguin/Viking.

Salmond, A. (1997). *Between Worlds: Early Exchanges Between Maori and Europeans 1773–1815*. Auckland: Viking.

Salmond, A. (2003). *The Trial of the Cannibal Dog: Captain Cook in the South Seas*. London: Allen Lane/Penguin Books.

Saunders, D. G. (2003). *Violence against women: Synthesis of research on offender interventions*. Washington, DC: National Institute of Justice.

Schechter, S., & Gary, L. T. (1988). A framework for understanding and empowering battered women. In M. B. Straus (Ed.), *Abuse and Victimization Across the Lifespan* (pp. 240–253). Baltimore: John Hopkins University Press.

Schuckit, M. A. (1995). *Drug and Alcohol Abuse: A Clinical Guide to Diagnosis and Treatment*, 4th ed. New York: Plenum Medical Book Company.

Schutz, A. (1972[1932]). *The Phenomenology of the Social World*. London: Heinemann Educational Books.

Searle, J. (1984). *Minds, Brains and Science*. Cambridge, MA: Harvard University Press.

Sedgewick, E. K. (1993). Epidemics of the will. In *Tendencies* (pp. 130–142). Durham: Duke University Press.

Seivewright, N., & Greenwood, J. (1996). What is important in drug misuse treatment? *The Lancet, 347*, 373–376.

Sexton, R. L. Ritualized inebriation, violence, and social control in Cajun Mardi Gras. *Anthropological Quarterly, 74*(1), 28–38.

Shaffer, H. J. (1997). The most important unresolved issue in the addictions: Conceptual chaos. *Substance Use and Misuse, 32*(11), 153–1580.

Shaffer, H. J. (1999). Strange bedfellows: a critical view of pathological gambling and addiction. *Addiction, 94*(10), 1445–1448.

Shaffer, H. J., Hall, M. N., & Vander Bilt, J. (1997). *Estimating the Prevalence of Disordered Gambling Behavior in the United States and Canada: A Meta-Analysis*. Boston: Presidents and Fellows of Harvard College.

Shaw, S. (1985). The disease concept of dependence. In N. Heather, Robertson & Davies (ed.), *The Misuse of Alcohol*. London: Croon Helm.

Sher, K. J., Walitzer, K. S., Wood, P. K., & Brent, E. E. (1991). Characteristics of children of alcoholics: putative risk factors, substance use and abuse, and psychopathology. *Journal of Abnormal Psychology, 100*, 427–448.

Shilling, C. (2003). *The Body and Social Theory*. London: Sage.

Shirres, M. P. (1997). *Te Tangata: The Human Person*. Auckland: Accent.

Sinclair, A. (1975). *Dylan Thomas: No Man More Magical*. New York: Holt, Rinehart & Winston.

Sisson, R. W., & Azrin, N. H. (1986). Family-member involvement to initiate and promote treatment of problem drinkers. *Journal of Behavior Therapy and Experimental Psychiatry, 17*, 15–21.

Smith, J. E., & Meyers, R. J. (2004). *Motivating Substance Abusers to Enter Treatment: Working with Family Members*. New York: Guilford Press.

Smith, J. W. (2000). Addiction medicine and domestic violence. *Journal of Substance Abuse Treatment, 19*(4), 329–338.

Stafford, L. L. (2001). Is codependency a meaningful concept? *Issues in Mental Health Nursing, 22*(3), 273–286.

Stanton, M. D., Todd, T. C., & Associates. (1982). *The Family Therapy of Drug Abuse and Addiction*. New York: Guilford Press.

Steinglass, P., Bennett, L. A., Wolin, S. J., & Reiss, D. (1987). *The Alcoholic Family*. New York: Basic Books.

Stith, S. M., Crossman, R. K., & Bischof, G. (1991). Alcoholism and marital violence: a comparative study of men in alcohol treatment programs and batterer treatment programs. *Alcoholism Treatment Quarterly, 8*(2), 3–20.

Szapocznik, J., Perez-Vidal, A., Brickman, A. L., et al. (1988). Engaging adolescent drug abusers and their families in treatment: a strategic structural systems approach. *Journal of Consulting and Clinical Psychology, 56*, 552–557.

Szasz, T. S. (1974). *The Myth of Mental Illness: Foundations of a Theory of Personal Conduct*. New York: Harper & Row.

Tamasese, K., Peteru, C., & Waldegrave, C. (1997). *O le Taeao Afua The New Morning: A Qualitative Investigation into Samoan Perspectives on Mental Health and Culturally Appropriate Services*. Wellington: The Family Centre and New Zealand Health Research Council.

Testa, M. (2004). The role of substance use in male-to-female physical and sexual violence: a brief review and recommendations for future research. *Journal of Interpersonal Violence, 19*(12), 1494–1505.

Thiesmeyer, L. (ed.). (2003). *Discourse and Silencing: Representation and the Language of Displacement*. Amsterdam: John Benjamins.

Thorberg, F. A., & Lyvers, M. (2006). Attachment, fear of intimacy and differentiation of self among clients in substance disorder treatment facilities. *Addictive Behaviors, 31*(4), 732–737.

Tolman, R. M., & Bennett, L. W. (1990). A review of quantitative research on men who batter. *Journal of Interpersonal Violence, 5*(1), 87–118.

Towns, A., & Adams, P. (2000). "If I really loved him enough, he would be okay": Women's accounts of male partner violence. *Violence Against Woman, 6*(6), 558–585.

Towns, A., Adams, P., & Gavey, N. (2003). Silencing talk of men's violence towards women. In L. Thiesmeyer (ed.), *Discourse and Silencing: Representation and the Language of Displacement.* Amsterdam: John Benjamins.

Tse, S., Wong, J., & Kim, H. (2004). A public health approach for Asian people with problem gambling in foreign countries. *Journal of Gambling Issues, 12,* 1–15.

Twain, M. (1955[1890]). *Huckleberry Finn.* Racine, WI: Whitman.

Vaillant, G. E. (1988). What can long-term follow-up teach us about relapse and prevention of relapse in addiction? *British Journal of Addiction, 83,* 1147–1157.

Vaillant, G. E. (1995). *The Natural History of Alcoholism Revisited.* Cambridge, MA: Harvard University Press.

Valverde, M. (1998). *Diseases of the Will: Alcohol and the Dilemmas of Freedom.* Cambridge: Cambridge University Press.

Velleman, R., & Orford, J. (1999). *Risk and Resilience: Adults Who Were the Children of Problem Drinkers.* Amsterdam: Harwood Academic.

Velleman, R., & Templeton, L. (2003). Alcohol, drugs and the family: a UK research programme. *European Addiction Research, 9,* 103–112.

Veysey, B. M., & Clark, C. (Eds.). (2004). *Sexual Abuse in Women with Alcohol and Other Drug and Mental Disorders: Program Building.* Binghamton: Haworth Press.

Walker, L. E. A. (1984). *The Battered Woman Syndrome.* New York: Springer.

Wallerstein, N. (1992). Powerlessness, empowerment, and health: Implications for health promotion programs. *American Journal of Health Promotion, 6,* 197–205.

Wallerstein, N. (2006). *What is the Evidence on Effectiveness of Empowerment to Improve Health?* Copenhagen: WHO Regional Office for Europe's Health Evidence Network (HEN).

Wampold, B. E. (2001). *The Great Psychotherapy Debate: Models, Methods, and Findings.* Northvale, NJ: Lawrence Erlbaum Associates.

Ward, J., Mattick, R., & Hall, W. (Eds.). (2000). *Methadone Maintenance Treatment and Other Opioid Replacement Therapies.* Amsterdam: Harwood Academic.

Weinrich, M., & Stuart, M. (2000). Provision of methadone treatment in primary care medical practices: a review of the Scottish experience and implications for US Policy. *Journal of the American Medical Association, 283*(10), 1343–1348.

Wekerle, C., & Wall, A.-M. (Eds.). (2002). *The Violence and Addiction Equation: Theoretical and Clinical Issues in Substance Abuse and Relationship Violenc*e. Philadelphia: Brunner/Mazel.

Welte, J., Barnes, G., Wieczorek, W., Tidwell, M. C., & Parker, J. (2001). Alcohol and gambling pathology among U.S. adults: Prevalence, demographic patterns and comorbidity. *Journal of Studies on Alcohol, 62*(5), 706–712.

West, M. O., & Prinz, R. J. (1987). Parental alcoholism and childhood psychopathology. *Psychological Bulletin, 102,* 204–218.

Whitfield, C. (1989). Co-dependence: our most common addiction—some physical, mental, emotional and spiritual perspectives. *Alcoholism Treatment Quarterly, 6,* 19–36.

Wilkinson, R., & Marmot, M. (2003). *Social determinants of health: The solid facts.* Copenhagen: World Health Organization, European Office.

Wittgenstein, L. (1974[1953]). *Philosophical Investigations* (G. E. M. Anscombe, Trans.). Oxford: Basil Blackwell.

Wong, J., & Tse, S. (2003). The face of Chinese migrants' gambling: a New Zealand perspective. *Journal of Gambling Issues, 9*(October), 1–11.

World Health Organization. (1952). Technical Report, Series No. 48, Expert Committee on Mental Health, Alcohol Sub-Committee, Second Report. Geneva: WHO.

World Health Organization Expert Committee on Mental Health. (1957). Addiction Producing Drugs: 7th Report of the WHO Expert Committee. Geneva: World Health Organization.

Yllö, K. (1993). Through a feminist lens: Gender, power, and violence. In R. J. Gelles & D. R. Loseke (eds.), *Current Controversies on Family Violence* (pp. 47–60). Newbury Park, CA: Sage.

Zakrzewski, R. F., & Hector, M. A. (2004). The lived experiences of alcohol addiction: Men of Alcoholics Anonymous. *Issues in Mental Health Nursing, 25*, 61–77.

Zinberg, N. E. (1984). *Drug, Set, and Setting: The Basis for Controlled Intoxicant Use*. New Haven: Yale University Press.

Author Index

Subject Index

Printed in the United States of America